"With cutting-edge information and critiques of theories and techniques of behaviour change, and methods of collecting and analysing data, this important go-to book is for all those wanting to understand, practise or teach the science of changing behaviour, especially in relation to health."

Susan Michie, *Professor of Health Psychology and Director of the Centre for Behaviour Change, UCL*

"Prestwich, Kenworthy and Conner have given the field a delightful gift – a thorough and thoroughly accessible soup-to-nuts look at the complexity of health behavior change. Their volume gives the reader all of the important facets of the behavior change conundrum – how to measure and intervene on relevant constructs, where those constructs fit in both conventional and newer theories, and how to consider the many environmental and contextual factors that are often just as if not more influential. This volume is one-stop-shopping for the student or health professional who wants a contemporary summary of all there is to know about theories of and approaches to health behavior change."

William Klein, *Associate Director of Behavioral Research, National Cancer Institute*

"What changes behaviour? How good are internet-based interventions? Do worry and rumination change behaviour? How can we reduce risk of bias in an experimental study? What is the right sample size? How do I quickly find useful literatures? These are just a few of the myriad questions this timely, authoritative compendium addresses that should prove indispensable to students, teachers and researchers alike."

Professor Dame Theresa Marteau, *Behavioural Scientist, University of Cambridge*

"The book is considered a cornerstone of information because it provides a comprehensive and up-to-date overview of the field, making it essential reading for students and researchers alike. Novice researchers can benefit from the book's clear explanations and practical examples, while seasoned researchers can use it as a reference tool to stay abreast of the latest developments in the field. It provides a wealth of information on various approaches to behavior change and offers practical guidance on how to design and implement effective interventions."

Prof. Dr. Ralf Schwarzer, *Freie Universität Berlin, Germany*

"I particularly like the discussion of key questions in the form of "Burning Issue Boxes". These boxes, in conjunction with the emphasis on critical skills toolkits, the overview of a wide array of methodologies as well as analytical choices for health behaviour change data, should equip the readers of this book with important critical skills to evaluate the evidence underpinning the various theories outlined in the book."

Nikos Ntoumanis, *Professor of Motivation Science,*
University of Southern Denmark

HEALTH BEHAVIOR CHANGE

The new and updated edition of *Health Behavior Change: Theories, Methods and Interventions*, provides a complete understanding of health behavior change, from its theoretical building blocks to the practical challenges of developing and testing an intervention. Based on the latest evidence in the field, the authors present a theory-driven, scientific approach to understanding and changing health behaviors, examining the theories that explain health behavior, the techniques that most effectively change health behavior, and the methods and statistical approaches essential to generating the underpinning evidence. This approach is presented in the context of both health promoting behaviors such as healthy eating, and health risk behaviors such as smoking, and considers not only the role of individuals but also other important influences on health behavior including the environment, policy and technology.

Among other additions, the revised edition includes the following features:

- More classic and modern theories explained and critiqued.

- Coverage of issues related to tackling COVID-19 through behavior change.

- Consideration of the replicability crisis, its causes, impact and potential solutions.

- Wider coverage of methods including different types of randomized trials, pilot studies, feasibility studies, consensus methods, N-of-1 studies and megastudies.

- Expanded critical skills toolkit.

Fostering a critical perspective, the book includes features to enable readers to better evaluate evidence and *Burning Issue Boxes* to highlight relevant, topical issues in the field. It will be essential reading for students and researchers of health psychology, public health and social work, as well as any professional working in this important area, particularly those tasked with reducing the high proportion of individuals failing to meet national health behavior targets.

Andrew Prestwich is a Senior Lecturer in Health & Social Psychology at the University of Leeds, UK. His research examines the impact of theory-based interventions on health behavior. He has previously held posts at the University of Oxford, University of Essex and University College London.

Jared Kenworthy is Professor of Psychology at the University of Texas at Arlington, USA. His research concerns social categorization and social influence in group processes, as well as intergroup relations and prejudice reduction. He was previously a post-doctoral researcher at the University of Oxford.

Mark Conner is Professor of Applied Social Psychology at the University of Leeds. His research focuses on understanding and changing health behaviors with a focus on the role of affect, attitudes, and intentions. He has published over 300 papers and edited a number of books in this area.

HEALTH BEHAVIOR CHANGE

THEORIES, METHODS AND INTERVENTIONS

SECOND EDITION

ANDREW PRESTWICH, JARED KENWORTHY
AND MARK CONNER

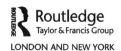

Routledge
Taylor & Francis Group

LONDON AND NEW YORK

Designed cover image: Getty Images

Second edition published 2024
by Routledge
4 Park Square, Milton Park, Abingdon, Oxon, OX14 4RN

and by Routledge
605 Third Avenue, New York, NY 10158

Routledge is an imprint of the Taylor & Francis Group, an informa business

First edition published by Routledge 2017

British Library Cataloguing-in-Publication Data
A catalogue record for this book is available from the British Library

Library of Congress Cataloging-in-Publication Data
Names: Prestwich, Andrew, 1978- author. | Kenworthy, Jared, 1973- author. | Conner, Mark, 1962- author.
Title: Health behavior change : theories, methods and interventions / Andrew Prestwich, Jared Kenworthy, Mark Conner.
Description: Second edition. | Abingdon, Oxon ; New York, NY : Routledge, 2023. | Includes bibliographical references and index. |
Identifiers: LCCN 2023027818 (print) | LCCN 2023027819 (ebook) | ISBN 9781032298610 (hbk) | ISBN 9781032298603 (pbk) | ISBN 9781003302414 (ebk)
Subjects: LCSH: Health behavior.
Classification: LCC RA776 .P8574 2023 (print) | LCC RA776 (ebook) | DDC 613--dc23/eng/20230710
LC record available at https://lccn.loc.gov/2023027818
LC ebook record available at https://lccn.loc.gov/2023027819

ISBN: 978-1-032-29861-0 (hbk)
ISBN: 978-1-032-29860-3 (pbk)
ISBN: 978-1-003-30241-4 (ebk)

DOI: 10.4324/9781003302414

Typeset in Bembo
by SPi Technologies India Pvt Ltd (Straive)

CONTENTS

7 BEHAVIOR CHANGE THROUGH TARGETING MECHANISMS OF ACTION: HEALTH PROMOTION, RISK AND DETECTION BEHAVIORS

PROLOGUE

Writing a book is hard work, very time consuming and we do not have a lot in the way of free time. Hence, when offered the opportunity to produce a second edition of this textbook by the publishing team, our motivation levels were not especially high. However, as you'll know, or will soon know upon reading this text, motivation (such as intentions) does not always translate into behavior: we do not always do what we are motivated (or intend) to do. In our case, our motivation to *not* update the book led to us actually updating the book. So, what changed? In short, the field; the field of health behavior changed since the publication of our original text in 2017.

The COVID-19 pandemic hit the world, and strategies were adopted to try to change people's behaviors to halt the spread of the disease and to help protect individuals themselves and those with whom they had contact. Common behaviors that research attempted to understand, predict and change far more than ever before included getting people to stay at home, socially distance, use hand gels and/or wash hands thoroughly, take vaccines and wear face masks. As a result, the new edition needed to consider many of these new behaviors.

A second important issue relevant to health behavior change was the replicability crisis that hit psychology and related disciplines. This crisis suggested that, due to a variety of reasons, a fair proportion of studies in the field are unlikely to replicate and produce equivalent results. While it means that we can have less confidence in relevant scientific studies in general, it has also been taken as an opportunity for the affected disciplines to consider how, collectively, things can be done better. Thus, within this new text, we consider the replicability crisis in-depth including its causes, impact and potential solutions, and have updated the "Science of Health Behavior Change: In Action" boxes accordingly.

In relation to theory, the Behavior Change Wheel and associated COM-B have emerged to become much more dominant. As such, the new edition provided us with an opportunity to describe and critique these, plus additional classic and more recent theories, alongside those theories covered in the original edition.

Perhaps the biggest change in this new edition is the "up-sizing" of the methods chapter. Feedback on the first edition suggested that readers liked

DOI: 10.4324/9781003302414-1

the fact that the book was helpful not just in terms of understanding health behavior change but was also for other areas. Methods and statistics, in particular, apply across many disciplines so the new edition enabled us to expand these more general sections. In this new edition, we now consider a much greater range of methods that are applied in health behavior change studies. The new methods considered include different types of randomized trials, pilot studies, feasibility studies, consensus methods, N-of-1 studies and megastudies.

Alongside a general update throughout, another key change has been the merging of two chapters related to health promotion and health risk behaviors. On balance, given that many theories and techniques are relevant to both (as well as to detection behaviors), plus changing health risk behaviors such as smoking are health promoting, a single (albeit much longer) chapter felt more appropriate.

In all, our original text was just over 100,000 words. Our initial target for the second edition was 120,000 words. It became apparent, however, that given the fundamental changes to the discipline, as well as the speed at which new research is being conducted, that increased word limit wasn't going to be enough. We are thus grateful to the publishing team for allowing us to revise this word limit upwards to 150,000. With some strict editing we managed to get within the revised target (just!). We hope that you enjoy the update. Should you have any feedback on the text, please feel free to contact us directly via email. You never know, there could be a third edition at some stage. Let's see how well our motivation predicts our behavior in the future…

Andrew, Jared and Mark

1

CHAPTER 1
INTRODUCTION

The idea that the behaviors we engage in might influence our health is not a new one. Over 40 years ago the Alameda County study followed nearly 7,000 people for a period of over 10 years and found that seven key behaviors were associated with increased levels of illness and shorter life expectancy (or morbidity and mortality as they are referred to in the research literature). The behaviors were smoking, high levels of alcohol intake, lack of exercise, being overweight, snacking, not eating breakfast, and sleeping less than 7–8 hours per night (Belloc & Breslow, 1972; Breslow & Enstrom, 1980). These behaviors (like smoking) and outcomes (like being overweight) are therefore, literally, a matter of illness and death.

Since the Alameda study, a large number of studies have confirmed these sorts of associations for various health promoting and health risking behaviors. Most of these studies have been conducted by epidemiologists or public health specialists and involve large numbers of people who are followed over a number of years and relate earlier behavior with later health outcomes like illness and death. So, for example, studies might look at the relationship between consumption of dietary fiber as reported by study participants at the beginning of the study with incidence of bowel cancer in the same individuals many years later. These studies, in order to achieve a clearer view of the relationship between dietary fiber and bowel cancer, will take into account statistically various other known influences on bowel cancer. The role of behavioral science has usually been in terms of understanding why individuals do or do not engage in these behaviors and how we might change these behaviors. These issues are the focus of this book.

To foster the understanding of these behaviors, including the factors that can influence them, several **theories** have emerged. These theories specify the key **constructs** (such as attitudes), their interrelationships and their links to behavior. In doing so, they provide suggestions about which targets (i.e., constructs) to try to change through intervention to promote health behavior change. Michie et al. (2014) identified 83 such theories. Interestingly, the same or similar constructs appeared in many of these theories. In Chapter 2, we overview and evaluate several of the most commonly used theories related to health behavior change. In Chapter 7, we focus on the key common constructs from these theories and look at the strength of their relationship to engaging in health behaviors and how the constructs might be changed to promote health behavior change.

DOI: 10.4324/9781003302414-2

Theories can be useful not just because they indicate constructs that should be targeted for intervention, but some theories also specify *how* these constructs should be changed. For instance, Bandura (1977) outlines different ways in which **self-efficacy** for a particular behavior can be enhanced and these have been integrated within Social Cognitive Theory – a popular theory which we introduce and evaluate in Chapter 2. In Chapter 3, we describe different **behavior change techniques (BCTs)** that can be used to change health behavior. Behavior change techniques are important aspects of interventions that represent what is done to the target participants/groups to facilitate behavior change. We also highlight and examine (in Chapter 10) the role of **behavior change taxonomies** which define and standardize behavior change techniques.

Theories also provide useful frameworks within which to accumulate evidence regarding health behavior change. Like taxonomies of behavior change techniques, theories provide a common language to describe different constructs and their impact on health behavior. Studies that test a particular theory can, in principle, be combined with other studies that do likewise to identify which theories are particularly useful and when. To do this, however, researchers need to ensure that their interventions are sufficiently theory-based so that the theory is applied and tested appropriately. Chapter 4 describes and discusses theory-based interventions and illustrates how a theory-based intervention can be designed and evaluated.

On the topic of research design and evaluation, in Chapter 5 we cover research methods, and in Chapter 6 we cover statistical analyses that are used to evaluate health behavior change interventions. Different methodologies have various strengths and weaknesses that have an impact on the overall quality of the evidence provided by any particular study. While there is no such thing as a perfect study, applying rigorous methods and appropriate statistics serve to minimize bias, enhance the quality of evidence and are fundamental aspects of a scientific approach to health behavior change. The scientific approach to health behavior change and how it is considered within this text book is illustrated in Figure 1.1. In this diagrammatic representation, the cyclical nature of the scientific process to health behavior change is emphasized, given the need to continuously use the best available evidence to refine/improve the better theories and to discard the theories that are of little use.

All sorts of behaviors are now known to influence health. These can usefully be split into the **health-promoting and health risking behaviors,** as well as **health checking behaviors**. Health promoting behaviors include things such as exercise, healthy eating and vaccination against disease. Health risk behaviors include smoking and excessive alcohol consumption. Health check behaviors include attending for health screening

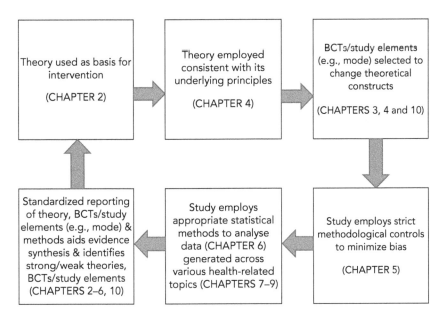

FIGURE 1.1 This book's scientific approach to health behavior change.

(e.g., for various types of cancer like cervical cancer and bowel cancer) and self-examination behaviors like breast or testicular self-examination.

A unifying theme across these different health behaviors is that each of them has immediate or longer-term effects upon the individual's health and are at least partially within the individual's control (see Burning Issue Box 1.1). One of the authors of this book loves to exercise and is careful that he eats healthy foods, but is partial to the odd alcoholic beverage. In this case, positive health outcomes may be promoted by exercise and eating behaviors but harmed by drinking, although engagement with each of these behaviors is controllable. Given the large amount of research on health behaviors, in Chapter 7 when looking at some of the key constructs that drive health behaviors, we look to health promoting, health risk and health check behaviors. Most of this research focuses on individual occasions of perform-ing a behavior like healthy eating. However, we should remember that the health consequences of healthy eating are usually based on performing the same behavior (e.g., choosing an apple over chocolate for a snack) over many occasions and over prolonged periods of time. Developing healthy habits and breaking unhealthy habits are important issues considered in Chapter 3.

Various features of the environment, such as the size of a plate or drinking glass, menus in restaurants, positioning of food and drink products in supermarkets, displays next to steps or elevators, can influence our health

BURNING ISSUE BOX 1.1

HOW HEALTH BEHAVIORS INFLUENCE HEALTH OUTCOMES

All sorts of behaviors influence health. These range from health-enhancing behaviors such as exercise participation and healthy eating, to health-protective behaviors such as vaccination against diseases like COVID-19 and condom use in response to the threat of HIV/AIDS. They also include health-detection behaviors such as health screening clinic attendance and breast/testicular self-examination, and avoidance of health-harming behaviors such as smoking and excessive alcohol consumption. Finally, they include sick-role behaviors such as compliance with medical regimens. A key question is how these behaviors influence health but to answer that question we also need to define health behaviors.

Several definitions of health behaviors have been suggested:

- "Any activity undertaken by a person believing himself to be healthy for the purpose of preventing disease or detecting it at an asymptomatic stage" (Kasl & Cobb, 1966).
- "Any activity undertaken for the purpose of preventing or detecting disease or for improving health and well-being" (Conner & Norman, 2015).

Behaviors encompassed in these definitions include medical service usage (e.g., physician visits, vaccination, screening), compliance with medical regimens (e.g., dietary, diabetic regimens) and self-directed health behaviors (e.g., diet, exercise, brushing and flossing teeth, contraceptive use).

These different health behaviors influence our health (morbidity and mortality) through three major pathways (Baum & Posluszny, 1999):

- generating direct biological changes such as when smoking cigarettes damages the lungs;
- changing exposure to health risks, as when the use of a sunscreen protects against skin cancer;
- ensuring early detection and treatment of disease, as when attending screening appointments leads to early detection of a cancer that can more easily be treated.

behavior in relatively automatic ways. In addition, policymakers can influence our health behavior, for instance through mandating warning labels on the front of cigarette packets, by banning smoking in public places or by taxing heavily unhealthy foods or sugary drinks. These environmental and policy-relevant influences on health behavior are covered in Chapter 8.

As well as an increased awareness around the role of the environment and the impact of different policies on health behaviors and outcomes, the last few years has also seen rapid technological developments that can be used to measure or track health behaviors, as well as to change them. As such, Chapter 9 considers the role of technology in health behavior change interventions. Chapter 10 draws the book to a close by highlighting three broad themes that represent key challenges for future research: identifying and characterizing factors that influence intervention success, achieving health behavior change at a population level to address significant challenges to global health, and accelerating the progress made by the science of health behavior change.

BOOK FEATURES

The book is separated into two parts. In the first part, we introduce the reader to the scientific approach underpinning health behavior change research. This involves the application of theory (Chapter 2) and behavior change techniques (Chapter 3) in the form of theory-based interventions (Chapter 4), adopting a strong methodological approach that minimizes the risk of bias that can unduly influence the findings of the study (Chapter 5) and applying appropriate statistical methods to evaluate the data (Chapter 6). The second part of the book focuses on the application of this scientific approach to different types of health behaviors and contexts: health behaviors and key constructs (Chapter 7), the environment and policy (Chapter 8) and technology (Chapter 9).

In this book, we use three core features: the Critical Skills Toolkit, Science of Health Behavior Change in Action, and Burning Issues Boxes. The Critical Skills Toolkit is applied in the first part of the text, while the Science of Health Behavior Change in Action feature is used in the second part of the text. The Burning Issue feature is applied across the book.

CRITICAL SKILLS TOOLKIT

Being critical is not a bad thing. In fact, it is a really good thing when done constructively because it challenges the status quo and can lead to refinements, improvements and innovation. Health behavior change needs to be underpinned by good science and good science needs criticism (as well as a rigorous, systematic approach). In our experience, being critical is something that people can find difficult; not necessarily because of politeness but more because they are unsure where to start. In this book, our aim is to arm the reader with a set of generic critical thinking skills that can be applied systematically to evaluate studies testing health behavior change interventions. As such, the reader can develop the ability to evaluate the strength of the evidence provided by any particular study.

SCIENCE OF HEALTH BEHAVIOR CHANGE IN ACTION

This feature illustrates how the scientific approach overviewed in the first part of the text, as well as the critical thinking skills developed via the Critical Skills Toolkit, can be applied to evaluate specific studies. As such, it is designed to illustrate how the reader can apply a systematic and rigorous approach to evaluating research concerning health behavior change.

BURNING ISSUE BOXES

In this feature, we introduce important issues that are either critical to the discipline, are being addressed by recent research or need to be examined more in the future. In some instances, this feature complements the main text by examining an issue in more detail; in other instances, the feature supplements the main text by covering a distinct topic.

OTHER FEATURES

In addition to the features already described, plus chapter overviews and summaries (included for all chapters except this one!), each chapter directs the reader to further readings which expand on some of the issues that we introduce in the text. Moreover, key terms are emphasized in bold and defined within a glossary section. In this edition, we have reframed and expanded critical evaluations of key theories in Theory Critique boxes in Chapter 2.

BURNING ISSUE BOX 1.2

PHYSICAL ACTIVITY AND HEALTH OUTCOMES

Physical activity is an important health behavior with clear consequences for health (Rhodes et al., 2017). For example, recent research suggests that at least 3% of cancers in the US are attributable to physical inactivity (Minihan et al., 2022). Other research suggests that over 100,000 deaths per year could be avoided if US adults aged 40 years or more increased their physical activity by as little as 10 minutes per day (Saint-Maurice et al., 2022). Many countries now have recommendations about the minimum levels of physical activity that individuals should engage in to benefit their health (Rhodes et al., 2017). Typically these recommendations focus on minimum amounts of moderate or vigorous levels of activity. However, engaging in any physical activity does appear to benefit health outcomes. Indeed research suggests that the greatest health benefit is for those who are inactive to start engaging in even modest amounts of activity (Rhodes et al., 2017). Some recent research has focused on number of steps taken per day, with evidence suggesting that although the greatest benefits (i.e., fewest deaths) are associated with engaging in the widely quoted 10,000 steps per day, even 3,500 steps per day were associated with better health outcomes (Paluch et al., 2022).

Despite these mostly well-known benefits of engaging in physical activity, the rates of engagement appear to be falling in many developed nations, particularly in adolescent groups (Conger et al., 2022). This points to the need for effective health behavior change interventions to promote engagement in physical activity (one of the things that we consider in this book).

FURTHER READING

The rest of this book! In Chapter 1, we couldn't really recommend anything else. But maybe we're biased.

GLOSSARY

Behavior change taxonomies: A classification system that represents and defines a set of behavior change techniques.

Behavior change technique (BCT): A systematic strategy used in an attempt to change behavior (e.g., providing information on consequences; prompting specific goal setting; modelling the behavior).

Constructs: A key concept or building block within a theory/model.

Health promotion behaviors: Behaviors that help protect or maintain health when engaged in such as exercise, healthy eating and vaccination against disease. **Health checking behaviors** also serve to protect or maintain health by looking for signs of ill health. These include attending for health screenings (e.g., for various types of cancer such as bowel cancer or cervical cancer) and self-examinations (e.g., testicular self-examinations). These behaviors are normally distinguished from **health risk behaviors** (e.g., smoking) where performance is associated with damage or risk to health.

Self-efficacy: Belief in one's capability to successfully execute the recommended courses of action/behaviors.

Theories: "A set of interrelated concepts, definitions and propositions that present a *systematic* view of events or situations by specifying relations among variables, in order to *explain* or *predict* the events or situations" (Glanz, Rimer, & Viswanath, 2015, p. 26).

REFERENCES

Bandura, A. (1977). Self-efficacy: Toward a unifying theory of behavioral change. *Psychological Review, 84*, 191–215.

Baum, A. & Posluszny, D.M. (1999). Health psychology: mapping biobehavioral contributions to health and illness, *Annual Review of Psychology, 50*, 137–163.

Belloc, N.B., & Breslow, L. (1972). Relationship of physical health status and health practices. *Preventive Medicine, 9*, 409–421.

Breslow, L., & Enstrom, J.E. (1980). Persistence of health habits and their relationship to mortality. *Preventive Medicine, 9*, 469–483.

Conger, S.A., Toth, L.P., Cretsinger, C. et al. (2022). Time trends in physical activity using wearable devices: A systematic review and meta-analysis of studies from 1995 to 2017. *Medicine and Science in Sports and Exercise, 54*, 288–298.

Glanz, K., Rimer, B.K., & Viswanath, K. (2015). Theory, research and practice in health behavior. In K. Glanz, B.K. Rimer and K. Viswanath (Eds.), *Health Behavior: Theory Research & Practice, 5th Edition*. San Francisco: Jossey-Bass.

Kasl, S.V., & Cobb, S. (1966). Health behavior, illness behavior and sick role behavior, *Archives of Environmental Health, 12*, 246–266.

Michie, S., West, R., Campbell, R., Brown, J., & Gainforth, H. (2014). *ABC of Behaviour Change Theories*. London: Silverback Publishing.

Minihan, A.K., Patel, A.V., Flanders, W.D., Sauer, A.G., Jemal, A., & Islami, F. (2022). Proportion of cancer cases attributable to physical inactivity by US State, 2013–2016. *Medicine and Science in Sports and Exercise, 54*, 417–423.

Paluch, A.E., Bajpai, S., Bassett, D.R., et al. (2022). Daily steps and all-cause mortality: a meta-analysis of 15 international cohorts. *Lancet Public Health, 7*, e219–228.

Rhodes, R., Janssen, I., Bredin, S., Warburton, D., & Bauman, A. (2017). Physical activity: Health impact, prevalence, correlates and interventions. *Psychology & Health, 32*, 942–975.

Saint-Maurice, P.F., Graubard, B.I., Troiano, R.P., et al. (2022). Estimated number of deaths prevented through increased physical activity among US adults. *JAMA Internal Medicine, 182*, 349–352.

2

CHAPTER 2
THEORY

OVERVIEW

Think of **theory** as "The General." Essentially it chooses its soldiers (**constructs** – or components of theory) and demands how these soldiers are organized. Specifically, the General will decide the rank of the soldier (its proximity to the key **outcome** – in health behavior change, this really is health behavior but could be improved health) as well as how the different soldiers should communicate with, or relate to, other soldiers under the General's control. If you don't want to talk about Generals and soldiers, perhaps you could draw upon a more formal definition of theory such as this: "A theory presents a systematic way of understanding events or situations. It is a set of concepts, definitions, and propositions that explain or predict these events or situations by illustrating the relationships between variables," Glanz and Rimer (2005, p. 4).

Over time, theories should be developed, tested and on the basis of the results refined into a better theory (or a more informed, efficient and practical General). This is how the science of health behavior change, and science in general progresses.

In Chapter 4, we will examine how theory can be used to develop interventions to change behavior. However, what are these theories? Which theories are the most popular in health behavior change? What are their strengths and weaknesses? After overviewing classic theories, we describe and evaluate more recent theories relevant to health behavior change, including the very popular COM-B model. Towards the end of the chapter, we consider the issue of behavior change maintenance as well as dual-process

DOI: 10.4324/9781003302414-3

models that combine automatic processes and slower, more reflective processing into a single umbrella or theory. We focus our attention on more general theories that can be applied across several health behaviors (and indeed outside the domain of health) rather than models that have been designed for one type of behavior (such as smoking). Although such models exist, they have typically been researched less often than the theories that we do consider.

CLASSIC THEORIES OF BEHAVIOR CHANGE

OPERANT LEARNING THEORY (SKINNER, 1953)

According to this theory, the likelihood or frequency a behavior is performed in the future is strongly influenced by the consequences of the behavior. If the consequences are positive, then the behavior is more likely to be repeated; if the consequences are negative, then the behavior is less likely to be repeated. These positive and negative consequences can be manipulated by the addition or removal of reinforcers (to increase behaviors) or punishment (intended to reduce behaviors).

Positive reinforcers involve the pairing of something desirable or rewarding with the behavior. For instance, Andrew (one of the authors of this book) used a sticker chart to reinforce good behavior by daughter, Milla, when she was younger. If Milla behaved well (e.g., helped to tidy the house or walked to the shops instead of insisting that she's too tired and wants to be carried – both behaviors linked to being more physically active), she received a sticker to add to her chart (see Figure 2.1a). These reinforcers do not need to delivered by a person; they can occur through other aspects of the environment. For instance, Andrew's youngest child, Sonny, used to have a "Jumperoo" (see Figure 2.1b), which encourages jumping by eliciting sounds and music after he jumps! Negative reinforcers involve the removal of something aversive (such as Milla tidying her room to prevent Andrew from nagging her). Positive reinforcement involves the introduction of a new stimulus to reduce the undesired behavior (such as Milla being told off if she is grumbling too much), while negative reinforcement reduces the undesired behavior by removing a desired stimulus. Returning to the sticker chart, if

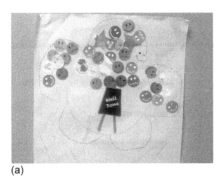
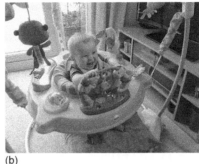

(a)   (b)

FIGURE 2.1 Operant Learning Theory in Practice. Milla's sticker chart (Figure
2.1a): a tried and tested example of positive reinforcement (and
negative punishment). Sonny's Jumperoo uses sounds, music and
lights as positive reinforcers to encourage jumping (Figure 2.1b).

Milla was naughty then a sticker was removed from her chart. Now that she
is 10, she is banned from all electronics★ (★correct at the time of writing!).

Over time, when reinforcers are no longer provided for a particular behavior, the frequency at which the behavior occurs should reduce through a
process termed operant extinction. If the behavior had been reinforced a lot
prior to extinction, then the process of extinction may be slow; if the
behavior had only been reinforced a few times prior, then extinction will
occur much more rapidly.

The reinforcement can be delivered for every instance of the desired
behavior or intermittently. Generally, intermittent reinforcement leads to
more persistent responding than rewarding every instance of desired behavior; intermittent reinforcement also leads to slower rates of extinction. Thus,
Milla did not receive stickers for every instance of good behavior! As Milla
is now older, stickers no longer appeal; the reward has to appeal. Nowadays,
the reinforcer can take many varied forms from a simple smile to a sweet
treat or time on an electronic device!

According to Skinner (1953), punishment is generally less effective than
reinforcement; punishment, even when severe and sustained, is argued to
lead only to a temporary suppression of the undesired behavior. It can also
generate negative emotions including fear, anxiety, rage or frustration that
can lead to illness. As such, alternatives to punishment are recommended.
These include (a) doing nothing (for instance, if it's a child going through a
developmental phase then they should grow out of it); (b) avoid situations

which can elicit the undesired behavior (for instance, if a person smokes cigarettes only in certain social environments then the person should avoid those social environments if they want to quit smoking); (c) undergo extinction (e.g., Milla's undesired behaviors could be ignored if the attention paid by Andrew is encouraging the behavior, so that Milla is no longer reinforced by the attention); (d) condition incompatible behaviors using positive reinforcement (e.g., reward instances in which Milla is calm when otherwise she may have become frustrated or upset).

SOCIAL LEARNING THEORY (BANDURA, 1971)

Behaviorism, which incorporates operant conditioning, sees behavior as being determined by the environment and, in particular, one's own direct experiences with the consequences of responses. Social Learning Theory differs from Operant Learning Theory by describing a reciprocal determinism between the environment and a person's behavior such that they influence each other. Moreover, it differs because the theory notes that, as well as learning by direct experience, behavior can be learned vicariously by observing others and seeing the consequences of these actions.

As an example, in the last edition, we mentioned about Andrew's daughter, Milla, and how she used to be scared of going down large slides before observing her dad go down a few times first (without injury and enjoying himself!) demonstrating both behavioral and emotional consequences. She has since become a very good swimmer and regularly competes in galas (see Figure 2.2). Her younger brother, Sonny, however, hates the water! Over the last few weeks, Andrew has deliberately taken Sonny along to watch his sister swim train with her friends. The other evening Sonny said to his dad, "Wow, Milla's fast!" recognizing that swimming isn't all that bad and, with practice, people get better. Also watching his sister swim backstroke, Sonny recently has learned to do this stroke and actually said that he quite likes swimming (which is a huge achievement for a boy who, not so long ago, really hated it!). Part of the transition was swimming on holiday around others who were having fun.

Key elements of Social Learning Theory include: attention (exposing people to models to help guide their behavior is only useful if the individual pays attention to the model and people pay more attention to certain models than others such as those with desirable qualities, like Sonny observing Milla swimming); retention (the individual need to have some memory of observing others to be influenced by their behavior in the future, and such memories can be strengthened either by rehearsing the sequence of behavior either mentally or behaviorally. To help Sonny to learn to swim backstroke, he's watched his sister a number of times and he

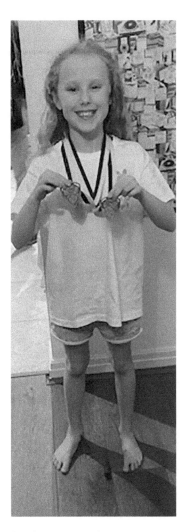

FIGURE 2.2 Milla after her first swim gala.

can practice backstroke arm movements at home, out of the water); motor responses (the individual must possess the sub-skills needed to put together the behavioral sequence; if not then the sub-skills need to be developed first through modeling and practice. Sonny's dad will swim with him to show him how to kick, etc.); and reinforcement/motivation (every time Sonny does a backstroke arm that neatly clears the water, his dad reinforces the action with a "good!" comment). The consequences for other people can serve to increase the behavior for the observer when the consequences are positive (vicarious rewards; e.g., Sonny seeing Milla having fun and swimming well) or reduce the likelihood of behavior for the observer when the consequences are negative (vicarious punishment). Thus, the same behavior that is observed in others may not be performed by the observer if they paid insufficient attention to the actions, failed to retain the information, do not possess the relevant skills or there is insufficient reinforcement or motivation.

Social Learning Theory also acknowledges that people can also make use of their cognitive abilities, for instance they can foresee the probable consequences (good or bad) of different actions and use this to guide their behavior. They can also learn about behavioral consequences through verbal or other types of communications so they do not need to try everything for themselves first! Furthermore, people can self-regulate their behavior. They can do this, in keeping with Social Learning Theory, by trying to change or alter the stimuli or cues preceding behavior and/or the consequences of their behavior.

GOAL-SETTING THEORY (LOCKE & LATHAM, 1990)

Locke and Latham joined forces in the 1970s as two relatively young, soon-to-be superpowers who had both worked independently beforehand on the impact of goal-setting on task performance. Locke had been inspired to conduct lab-based work around this topic by work from the 1930s that had suggested (albeit not statistically tested) that employees given a specific daily goal to achieve outperformed those who were simply told to do their best (Mace, 1935). Latham had been conducting applied work discovering that pulpwood crews that set specific goals regarding how much wood to harvest in a day or week were more productive than those that did not (see Locke & Latham, 2019).

Over time, they found that setting specific, high/difficult goals can give people a sense of purpose, challenge and accomplishment that they may not otherwise have. It can influence attention, effort, persistence and encourage the use of existing strategies or the drive to find new, better strategies which serve as key mediators of the effect of goal-setting on performance. They can also lead to more positive feelings (e.g., pride) and external rewards than setting easy goals.

A number of moderators have emerged representing the boundary conditions for which goal-setting works best, including receiving feedback so that progress against the goal can be tracked (similar to Control Theory, see later in this chapter), goal commitment (higher commitment is beneficial), having the requisite knowledge and skill to be able to achieve the goal, and the level of support or obstruction within the environment. When a set task is beyond the skill or knowledge of an individual or team, setting specific, challenging *learning* rather than *performance* goals might work best. There have been some seemingly contradictory findings on whether being assigned goals or being involved in the setting of one's goals (i.e., participatively set goals) is most beneficial. Participatively set goals might be helpful at times, in part, because they can lead to setting more challenging, difficult goals. Research suggests being assigned goals *with a rationale* (rather than a simple call "to do this") are as effective as participatively set goals (Latham et al., 1988).

While setting challenging goals is important, identifying the factors that influence how challenging goals are set (e.g., an individual's level of competitiveness; receiving positive feedback for previous goal attempts can encourage one to set even more challenging goals next time, see Locke & Latham, 2020) is also useful. This is useful because setting challenging goals can help to improve performance.

Based on around 400 studies, Locke and Latham ultimately published their book on goal-setting (Locke & Latham, 1990) that was later refined and further developed (e.g., Locke & Latham, 2002; Locke & Latham, 2019). Although it was developed and applied largely in work contexts, the theory has been utilized effectively in other contexts including the promotion of health behaviors such as physical activity (Swann et al., 2021).

THEORY CRITIQUE BOX 2.1

ADVANTAGES AND DISADVANTAGES OF GOAL-SETTING THEORY

Advantages

1. It is very practical offering clear recommendations regarding how best to set goals to maximize performance.
2. Underpinned by a wide-range of research in both laboratory and field settings and utilizes a relatively high proportion of experimental evidence and objective outcomes.
3. Generality. Supportive evidence can be found not only in organizational settings (where a lot of research has been conducted) but also in other fields including sports, exercise and other forms of health behavior change.
4. There are recommendations regarding how the theory should be tested in lab and field settings (Locke & Latham, 1990).
5. The theory has been developed inductively, observing findings and then developing ideas and theory that may explain these findings. Locke and Latham (1990) developed their theory based on about 400 studies and 25 years of prior research.

6. Related to point 5, given the theory has evolved as the literature expands rather than the other way around (theory first, findings second), it has evolved more easily to incorporate new findings.
7. The theory specifies both moderators (the conditions in which goal-setting works best/does not work) and mediators.

Disadvantages

1. May work less well in the long-term.
2. Comparisons of difficult vs. easy goals may reflect a benefit of difficult goals not because difficult goals are motivating but because easy goals can become demotivating (Vancouver, Ballard & Neal, 2022).
3. Further meaningful moderators need to be tested (e.g., goal conflict; Locke & Latham, 2020).
4. There are instances in which setting specific, challenging goals can be detrimental such as in the early stages of learning a new, complex task (where learning goals are more appropriate) or when the individual finds the goal threatening or anxiety-inducing. Swann et al. (2021) have argued that the theory and its subsequent evolution can be misapplied reasonably often in certain contexts such as prompting the wrong type of goal for the wrong people (e.g., performance goals to promote physical activity in inactive people given such goals can backfire when people don't have the necessary knowledge, commitment, resources, etc.).
5. By specifying a goal up-front, there may be increased risk of misreporting behavior at follow-up so that it is in-line with the original goal (though it is important to note that many studies have supported the theory using objective measures of performance/ behavior).
6. There is a risk that failing to achieve a set-goal has a negative impact on the individual (e.g., they experience negative emotions, reduced self-efficacy; Swann et al., 2021).

CONTROL THEORY (CARVER & SCHEIER, 1982)

Like goal-setting theory, control theory incorporates goal setting and considers how the discrepancy between set goals and actual performance can drive performance. While this is viewed in a more favorable light in goal-setting theory, in control theory, it is described more as leading to an adverse state in which an individual increases behavior in line with the set-goal to remove the adverse feelings arising from the initial discrepancy. When the behavior changes, it is re-assessed against the goal/standard and as such represents a negative feedback loop. Carver and Scheier (1982) present this feedback in the context of a five-level hierarchy of feedback systems where higher level systems trigger setting of standards/references at lower levels of the hierarchy. Comparison of one's actions against a set goal or standard necessitates some form of monitoring (e.g., of behavior) and feedback (e.g., how well one is doing vs. the goal/standard). Moreover, if one expects they have a reasonable chance of success, they are likely to continue with their attempts to reach the standard but as their perceptions of success subside, they become likely to disengage.

Taken together, goal-setting, self-monitoring and feedback might represent a useful combination of behavior change techniques on the basis of this theory. Some support for this comes from a review by Michie et al. (2009) which found that combining self-monitoring with at least one other technique from control theory led to larger changes in physical activity or dietary behaviors than the other interventions included in the review. However, none of the studies that were eligible for this review were explicitly based on control theory. In a more direct test of the theory, Prestwich et al. (2016) randomly allocated participants to one of three groups that incrementally involved more techniques affiliated with control theory (goal-setting alone vs. goal-setting + self-monitoring vs. goal-setting + self-monitoring + feedback) in an attempt to increase objectively measured levels of physical activity. Participants in the goal-setting + self-monitoring + feedback condition performed better than those who were only asked to set physical activity goals. As a result, there is some direct evidence that the theory can be used to develop effective health behavior change interventions.

Together, these classic theories have influenced many of the theories considered in the next section of this chapter, as well as a number of **behavior change techniques** considered in Chapter 3 such as the use of rewards. In the next section, we consider more recent theories related to health behavior change. While we are unable to cover all theories, we have tried to describe and evaluate many of the most popular and often used theories.

MODELS OF SOCIAL/HEALTH COGNITION

These more recent theories of behavior comprise constructs which are interrelated with one another and are linked either directly, or indirectly (via other constructs), with behavior. They are essentially models of prediction having been built predominately upon correlational research (see Chapters 5 and 6 for more information about correlational research).

In this type of research, participants typically complete questionnaires assessing each of the constructs or components of the model. For example, to test the Theory of Planned Behavior, participants would complete questionnaire items assessing an individual's attitudes towards the behavior (e.g., "My using condoms is: good/bad, beneficial/harmful," etc.), subjective norms (e.g., "My friends would approve of my using condoms": strongly agree/strongly disagree), perceived behavioral control (e.g., "If I wanted to, I am capable of using condoms"), intentions (e.g., "I will use condoms") and behavior (e.g., "I use condoms"). Responses on these questionnaires are subsequently analyzed to see how strongly they correlate with each other. If the correlations between the constructs are high and they explain lots of variance in behavior (see Critical Skills Toolkit 2.1), then the model is said to be useful in understanding behavior and that it has a good level of predictive validity (see Chapter 5 for overview of predictive validity).

Across the theories, the same (or similar) constructs appear in several theories (e.g., intention/motivation, perceived behavioral control/self-efficacy) suggesting these are important constructs. However, each model has some element that makes it unique from the other theories. Each theory in this section is a model of social/health cognition containing constructs that underlie one's motivation to perform a particular behavior. They can be used to differentiate between those individuals that perform the behavior in question and those that do not.

Is one theory better than another? This is an interesting question of which there is no definitive answer. Each model has its own strengths and weaknesses which are highlighted in the following section. One way in which models can be compared is on the amount of variance that the model explains in behavior (see Critical Skills Toolkit 2.1).

CRITICAL SKILLS TOOLKIT 2.1

THE CONCEPT OF EXPLAINING VARIANCE AND THE TRADE-OFF BETWEEN PARSIMONY AND EXPLAINING MORE VARIANCE

Imagine a box representing all the reasons why people exceed the driving speed limit. The more reasons you put into the box, the more the box fills up (in other words, the more variables in your model of behavior, the more variance in speeding you explain).

The more variance your model explains, the more you might understand why somebody exceeds the driving speed limit/or at least the factors associated with their speeding (meaning your model gets better and so you can use it to make better (more reliable/accurate) predictions). If your model explained 100% of variance in speeding, then you'd be able to use your model to perfectly predict how much any individual speeds.

In Model 1 (comprising only what a person intends to do (i.e., intentions)), intentions explain 15% of the variance in speeding, so your box becomes 15% full (see below).

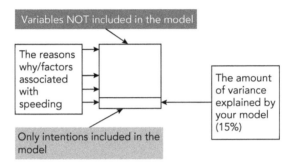

MODEL 1 Intentions as a Predictor of Speeding.

In Model 2 (comprising what a person intends to do (i.e., intentions) and their perceived behavioral control), 35% of the variance in speeding is explained, so your box becomes 35% full (see below). Obviously, you can never explain more than 100% variance in your outcome variable, so variance explained will always range between 0%–100%.

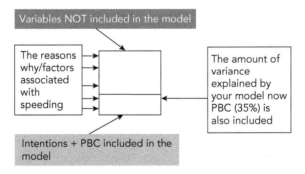

MODEL 2 Intentions & PBC as Predictors of Speeding.

Please note that this doesn't necessarily mean that intentions explain 15% of variance in speeding in total, and PBC explain 20% in total – remember intentions and PBC will correlate with each other to some extent – thus, they *share some variance*. You know that intention and PBC together explain 35% of variance and that PBC explains 20% of *unique* variance (i.e., the variance that isn't explained by intentions). The aim of developing models, conceptually speaking, is to fill up this box by explaining more and more *unique* variance (i.e., the proportion of variance in speeding that is unexplained by the other predictors in the model) because by doing so, we can predict with more accuracy the amount that an individual speeds when they drive.

However, there is a trade-off. If we measure more and more variables, then we'd explain more variance in speeding (which is good). However, measuring lots of variables (or manipulating lots of variables) is cumbersome and time consuming, and makes our model of prediction really complex (which is bad). Ideally, your model of prediction would explain most of the variance in the outcome (dependent) variable using as few variables as possible (i.e., it has parsimony).

So, to critique models or theories, ask yourself the following questions:

1. Does the model explain large portions of variance in key outcomes such as behavior?
2. Is the model parsimonious (i.e., it explains lots of variance in key outcomes using few variables) or does it contain variables that relate only weakly to key outcomes and other variables in the model?
3. Are any important variables missing such as those which would explain large portions of variance in key outcomes?

THEORY OF PLANNED BEHAVIOR (TPB; AJZEN, 1991)

The TPB, considered also in Chapters 4, 7 and 8, is a model that can be used to predict an individual's behavior. According to the TPB, the direct precursor to behavior is one's underlying behavioral **intentions**. One's behavioral intentions are jointly determined by one's attitudes towards the behavior (whether the individual views their own performance of the behavior as positive or negative), subjective norms (whether the individual perceives other people, who are important to the individual such as friends and family, would approve of their engaging in the behavior) and perceived behavioral control (PBC; the extent to which the individual feels that they have the capabilities to enact the behavior). As well as predicting one's intentions, PBC also moderates the link between intentions and behavior such that intentions are more likely to lead to behavior when an individual possesses high (rather than low) levels of PBC.

PBC has also been proposed to moderate (i.e., increase or decrease) how strongly subjective norms and attitudes each correlate with intentions: the proposal being that more favorable norms and attitudes are more likely to correspond with stronger intentions to perform the behavior when an individual has stronger PBC as opposed to weaker PBC. While there is support for the moderating role of PBC on intention-behavior relations, there appears insufficient support, at this stage, that PBC moderates the other relations (norms-intentions; attitudes-intentions; Hagger et al., 2022). This model is outlined in Figure 2.3. It originates from the Theory of Reasoned Action (TRA; Ajzen & Fishbein, 1980). The key difference between the two models is the inclusion of PBC in the TPB.

The TPB has been widely tested and successfully applied to the understanding of a variety of behaviors. For example, in a meta-analysis of the TPB (McEachan et al., 2011) intentions emerged as the strongest predictors of behavior, while attitudes and PBC were the strongest predictors of intentions, with subjective norms also related to intentions. In support of its use in the development of interventions to change behavior, Steinmetz et al. (2016) reported that behavior change interventions based on the TPB generate medium sized effects (d = .50, see Chapter 6 for an explanation of effect sizes).

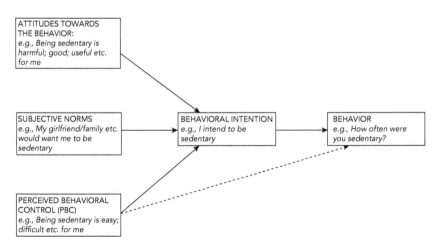

FIGURE 2.3 Theory of Planned Behaviour (Ajzen, 1991). Applied to being sedentary (dashed line denotes that PBC directly predicts behaviour when it reflects actual behavioural control).

THEORY CRITIQUE BOX 2.2

ADVANTAGES AND DISADVANTAGES OF THE THEORY OF PLANNED BEHAVIOR

Advantages

1. Many studies support the model (however, these studies are primarily correlational providing evidence for the model as a model of *predicting* behavior).
2. Clear definitions of constructs.
3. Standardized measures (i.e., clear direction regarding how to measure constructs, see https://people.umass.edu/ aizen/tpb. html).
4. Viewed as a parsimonious model; it explains relatively high proportions of variance in intentions and behavior with few constructs (see Critical Skills Toolkit 2.1).

Disadvantages

1. It was not designed as a model of behavior *change*. Although studies have tested TPB-based interventions (see review by Steinmetz et al., 2016) it is not clear how many of these interventions target all of the constructs within the TPB.
2. It assumes the influences of many other predictor variables are subsumed by the constructs specified in this model (attitudes, subjective norms, PBC). Recent work suggests that a range of predictors can influence one's underlying intentions and behavior over and above the constructs specified in the TPB (e.g., moral norms, goals, etc.). Consequently, other key variables are not specified in the model. Thus, on the flipside of Advantage 4, the model has been argued by Sniehotta et al. (2014) and others to be *too* parsimonious.
3. Specific aspects of the model, particularly whether the strength of individuals' perceived behavioral control can increase or decrease the size of the relationships between attitudes and intentions as well as subjective norms and intentions, require stronger evidence.

REASONED ACTION APPROACH (RAA; FISHBEIN & AJZEN, 2009)

The RAA is really an extension of the TPB which distinguishes between different subcomponents of attitudes (**experiential attitudes**; **instrumental attitudes**), perceived behavioral control (**capacity**; **autonomy**) and perceived (labelled subjective norms in the TRA/TPB) norms (**descriptive** norms; **injunctive norms**). According to this model, intentions predict behavior as long as the individual has the skills and abilities to do the behavior and there are no environmental constraints (e.g., tempting TV shows) that get in the way of translating your "oh so good" intentions (e.g., I intend to run 10km three times this week) to actual behavior (I ran 10km once and watched the latest season of *Cobra Kai*).

While models such as the RAA and TPB have often been interpreted as presenting behavior at the end of a slow, deliberative, rational decision-making process, Fishbein and Ajzen (2009, p. 23–24) make clear that their models do not suggest this. Instead, the models allow for irrational beliefs and also that intentions can arise quite automatically on the basis of the underlying beliefs. In new or particularly important situations, individuals might engage in careful consideration of factors, such as what others might think and how easy or difficult the behavior is, but this is unlikely for behaviors that are more commonly performed and/or less important.

The RAA can be used to identify what to target for intervention via two phases. In the first phase, one needs to identify/define the target behavior and population, representatively sample from this target population and identify salient beliefs related to doing the behavior (usually with qualitative methods) before assessing the relationships between the theory variables to identify which variables predict intentions and behavior. In the second phase, one considers the relationships between the main constructs (e.g., perceived norms) and underlying beliefs (e.g., injunctive norms) to further identify which elements of the theory to target for intervention. Selection of what to target can be based on correlations, whether mean scores for the constructs are low or high, as well as how easy or difficult the construct is to change (see Burning Issue Box 4.1).

THEORY CRITIQUE BOX 2.3

ADVANTAGES AND DISADVANTAGES OF THE REASONED ACTION APPROACH

Advantages

1. Support for many aspects of the model has been provided via meta-analytic review (McEachan et al., 2016).
2. Unlike many other theories, the RAA distinguishes between different subtypes of constructs (e.g., descriptive vs. injunctive norms).
3. Guidance is available regarding how to construct a RAA question-naire (Fishbein & Ajzen, 2009).

Disadvantages

1. While the theory can be used to identify what to target and highlights the important role of techniques designed to change beliefs (e.g., persuasive communication) and to translate intentions to action (e.g., implementation intentions), it does not directly specify which techniques (or combination of techniques) to use.
2. Evidence for the moderating roles of PBC can be quite weak.
3. While Fishbein and Ajzen (2009) point out that their model should not be conceived as a model that cannot account for spontaneous, more automatic behaviors, research is needed (e.g., using ecological momentary assessment, see Chapter 5) to see how key determinants of the model such as intentions are activated or change in particular social situations to influence subsequent behavior.
4. For certain types of behavior (e.g., those with a moral component), alternative measures of norms (e.g., moral norms) may explain additional variance which raises questions about the utility of the RAA across different types of behavior.
5. Anticipated affective reactions (e.g., If I did not run 10km three times this week, I would regret it) have been argued to be a potentially valuable addition to the model. Fishbein and Ajzen (2009), however, argue that these measures may overlap with other elements of their attitudes construct and that the potential value of such measures might lie in the fact that these measures tend to be framed differently from others (i.e., in relation to not doing the behavior rather than doing the behavior). They argue that while also assessing individuals' beliefs about alternative behaviors might improve prediction of the main/focal behavior, doing so would take participants a lot of time.
6. For behaviors/individuals where they do not have control over their behavior (e.g., drug taking in drug addicts; phobic reactions in individuals with phobias), the model is of less value.

PROTECTION MOTIVATION THEORY (PMT; ROGERS, 1983)

At a basic level, this theory suggests that people engage in two types of appraisal: threat appraisal (how severe a negative outcome is and how vulnerable one is to this negative outcome) and coping appraisal (how effective and easy it is to perform a behavior that will reduce the negative threat). These two appraisals interact to determine one's level of protection motivation (how motivated one is to engage in a behavior that will help to minimize their risk).

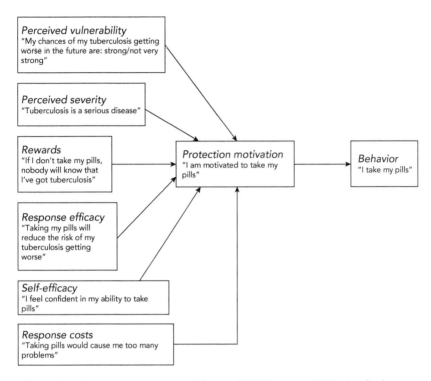

FIGURE 2.4 Protection Motivation Theory (PMT; Rogers, 1983). Applied to taking medication.

This theory has been applied within interventions designed to change behavior. According to this theory, to change behavior, people need to be threatened by feeling vulnerable (perceived vulnerability) to a severe consequence (perceived severity) and then identify a new behavior that one is capable of (self-efficacy), has little cost (response costs), and is something that is effective at reducing the threat (response efficacy). Interventionists take note. According to this theory, to make people change their health behavior (e.g., start exercising) we need to make people worry about a gruesome illness (e.g., their risk of heart disease) and then present the healthy behavior (e.g., exercise) as an easy-to-perform, effective means, with little cost, to reduce their risk of the illness.

PMT has been successfully applied to the prediction of a number of behaviors (see Norman et al., 2015). For example, in a study of over 750 health-care workers in Iran, protection motivation to adopt recommended protective behaviors against COVID-19 were correlated with the various components of PMT (Bashirian et al., 2020). Specifically, those who felt more vulnerable (perceived vulnerability), deemed coronavirus to be more severe (perceived severity) and that protective behaviors are more effective at protecting against coronavirus (response efficacy) were more motivated to engage in relevant protective behaviors. Surprisingly, however, those who felt there were more response costs to engaging in these protective behaviors were also more motivated although the relationship was weak. Higher threat and coping appraisal were also related with more regular adherence to protective behaviors. Meta analytic reviews of PMT (e.g., Milne et al., 2000) indicate intentions and self-efficacy to be the most powerful predictors of behavior, while self-efficacy and response costs were most strongly associated with intentions (see Chapter 7 for more detail about the model).

THEORY CRITIQUE BOX 2.4

ADVANTAGES AND DISADVANTAGES OF PROTECTION MOTIVATION THEORY

Advantages

1. A fair proportion of evidence supporting the model is experimental.
2. Manipulations of PMT constructs have been shown to lead to health behavior change (Milne et al., 2000).
3. Threat and coping appraisals have been shown to both play a role in influencing intentions (although coping seems likely to be more important, Milne et al., 2000; see also Disadvantage 1).
4. As noted by the PMT, intentions seem to be the strongest predictor of behavior compared to other PMT constructs (Milne et al., 2000).

Disadvantages

1. Threat-based models have been criticized as threat is not a consistent determinant of behavior (e.g., Albarracin et al., 2005).
2. The role of perceived vulnerability on motivation/intentions might be via other constructs rather than direct as specified in the PMT (Milne et al., 2000).
3. While the rewards component was added to the model in 1983 (not appearing in the original model), it is often not included within tests of the model thus little is known about its role and importance.
4. Does not include normative belief elements.
5. In their PMT review, Kothe et al. (2019) highlight a number of measurement issues: a) some studies collapse perceived

vulnerability and severity into a single measure; b) there have been relatively few tests of the model in full; and c) few studies use belief elicitation methods to ensure that the beliefs being assessed at the most relevant/salient beliefs.

6. Response costs may be difficult to change, at least in some contexts. In Milne et al.'s (2000) review, this was the only reported construct of PMT that was not changed significantly by manipulations, though only one study had attempted to do so.

7. Refinements to the model have been suggested including the order of the PMT being structured, such that threat appraisal precedes coping appraisal and some effects can be bidirectional (e.g., changes to behavior reduce perceptions of threat and vice-versa) (e.g., Plotnikoff & Trinh, 2010).

HEALTH BELIEF MODEL (HBM)

The HBM is based on a set of core beliefs relating to threat (perceived susceptibility and perceived severity) and perceived benefits (one's belief in the efficacy of the recommended action to reduce the risk or seriousness of the consequence). Sound familiar? In these respects, it is very similar to the PMT. In addition, it has a perceived barriers construct, cues to action (e.g., a close relative dying of a particular illness) and self-efficacy (which was added by Rosenstock et al., 1988).

In Janz and Becker's (1984) review of 18 prospective studies, of the four core beliefs (perceived severity, perceived vulnerability, benefits, barriers), severity was the least consistent predictor and barriers the most consistent. There is some experimental support for the model. For example, in a review of studies by Jones, Smith and Llewellyn (2014) that used the HBM to develop an intervention to promote adherence behaviors such as adherence to antibiotics or uptake of vaccinations, 14 out of 18 studies demonstrated a significant effect of the intervention; and seven studies produced medium or large effect sizes. However, as is the case for many experimental tests of theory, few studies (only six) targeted all constructs in the HBM (excluding the self-efficacy component added in 1988), and the HBM-based interventions were typically compared against no-intervention or usual care control groups rather than against other theory-based interventions. Thus, whether the interventions benefited from being based on the HBM rather than on any particular theory is not clear.

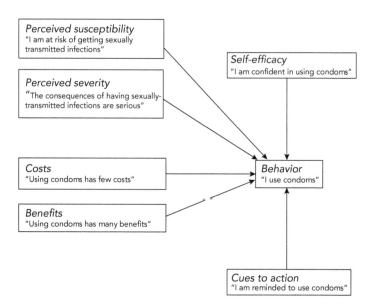

FIGURE 2.5 Health Belief Model. Applied to condom use.

THEORY CRITIQUE BOX 2.5

ADVANTAGES AND DISADVANTAGES OF THE HEALTH BELIEF MODEL

Advantages

1. Rosenstock et al.'s (1988) addition of the self-efficacy construct has improved the predictive validity of the model.
2. Generated a lot of research interest (particularly in the 1980s and 1990s).

Disadvantages

1. Threat-based models have been criticized as threat is not a consistent determinant of behavior (e.g., Albarracin et al., 2005).
2. Suffers from a lack of clear operational definitions of the constructs within in the model (Abraham & Sheeran, 2015).
3. The model does not specify the ordering of the predictor variables (Champion & Skinner, 2008). How are the predictor variables related to one another? Are some predictors "closer" to behaviors than others? Are all predictors equivalent, or is there some form of

sequence? Do any of the predictors interact? For example, does perceived severity and susceptibility both need to be high to influence behavior?

4. While studies show that the model predicts behavior, the effects tend only to be small (Abraham & Sheeran, 2015).

5. As a cognitive-based model, affective influences on behavior are underplayed (e.g., Champion & Skinner, 2008).

6. Comparisons across studies are difficult as, when the model has been tested, there have been inconsistencies in which constructs have been tested and which have not been tested (Abraham & Sheeran, 2015). Relatedly, not all of the HBM constructs are typically targeted within interventions (Jones et al., 2014).

7. Within analyses, rather than test the individual effects of each construct, authors have sometimes combined constructs (e.g. by adding or multiplying them, Quine et al., 1998). These different analytic approaches make it difficult to compare across studies.

SOCIAL COGNITIVE THEORY (SCT; BANDURA, 1986, 1997)

According to Bandura (1986), there are three interacting sets of factors that each influence one another: *personal factors* (like one's goals and how well people see themselves to be working towards those goals; their confidence in performing a particular behavior [self-efficacy]; the perceived consequences of an action [labelled action–outcome expectancies]); *environmental factors* (including people who might influence an individual and the rewards, feedback, guidance and standards within the environment); and *behavioral factors* (including the choice of behaviors, effort and persistence). As an example of how these factors can interact, imagine an individual who observes a high status person in an environment performing a particular behavior (environment factor). This environment factor can influence the self-efficacy or action–outcome expectancies related to that behavior (personal factors) which influences the effort and persistence that an individual invests in performing the behavior (behavioral factors). These three processes interact in various ways. For example, it's not just the environment influencing personal factors or behavioral factors; personal factors can influence the environment with individuals choosing which environments to submerge themselves within. For instance, an individual can choose to go a pub or to the gym based on their personal factors, and this in turn can influence behaviors and may also influence their initial personal factors (e.g., increase self-efficacy further).

Within SCT, self-efficacy is seen as an important construct. Self-efficacy reflects a person's confidence in performing a particular behavior and is linked with one's behavioral capability, the knowledge and skill that an individual has to perform a given behavior. Bandura (1977) has outlined four sources of information that can be used as methods to change self-efficacy:

- *Mastery experiences*: having the opportunity to practice a behavior (or sub-set of skills necessary to perform the behavior) and then master them.

- *Modelling (vicarious experience)*: observing others successfully perform the behavior. The qualities of the person being modelled matters. Models who are perceived to be more competent, more similar to the observer and of higher status are likely to be more influential.

- *Social/verbal persuasion*: others expressing confidence in your ability to perform a particular behavior; remembering positive comment from somebody.

- *Physiological experience*: correcting potentially harmful emotional beliefs such as butterflies in the stomach which should be seen as normal/useful.

In a meta-analysis (see Chapter 6 for a detailed look at meta-analyses) examining the best means to change self-efficacy (Ashford, Edmunds, & French, 2010), feedback on one's past behavior or the behavior of others, as well as modelling/vicarious experience were the most effective. Persuasion, mastery experiences and barrier identification were less successful.

The second major construct within the theory are action-outcome expectancies (the outcomes anticipated from the behavior and the extent that one's actions help one to achieve the outcomes). The outcomes could be physical (e.g., get healthier), social (e.g., approval from others) or self-evaluative (e.g., feeling good about oneself) thus they represent a mixture of attitudinal and subjective norm beliefs.

The third key construct within the model are barriers (including changes to the environment, emotional barriers or one's perceptions of them). Other variables such as self-control (how well an individual can personally regulate their behavior) and goals, which can energize behaviors, have been linked to the theory. To illustrate the role of these variables, imagine setting yourself the goal, as Andrew recently did, to run 5km in under 20 minutes.

Aside from giving impetus and drive to actually get out of the house and run, strategies to help achieve this goal can be implemented (e.g., planning to run three times a week, running shorter distances to build speed, running longer distances to build stamina, etc.) and progress towards the goal can be monitored to check how well you're doing in relation to the set-goal. Depending on progress, the strategies can be modified as needed (Schunk & DiBenedetto, 2020). Blaming a series of injuries and general aging, Andrew didn't quite reach his goal though he did come close (and there is still time!). Bandura's model accommodates such factors having more recently added socio-structural factors (such as one's living conditions; their health, political, economic and environmental systems) which can impede or facilitate behavior (see Chapter 7 for further model description).

SCT has been successfully applied to predicting various health behaviors, although as yet there is no general systematic review of its application to predicting a range of health behaviors. Instead, there have been non-systematic reviews (e.g., Luszczynska & Schwarzer, 2015) or systematic reviews focused on specific health behaviors. In one such review, Young et al. (2014) suggested that some components of SCT (self-efficacy and goals) were consistently associated with physical activity but others were not (socio-structural factors and outcome-expectancies).

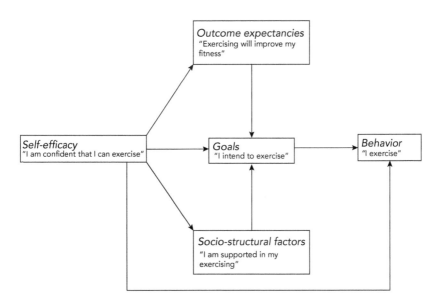

FIGURE 2.6 Social Cognitive Theory. Applied to exercise.

THEORY CRITIQUE BOX 2.6

ADVANTAGES AND DISADVANTAGES OF SOCIAL COGNITIVE THEORY

Advantages

1. Brings self-efficacy to the forefront; this is undoubtedly an important construct that is related to behavior.
2. Bandura has outlined methods to build self-efficacy; theories do not always explain how to change central constructs.
3. Attempts to integrate the role of the environment which other models have tended to overlook.

Disadvantages

1. Model clarity. As various constructs have been linked to the theory and not all of the constructs within the model are specifically well-defined, this has led to inconsistencies in the testing of the model. This lack of consistency in the implementation of the theory makes it difficult to pool evidence/generalize across studies.
2. Issues with measures and methods. Measures of self-efficacy (phrased as whether an individual "can do" the behavior) have been argued to strongly overlap with or even reflect motivation rather than somebody's perceived capability. As such, authors such as Williams and Rhodes (2016) have argued that self-efficacy may reflect motivation rather than be a factor that determines motivation. More broadly, measures and methods used to typically evaluate the model fail to capture the dynamic interplay between factors that the model presents; instead, it is typically assessed cross-sectionally or before and after an intervention, not capturing changes to key variables in-between or in the longer-term. Aside from illustrating the limitations with the measures and methods, this has limited the body of evidence that the model can be used to support long-term changes in behavior (Schunk & DiBenedetto, 2020).
3. Consistency across cultures. While there has been some support for aspects of the model across at least some countries (e.g., Williams & Williams, 2010), Schunk and DiBenedetto (2020) argue that there are reasons to expect that the model does not work across all cultures. This can be for a variety of reasons, including people in Western countries tending to overestimate their self-efficacy more.

HEALTH ACTION PROCESS APPROACH (HAPA; SCHWARZER, 1992)

There are three key features of the HAPA model that mark it out from many other theories of behavior or behavior change. First, it incorporates (coping and action) planning which helps to bridge the "intention-behavior gap" (a gap considered in detail later in this chapter). Second, it is a hybrid model between stage and non-stage-based models. Third, it incorporates three different types of self-efficacy (task, coping and recovery) that predominate at different stages of the behavior change process.

1. *Incorporation of planning to reduce the intention-behavior gap*
   While many other theories of behavior or behavior change specify intention as being a direct predictor of behavior, the HAPA model inserts planning between intention and behavior (see Figure 2.7) to overcome, to some extent, the intention-behavior gap (the problem that people who intend to perform a specific action do not always do it).

   According to the model, people who intend to perform an action are more likely to plan how they will act either in the form of action plans or coping plans. It is forming these plans that help an individual to do what they intend to do (in other words, these plans mediate the relationship between intentions and behavior, see Mediation Analysis, Chapter 6).

   Within the model, there are two types of plans. When forming action plans, individuals decide the situation (when and where) they

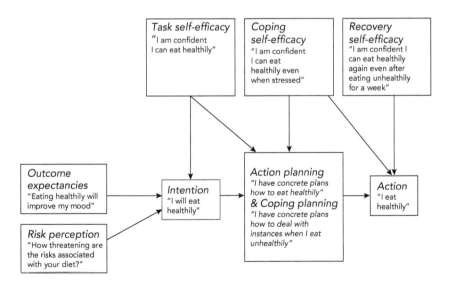

FIGURE 2.7 Health Action Process Approach. Applied to healthy eating.

will perform a specific behavior (e.g., "When I'm in my local super-market, I will buy vegetables"). Coping plans are similar but link specific coping responses to situations that threaten to disrupt one's goal achievement (e.g., "If I'm shopping and tempted to buy a food high in calories, I will tell myself that I want to stay slim!"). Action plans and coping plans are analogous to implementation intentions considered in Chapters 3 and 7.

The HAPA model posits that forming an intention is not necessarily sufficient to lead to behavior; other (planning) processes are often required. Thus, according to the HAPA, there are distinct phases to achieving one's goal – a goal-setting/motivational phase and a goal-striving/volitional phase.

2. *A hybrid model*

As well as being described as a two-stage/process model, the HAPA has also been dissected into a three-phase model representing non-intend-ers, intenders and actors. The constructs relevant to non-intenders are the constructs to the left-hand side of the model (i.e., risk perceptions, outcome expectancies, task self-efficacy and intention, see Figure 2.7). The constructs relevant to intenders are the constructs in the middle of the model (planning, coping self-efficacy, plus task self-efficacy-again). The constructs relevant to actors are action, recovery self-efficacy, plus coping self-efficacy again. By incorporating such features (see Lippke, Ziegelmann, & Schwarzer, 2005), the model flexibly shifts between a non-stage based model (like the TPB, HBM, PMT, etc.) to a stage-based model (like the Transtheoretical Model, TTM, considered later in this chapter).

3. *Three types of self-efficacy*

As outlined above (and also in Figure 2.7), the model explicitly differ-entiates between various types of self-efficacy, unlike other models that incorporate self-efficacy (such as TTM) or related constructs such as PBC (like the TPB).

- Task (motivational) self-efficacy: one's confidence in being able start to engage in the behavior even when one doesn't feel like doing the behavior (e.g., lacking in some form of motivation)

- Coping (volitional) self-efficacy: one's confidence in continuing to perform the behavior in instances when time is needed (e.g., when one does not see immediate benefits; or when the behavior takes a while to become routine)

- Recovery self-efficacy: one's confidence in re-engaging in the behavior after set-backs.

THEORY CRITIQUE BOX 2.7

ADVANTAGES AND DISADVANTAGES OF THE HEALTH ACTION PROCESS APPROACH

Advantages

1. Actively addresses the intention-behavior gap through the inclusion of planning and various forms of self-efficacy.
2. There is some experimental evidence demonstrating that manipulating motivation and planning leads to stronger changes in behavior than manipulating only motivation or only planning components (see review by Prestwich & Kellar, 2014). This supports the premise that there are distinct motivational and volitional components to goal-striving.
3. The maintenance of behavior (change) is often neglected by behavioral scientists who like to focus on promoting behavior (change). In fairness, it is much more expensive to run studies (particularly experimental studies) targeting behavior change in the long-term. However, there is evidence that components of the model not explicitly featured in other models – maintenance self-efficacy and recovery self-efficacy – are useful in understanding behavior maintenance (Scholz, Sniehotta & Schwarzer, 2005). A review of studies that have applied the Health Action Process Approach provides support particularly for the role of maintenance self-efficacy (Zhang et al., 2019) with the authors arguing that recovery self-efficacy is only likely to be important when people have a lapse in their behavior.
4. The stage-based version (more so than the continuum-version) could be seen as good for behavior change interventions. The continuum (non-stage-based) version could be seen as better for predicting behavior.

Disadvantages

1. More experimental tests needed (a lot of the research testing the model has been correlational) to examine whether changes in one construct causes changes in a related construct.
2. To support the stage-based element of the theory, more experimental evidence is needed to show that stage-matched interventions are more effective than stage mismatched interventions.
3. More research is needed to validate the role of recovery self-efficacy to identify when it is and when it isn't an important factor in influencing behavior.
4. As with several other models, there is scope to explain more variance in behavior by the inclusion of constructs related to nonconscious, more automatic processing such as habits.

Zhang et al. (2019) showed in a review of 95 studies that these three forms of self-efficacy relate differently to other variables in the model suggesting that they are distinguishable. They also provided statistical support for the other relationships between the HAPA variables (e.g., outcome expectancies-intentions) although evidence for the role of risk perception and recovery self-efficacy were weaker.

TRANSTHEORETICAL MODEL (TTM; PROCHASKA & DICLEMENTE, 1983)

The most popular stage-based model, the TTM, proposes five qualitatively distinct stages of behavior change: Pre-contemplation (where an individual has not considered performing the behavior), contemplation (where the individual considers the pros and cons of the behavior but not made formal plans to do so), preparation (where an individual plans and makes preparations for the behavior), action (where an individual has started to perform the behavior, not performing the behavior regularly), and maintenance (where an individual has sustained behavior change).

Ten processes of change (e.g., rewarding oneself, finding out more about the behavior) have been described as useful techniques to change behavior/move people from one stage to another. Different processes are thought to be useful at different stages. For example, finding out more about the behavior (consciousness raising) should be particularly useful for those in the pre-contemplation stage while rewards (contingency management) should be more useful for those in the action or maintenance phases. Changes in self-efficacy and decisional balance (one's evaluation of the positive and negative aspects of performing the behavior) underlie the effects of these processes of change and translation from one stage to another. Increasing levels of self-efficacy and an increasingly favorable decisional balance promote positive changes in stages.

THEORY CRITIQUE BOX 2.8

ADVANTAGES AND DISADVANTAGES OF THE TRANSTHEORETICAL MODEL

Advantages

1. By specifying processes of change, it gives some reasonable guidance regarding how to change behavior.
2. If there are distinct qualitative differences between people at the different stages, it could be used to effectively tailor behavior change interventions to the needs of the individual.

3. TTM questionnaires applied to physical activity have been validated in over 10 different languages (see Romain et al., 2018) enabling widespread testing of the model in this context.

Disadvantages (see West, 2005, 2006)

Robert West has argued that the theory does not provide a particularly complete or accurate description of behavior change. So unimpressed with the model, West (2005) has stated "reverting back to the common sense approach that was used prior to the Transtheoretical Model would [be] better than staying with the model" (p. 1036).

1. It has been argued that there are no stages of change. Instead, by devising stages of behavior change, the theory has taken continuous variables of motivation (desire and ability to change) and chopped it up into separate, arbitrary stages. As a result these stages are unstable and there is a continuous cycle of change.
2. TTM constructs have been argued to be no better than desire or intention as predictors of behavior.
3. The model needs to explain how people can "change" with sudden, minimal triggers. There is only a small body of evidence looking at the transitions between stages and the factors that underlie them (Armitage, Sheeran, Conner & Arden, 2004; Armitage, 2006).
4. It falsely makes the assumption that people always make formal plans and by focusing on conscious decision-making processes, it neglects more automatic (less conscious) determinants of behavior such as habits.
5. By categorizing people in arbitrary, unstable stages, it gives a false sense of diagnosis. By presenting such a "diagnosis" the model has been seen by some people as an appealing theory.
6. Describing people as being within a particular stage gives the impression that moving one step in stage is "good." We need to go the "whole hog," do the "Full Monty," and strive for sustained behavior change.
7. It is not clear that basing an intervention on the TTM leads to greater changes in behavior. In a review, Bridle et al. (2005) demonstrated that there was little evidence that interventions based on TTM were particularly effective in changing health behaviors (11 comparisons showed a benefit of using the TTM; 20 showed no difference between the intervention based on the TTM and the control; 11 were inconclusive as they showed mixed effects). Kleis et al. (2020) showed similar mixed evidence in relation to the use of the TTM to promote physical activity.

In addition, according to a review by Conn et al. (2008) interventions based on the TTM were less effective than interventions that were not based on TTM. A more recent review has shown that interventions based on the TTM (or the SCT) were no more effective than interventions not reporting a theory base (Prestwich et al., 2014).

8. A possible reason for limited effects is that given the many aspects to the model, different researchers apply the model in different ways and often fail to apply the theory in full.

CRITICAL SKILLS TOOLKIT 2.2

GENERAL CRITICISMS OF HEALTH/SOCIAL COGNITION MODELS

1. They have typically been designed as models of predicting behavior rather than models of behavior change. For example, in their meta-analysis of longitudinal studies concerning the TPB, Sutton and Sheeran (2003, cited in Sheeran et al., 2005) reported past behavior explained 26% of variance in future behavior, while intentions explained an additional 7% of variance over and above past behavior. In other words, intentions explain little variance in behavior change.

2. They have been developed with the aim of predicting as much variance in behavior as possible and as such have been built upon correlational rather than experimental evidence. Due to the correlational nature of the data it is difficult to infer causation and weaknesses of correlational methods apply (see Chapter 5).

3. Few studies have demonstrated *how* these models can be used to inform behavior change *interventions*.

4. Relatedly, models typically do not specify in what contexts (e.g., when, for whom) targeting particular constructs or determinants is likely to be effective or ineffective (Sheeran et al., 2017). Intensive within-participant forms of data collection where the same constructs are assessed multiple times (e.g., every few hours) may help identify when certain constructs are likely to impact behavior or not.

5. The models are not specific about which behavior change techniques should be used to change the theoretical constructs (but see TTM and SCT).

6. These models tend to view intentions as the direct precursor of behavior (see "Intention-Behavior gap" section of this chapter).

7. None of these models are comprehensive, other constructs can always be added to the model to explain additional variance.

8. Many of the models are difficult to refute (Noar & Zimmerman, 2005). As they are built on correlational evidence, at what point are the intercorrelations between the constructs too weak?

9. These models primarily treat individuals as rational actors in which we consider and subsequently use our explicit cognitions (e.g., perceived behavioral control, response costs) to direct our behavior which overlooks many of the more automatic processes influencing behavior (see Dual Process Models later in this chapter for an alternative approach).

10. Across theories, equivalent constructs are labelled with different terms (e.g., TPB: attitudes; HAPA: outcome expectancies; TTM: pros and cons) and this could potentially slow down or hinder the accumulation or synthesis of related evidence.

11. Health behavior theories often fail to consider sub-categories or sub-types of constructs, failing to distinguish, for example, injunctive (beliefs about what other people think you should do) and descriptive (beliefs about how much of the behavior other people do) norms or affective (how one feels regarding a behavior) and instrumental (whether one feels that performing a behavior is beneficial) attitudes (Sheeran et al., 2017).

12. These models are often tested in WEIRD (Western, Educated, Industrialized, Rich, Democratic) countries and, as such, the empirical evidence for the utility of these models in other countries (e.g., where one's actions might be more collectivist and less individualist) is relatively limited.

A COMMON PROBLEM FOR MANY OF THESE THEORIES: THE INTENTION-BEHAVIOR GAP

WHAT IS IT?

According to many of the theories described above, intentions are seen as the main, immediate determinant of behavior and thus there should be a strong relationship between intentions and behavior. In other words, if a person intends to eat healthily, then they should eat healthily. Similarly, if a person does not intend to speed while driving, then they should not speed.

However, this does not always happen. Sometimes people who intend to eat healthily do not do it, and sometimes people who do not intend to speed actually do it. The former group in particular represent the most common scenario underlying what is called the intention-behavior gap (Orbell & Sheeran, 1998). The intention-behavior gap is a term used to reflect the fact that, sometimes, people do not always do what they intend to do.

WHY DO PEOPLE FAIL TO ACT ON THEIR INTENTIONS?

One reason why intentions fail to predict behavior is that individuals may struggle, when they complete measures of intentions, to accurately consider how they would actually feel in that situation (e.g., whether or not to engage in unprotected sex during a night out when neither partner has condoms). Sheeran and Webb (2016) suggest a wide range of other factors that can lead to people failing to act on their intentions (see also Chapter 7, Intentions and Health Behavior section). These can relate to *getting started* with the behavior in the first place (e.g., they forget to do it; they miss good opportunities to act), failing to *keep on track* with the behavior (other things get in the way such as more tempting, competing goals ("Oh, that packet of cookies looks nice…"), bad habits ("I eat cookies whenever I'm bored at home") or bad influences ("I'm having half a pack of cookies, do you want the other half?!").

Reviews by Conner and Norman (2022), Cooke and Sheeran (2004), as well as Sheeran and Webb (2016), highlight a range of moderators, largely relating to the qualities or strength of intention, that influence the relationship between intentions and behavior. Moderators are variables that influence the strength of the relationship between two other variables (see Chapter 6 for more details). Effectively, stronger intentions are more likely to be fulfilled and certain factors can influence how strong one's intentions are, many of which are listed here:

> *Intention stability*: the extent to which intentions do not change over time. Intentions are more strongly associated with behavior when intentions remain stable across time (e.g., Conner, Sheeran, Norman & Armitage, 2000). Put another way, one reason that intentions might not predict future behavior is that intentions might change between the measurements of intention and behavior.
> *Accessibility*: intentions more strongly predict behavior when intentions are more highly accessible (e.g., more easily come to mind in certain, critical situations).
> *Intention certainty* (e.g., I am certain that I intend to eat five portions of fruit and vegetables): refers to being unbudgeable on an issue (Bassili, 1996).

Anticipated regret (e.g., I would regret not eating five portions of fruit and vegetables): beliefs regarding whether or not feelings of regret will arise when one fails to act. If one anticipates that they will regret not performing a specific behavior then they are more likely to perform their intended behavior. There are at least three possible reasons for this (Sheeran & Orbell, 1999). First, anticipated regret might increase the accessibility of intentions thus increasing the likelihood that these intentions are activated and subsequently acted upon. Second, anticipated regret could encourage people to plan more how they will act thus influencing intention elaboration, or third, by associating inactivity with negative affect anticipated regret might bind people to their intentions.

Identity (e.g., I'm the kind of person who eats five portions of fruit and vegetables each day): when an individual sees doing the behavior as being part of who they are, intentions to do the behavior are more likely to lead to performing the behavior.

Intentions based on attitudes (vs. norms), especially affective attitudes (vs. cognitive attitudes): Sheeran and Webb (2016) highlight evidence that basing an intention on personal beliefs (attitudes) rather than perceptions of what others may want you to do (norms) leads to intentions that are more likely to translate to behavior. This is particularly likely to be the case for affective attitudes (feelings about doing the behavior) than cognitive attitudes (what one thinks are the consequences of performing the behavior).

Goal prioritization: when the behavior is prioritized over other competing behaviors then intentions are more likely to be predictive of behavior. For example, Conner et al. (2016) demonstrated that a measure of goal priority (e.g., I would be prepared to give up many other goals and priorities to exercise vigorously at least three times per week over the next two weeks) influenced the extent to which intentions to exercise vigorously predicted levels of vigorous exercise. Specifically, those individuals who prioritized vigorous exercise over other goals were more likely to follow through on their intentions to do vigorous exercise.

More recent work has demonstrated that goal prioritization can be manipulated. Conner et al. (2022) asked participants in two intervention groups to choose health behaviors to prioritize from a choice of six (e.g., physical activity, dental flossing). One intervention group prioritized one behavior and the other prioritized two. Afterwards, they wrote down how they would prioritize these behaviors. They found that those participants randomized to the goal prioritization groups reported performing their chosen behaviors more than those in the control groups. Importantly, this happened without a detrimental impact on the remaining behaviors on the initial list of six. It is not known, however, whether there were any detrimental effects on health behaviors or other behaviors not on the initial list.

Habits: when behaviors are performed consistently in the same (non-changing) context then they become habitual and are guided not by conscious decision making but by automatic processes (Ouellette & Wood, 1998). Consequently, intentions can correspond with behavior more strongly when habits are weak than when habits are strong (e.g., Verplanken et al., 1998).

MODERN APPROACHES

THEORY INTEGRATION

As you can see, there are a large number of theories of behavior; only some of which have been outlined above. A problem one faces when trying to understand, predict or change behavior is which theory should I choose? One way of getting around this problem is to try to integrate these key theories into one "super-theory."

There have been two independent attempts, based on expert consensus, that have identified the most important determinants of behavior (Fishbein et al., 2001; Michie et al., 2005). Looking through the overviews of the theories above, you'll notice that a number of constructs (elements within a theory), or very similar constructs (e.g., perceived behavioral control and self-efficacy; attitudes and outcome expectancies), appear in more than one theory. This overlap between the theories provides the basis for attempting to combine or integrate the theories.

FISHBEIN'S APPROACH

A team of leading psychologists led by Martin Fishbein first attempted to identify the key determinants of behavior from the leading theories of health/social behavior. They concluded there were eight key determinants of any behavior:

1. *Intentions*: how committed individuals are to performing the behavior
2. *Environmental constraints*: preventing behavior (e.g., not having sports facilities near to where one lives might be viewed as an environmental constraint hindering exercise)
3. *Skills*: whether the person has the *actual* ability or skills to perform the behavior
4. *Self-efficacy*: whether the person *thinks* they have the ability to perform the behavior in a variety of situations

5. *Emotional reactions*: to the behavior and whether these are positive or negative
6. *Self-standards and sanctions*: whether the person sees their performing the behavior as being consistent or inconsistent with how they see themselves
7. *Perceived normative pressure*: whether individuals feel that important people want them to perform the behavior or not; peer pressure could be seen as a fairly strong example of this
8. *Anticipated outcomes*: attitude towards performing the behavior.

These determinants should help explain why some people perform a given behavior while others do not. The first three determinants are viewed as necessary (i.e., if a person does not have positive intentions *or* there are environmental constraints *or* the person does not have the skills needed to perform the behavior then the behavior will not be performed) and sufficient (if an individual has the intention to ask for a pay raise); there are no environmental constraints (e.g., a poor financial climate) and the skills to ask for a pay raise, the individual is very likely to ask for a pay raise). Determinants 4–8 are seen as influencing intention.

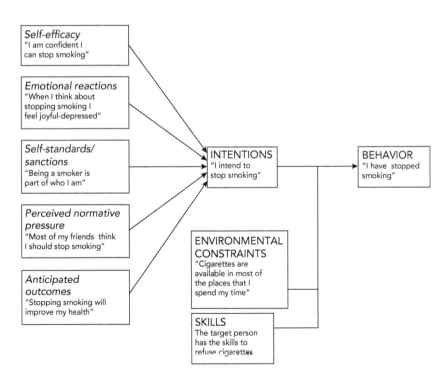

FIGURE 2.8 Fishbein et al.'s Theoretical Integration of Key Behavioural Determinants. Applied to stopping smoking.

THEORETICAL DOMAINS FRAMEWORK (TDF)

A second attempt (Michie et al., 2005) used a similar consensus approach to identify key determinants of changing the behavior of health professionals such that they act in line with the best practice. The final list of 128 constructs identified from 33 theories were grouped into 12 domains to constitute the original Theoretical Domains Framework (TDF). This original version overlapped significantly with the determinants of Fishbein et al. As these projects were conducted independently, there is some level of confidence that these are key determinants of behavior. In addition to the eight determinants identified by Fishbein et al. (2001), the four additional domains identified by Michie et al. were: (1) knowledge (e.g., regarding particular illnesses/risks associated with performing/not performing the behavior – knowing how to perform the behavior); (2) memory, attention, and decision processes (e.g., will an individual remember to perform the behavior or be distracted by features of the environment); (3) behavioral regulation (largely related to tackling the intention-behavior gap through strategies such as planning and self-monitoring); and (4) nature of the behaviors (e.g., whether it has become part of one's routine or whether it is a behavior that the individual has not performed before). More recently, the TDF has been revised to include new domains (e.g., optimism) or to refine or remove other domains (Cane et al., 2012). This 14 domain version is summarized in Figure 2.9 illustrating how the domains map onto a simpler model called the COM-B and takes us on, quite nicely, to our next section.

COM-B AND THE BEHAVIOR CHANGE WHEEL

The Capability Opportunity Motivation–Behavior model (COM-B; Michie, van Stralen & West, 2011) states that behavior is influenced by a combination of (1) physical and (2) psychological capability (covering things such as strength, knowledge and skills), (3) physical and (4) social

CAPABILITY		MOTIVATION		OPPORTUNITY	
Psychological	Physical	Automatic	Reflective	Social	Physical
1. Knowledge 2. Memory, attention and decision processes 3. Behavioural regulation	4. Physical skills	5. Reinforcement 6. Emotion	7. Social/professional role and identity 8. Beliefs about capabilities 9. Beliefs about consequences 10. Optimism 11. Intentions 12. Goals	13. Social influences	14. Environmental context and resources

FIGURE 2.9 Theoretical Domains Framework (green)/COM-B (yellow) relationship.

(Based on Michie, Atkins & West, 2014).

opportunity (e.g., the behavior does not have physical barriers and is socially acceptable) and motivation, broadly construed to include (5) reflective/decision-making, reflecting on what's good and bad about performing/not performing the behavior and more, (6) automatic/impulsive/emotional reaction types. According to this model, all of these components, with the exception of reflective motivation, are needed for behavior to occur. Opportunity and capability also influence motivation.

COM-B has been integrated in a wider framework called the Behavior Change Wheel (BCW). The BCW guides interventionists (researchers, policymakers, etc.) on how to select particular interventions and the policies that can be implemented to deliver the interventions. At the heart, or the inner wheel, of the BCW is the COM-B which can be used to identify the key factors (capability, opportunity, motivation) that should be targeted to change the behavior. On the next (middle) wheel, are the nine intervention types or functions (e.g., persuasion, education, environmental restructuring) that can be used to change the various COM-B components. The outer wheel of the model comprises the seven policy options that can be used to implement the intervention types (see Figure 2.10).

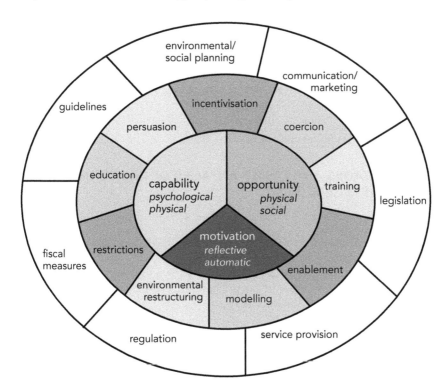

FIGURE 2.10 Behaviour Change Wheel/COM-B.

Adapted from Michie et al. (2011).

The starting point for using the BCW to develop an intervention is to consider which behavior(s) need to change in whom before considering which aspects of capability, opportunity and/or motivation need to be targeted. Should you wish to use a more detailed approach to understanding behavioral determinants than the COM-B, the TDF (see previous section in this chapter) can be used instead.

Once you have figured out what needs to change, the relevant COM-B or TDF components can be mapped to intervention types and, in turn, policy options using the recommended intervention types for each COM-B component and the recommended policy options for each intervention type. As the intervention types are quite broad, the intervention functions can be mapped to more specific behavior change techniques (as included in the Behavior Change Techniques Taxonomy v1, see Chapter 3) or such mappings can be made directly from the TDF domains to behavior change techniques. At the final step, how the intervention is to be delivered (mode, intensity, etc.) needs to be decided.

When developing the intervention, the intervention elements, such as the intervention functions, behavior change techniques or policy options, can be evaluated using the APEASE criteria (Affordability, Practicability (i.e., whether it can be delivered to the target population as intended), Effectiveness/cost-effectiveness, Acceptability, Side-effects/safety, Equity (i.e., do different groups of people benefit equally?)) to narrow down choices regarding what the intervention should include/not include.

THEORY CRITIQUE BOX 2.9

ADVANTAGES AND DISADVANTAGES OF THE BEHAVIOR CHANGE WHEEL (BCW)

Advantages

1. The COM-B elegantly and simply represents the key determinants of behavior.
2. Compared to many other models or frameworks, the BCW more explicitly specifies how behavior change can be achieved with direct guidance for interventionists.
3. Related to point 2, the BCW directly links interventions to theory (COM-B) with guides regarding which types of interventions should change capability, opportunity and motivation.
4. The BCW helps bridge the gap between theory, interventions and policy and as such can be used by policymakers (and others) to

make choices about how to address particular issues related to behavior and their associated outcomes such as reducing obesity in children. It provides guidance regarding which types of policies are best used to deliver which types of interventions.

5. As it was derived from a host of frameworks, the BCW is regarded as comprehensive in terms of its coverage of intervention types and policy options.
6. By incorporating "opportunity," the BCW considers behavior in context rather than in isolation of context.
7. It incorporates automatic, as well as reflective, processes like dual-process models.
8. Guidance is provided regarding how interventionists can identify the root problem/s (i.e., whether capability, opportunity and/or motivation should be targeted). This can be achieved using interviews or focus groups, questionnaires and worksheets (and ideally a combination of these to enable triangulation of results; i.e., do the methods lead to the same findings?) with recommendations provided for each.
9. A formal means of selecting intervention components (e.g., behavior change techniques, policy options) is provided via the APEASE criteria.
10. Guidance is provided on how to evaluate BCW-based interventions including identifying mechanisms/processes and fidelity.

Disadvantages

1. The body of evidence to show that the BCW can be used to develop effective interventions is still emerging.
2. Links between the COM-B components and intervention types, and between the intervention types and the policy options, were derived through expert opinion/small-sized consensus methods rather than data-driven experimental evidence.
3. It may not always be obvious which combination of capability, opportunity and motivation is interfering with the target behavior and other elements of the process (e.g., evaluating different components using APEASE criteria) can be subjective.

FOGG BEHAVIOR MODEL

B.J. Fogg presents a model that is similar in some ways to that of the COM-B in that three factors – motivation, ability and prompts/triggers – must come together for behavior to happen. According to this model, for behavior to occur, an individual must have at least some motivation to perform the target behavior, have at least some ability to perform it and be prompted at the right time.

The model also describes motivation and ability as a trade-off: if motivation is particularly high, then ability does not need to be very high initially (individuals may be so motivated that they figure out a solution to aid their ability to do the behavior: Andrew's younger child, Sonny, is motivated to do well on a math game called TimesTables Rockstars so he persisted, despite his initial lack of ability, to do well on the game and master his times tables) and vice-versa (Andrew's older daughter, Milla, is good at the game but isn't particularly motivated to do it; sometimes she'll play it simply because it is easy for her and doesn't require much effort). The combination of motivation and ability levels will put individuals above or below a behavior activation threshold. Receiving a trigger when the individual is above the behavior activation threshold can lead to the behavior. If the wrong type of trigger arrives at the wrong time, then these can lead to adverse outcomes such as feeling frustrated (prompted when ability is too low) or distracted (prompted when motivation is too low).

So how is motivation and ability increased and what types of triggers are needed and when? Motivation can be increased by influencing pleasure/pain; hope or fear in anticipation of an outcome; promoting social acceptance or helping to avoid social rejection. For ability, the model resists recommending teaching or training, arguing these require effort and energy and that people prefer methods that make the behavior easier to do. Ease can be enhanced through (1) time (making things quicker to do), (2) cost (ensuring the behavior (e.g., buying fresh fruit and vegetables) is affordable for the target population, requiring (3) less physical effort and (4) thought, (5) does not break social conventions and (6) the behavior being routine (i.e., that they do repeatedly). Interventionists should identify which of these six factors is in the shortest supply, at the point that the behavior is triggered (e.g., time), and work to address this (e.g., can the behavior become quicker to do?).

Fogg describes three types of trigger needed depending on whether the individual has high motivation but low ability (*facilitator* triggers which indicate the behavior is simple in some way (i.e., quick, requires little physical effort, etc.), low motivation but high ability (*spark* triggers of pleasure/pain, hope/fear or social rejection/approval), or high motivation and high ability (*signal* triggers that serve as reminders, e.g., signs in the environment to remind people to walk up steps rather than using escalators can remind those who are motivated and have the ability to use the steps).

If the target behavior is not happening then, according to this model, researchers can try to identify whether this is due to a lack of motivation, lack of ability or inappropriate or ineffective prompts. Conversely, if an unwanted (e.g., unhealthy) behavior is occurring, Fogg argues that figuring out ways to take away motivation or ability or to remove triggers/prompts for the behavior can be an effective means of preventing the behavior from happening.

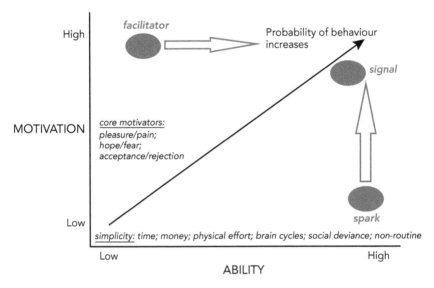

FIGURE 2.11 Fogg Behavior Model (note: red ovals reflect the three forms of trigger).

Adapted from Fogg (2009).

THEORY CRITIQUE BOX 2.10

ADVANTAGES AND DISADVANTAGES OF FOGG'S BEHAVIOR MODEL

Advantages

1. Intuitively appealing as a potential means of explaining how behavior can be triggered in certain situations as well as explaining variability in individuals (how or why individuals may do certain behaviors sometimes but not others).
2. Suggests how different types of prompts can work for different people depending on their level of motivation and ability – as such it is useful for underpinning tailored interventions and can be

applied within technology-based interventions (e.g., apps) that can provide tailored forms of persuasion more easily.

3. Can inform interventions for both increasing healthy behaviors and reducing unhealthy behaviors.
4. Specifies triggers for increasing motivation and ability, as well as triggers for when both motivation and ability are high – as such, the model is helpful for behavior *change* as well as prediction.

Disadvantages

1. Few experimental tests of the model and those that do use experimental methods do not provide much support (e.g., Plak, van Klaveren & Cornelisz, in press).
2. At least for healthcare behaviors, it has been claimed that facilitator triggers may not be particularly effective (Krejany, Kanjo, Dadich & Jiwa, 2020).
3. Emerged particularly in the context of technology-driven online behaviors rather than health behaviors directly.
4. May work better for simple behaviors (e.g., getting people to visit certain websites, click on certain links, etc.) than more complex or effortful behaviors.

DUAL PROCESS MODELS

While the models above have tended to focus predominately on explicit cognition that one is consciously aware of and requires effort to process relevant information (i.e., thoughts and feelings about a behavior), more recent theories have also sought to incorporate implicit cognition that which occurs quickly, efficiently, with little or no effort and happens outside of one's conscious awareness. Models that take into account both explicit and implicit processes have been labelled dual process models.

There are a fairly large number of dual process models that have been referred to within the psychological literature. These tended, at least initially, to emerge in the sub-disciplines of social psychology and cognitive psychology (see Smith & DeCoster, 2000, for a review) though others have emerged in health and clinical psychology such as PRIME Theory (West & Brown, 2013). One of the more most popular dual process models is Strack and Deutsch's (2004) Reflective & Impulsive Model (RIM).

The RIM (see also Chapters 7 and 8) describes behavior as being influenced by two distinct systems of processing – a reflective system and an impulsive system. The reflective system is analogous to the type of systems and processes outlined in many of the theories that we have considered in this chapter with a decision process that results in intending. For example, once an individual sees an object such as a piece of fruit, classifies it as a piece of fruit, draws on factual (e.g., it is an apple) and evaluative (e.g., I like apples) information, they come to the point of forming an intention relating to whether they will buy/approach or not buy/avoid this particular piece of fruit. The impulsive system operates through a process of spreading activation whereby activation of particular concepts (e.g., apples) following perceptual input (e.g., seeing the apple) leads to the quick-fire activation of associated concepts (e.g., love, tasty). These two systems can interact and jointly activate behavioral schemata that directly precede action. Consequently, both impulsive and reflective systems can jointly influence action and their relative contributions can vary as a function of different factors.

Hofmann, Friese and Wiers (2008) classified three groups of factors that influence the extent to which implicit attitudes relate to behavior: 1) availability of control resources, 2) reliance on impulses, and 3) motivation to control one's behavior. Implicit attitudes are argued to be more strongly predictive of behavior when control resources are not available and/or one is not motivated to control their behavior (e.g., when doing so is too effortful, there are few costs in relation to performing the behavior) or when one relies on impulses.

Implicit attitude research is currently an emerging topic in health behavior change having received much attention in social psychology and applied areas such as consumer psychology. As well as correlational evidence that implicit attitudes can predict product choice (e.g., Friese et al., 2006; Perugini, 2005; Richetin et al., 2007), there is some experimental evidence supportive of the role of implicit attitudes in determining consumer behavior. In a study by Strick et al. (2009), participants exposed to humorous cartoons related to a novel energy drink or household products were more likely to choose these products when given the choice. Changes in implicit attitudes explained (mediated, see Chapter 6) the effect of these cartoons on product choice suggesting that implicit attitudes can be important in determining behavior. Hollands et al. (2012) have also shown, in the context of health behavior change, that exposing individuals to images illustrating the adverse consequences of an unhealthy diet can promote healthier implicit attitudes and healthier food choices. However, reviews of the evidence provide a mixed picture regarding the impact of changing implicit attitudes on behavior change (Aulbach et al., 2019; Forscher et al., 2019).

BURNING ISSUE BOX 2.1

DO INDIVIDUALS RESPOND TO INFORMATION PRESENTED AS GAINS OR LOSSES DIFFERENTLY?

In simple expectancy-value models, we might expect gains and losses to be given similar weights in deciding how we act. Prospect Theory (Tversky & Kahneman, 1981) suggests that losses are actually more painful than gains are pleasurable (i.e., they are not simple opposites). For example, people are more upset by a loss of £100 than they are pleased by a gain of £100. Indeed individuals want approximately one and a half times as much gain to balance a loss (e.g., to be prepared to bet and lose £10 on a coin toss they want to be able to potentially win £15 to think it is a worthwhile bet).

As well as showing that a loss is more significant than the equivalent gain, Prospect Theory also shows that a sure gain is favored over a probabilistic gain, and that a probabilistic loss is preferred to a definite loss. This difference between gains and losses also shows up in framing studies. The framing effect is an example of a cognitive bias, in which people react differently to a particular choice depending on whether it is presented as a loss or as a gain. People tend to avoid risk when a positive frame is presented but seek risks when a negative frame is presented. The classic example is one where people were asked to imagine that they are responsible for deciding between two policies in the face of a flu epidemic that was expected to kill 600 people. In the positive frame presented below, 72% chose option A and 28% choose option B. In the negative frame presented below, 78% choose option B and 22% choose option A. Clearly the differing options present the same net outcome but the framing drives the choices made.

	Option A	Option B
Positive Frame:	200 lives saved	One-third chance 600 lives saved, two-thirds chance 0 lives saved
Negative Frame:	400 lives lost	One-third chance 0 lives lost, two-thirds chance 600 lives lost

Such framing effects can be used to influence how decisions are made and are one example of the fact that we do not always act as rational decision makers but show systematic biases in the way we use information.

PROTOTYPE-WILLINGNESS MODEL (PWM; GIBBONS & GERRARD, 1995)

The PWM is a different type of dual-process model and was developed to try to explain why many young people engage in health risk behaviors such as unprotected sex. They argue that young people (and presumably others, as risk behaviors are in no means restricted by age!) are likely to experience situations in which the opportunity to engage in different health risk behaviors presents itself. Despite not intending to engage in the risk behavior, as an individual encounters a situation that could make the behavior more likely (e.g., being intoxicated and not having condoms for risky sex; being late and speeding while driving), an individual may be "willing" to engage in the behavior given the opportunity to do so. Their behavior is assumed to reflect a reaction to the social situation rather than a premeditated intention or plan to engage in a health risk behavior.

The PWM is based on three key assumptions. First, that many of the health risk behaviors performed by young people in particular are not best thought of as intentional or planned. Rather, they can be considered to be the result of reactions to "risk-conducive situations" that many young people encounter. Second, many health risk behaviors are typically performed with, or in the presence of, others. So, Mark might be more likely to have too many alcoholic drinks when out with friends or when having dinner with his partner Sarah. The social nature of these events is key and so social comparison processes are likely to have an important impact on performance of the health risk behavior. Third, young people tend to be more concerned about their social images and, as a result, are likely to be aware and react to the social implications of their behavior. This is likely the case for behaviors that are performed with others in social settings and that are associated with vivid/salient images. These images might include the "typical drinker" or the "typical smoker" (Blanton et al., 2001). As a result, performing a health risk behavior likely has important social consequences, i.e., an acceptance of the image associated with the behavior.

PWM describes two "pathways" to health risk behavior among adolescents and young adults. First, a "reasoned pathway," reflects the operation of more or less rational decision making processes as outlined by models such as the TPB. In this pathway, health risk behavior is based on a consideration of the pros and cons of performing the behavior. Consequently, behavioral intention is seen to be the key proximal predictor of health risk behavior in this pathway. Gibbons and Gerrard (1995) use measures of behavioral expectations rather than of behavioral intentions to predict health risk behavior (see Sheppard et al., 1988), arguing that adolescents may be more likely to acknowledge that they are likely to perform a health risk behavior in the future than they are to admit that they intend to do so.

Second, a "social reaction pathway" is what makes the PWM distinct from models such as the TPB. This is the pathway likely to drive behavior in risk-conducive situations and describes four factors that impact on individuals' willingness to engage in health-risk behaviors when they encounter risk-conducive situations. Number one is *subjective norms* that focus on perceptions of whether important others engage in the behavior and whether they are likely to approve or disapprove of the individual performing the behavior. In this way, Gibbons and Gerrard (1995) highlight the importance of both descriptive and injunctive social norms (Cialdini et al., 1990). Number two is *attitudes* that are primarily concerned with the perceived likelihood of negative outcomes (e.g., perceived vulnerability). In particular, a willingness to perform a health-risk behavior in a risk-conducive situation may be associated with a downplaying of the risks associated with the behavior. Number three is *past behavior*. Given that many health-risk behaviors attract social approval and are enjoyable, having performed a health-risk behavior in the past may be associated with more positive subjective norms (Gerrard et al., 1996), more positive attitudes (Bentler & Speckart, 1979) and a greater willingness to perform the behavior again in the future (Gibbons et al., 1998). Number four is the *prototype* associated with the health-risk behavior, i.e., the image that people have of the type of person who engages in a certain behavior (e.g., the "typical ecstasy user"). According to the PWM, prototype favorability (i.e., the extent to which the image is positively evaluated) and prototype similarity (i.e., the perceived similarity between that image and how you view yourself) interact to impact on individuals' willingness to engage in a health-risk behavior. The four factors identified in the "social reaction pathway" have their influence on behaviors through **behavioral willingness**. Gibbons and Gerrard (1995) argue that the willingness to engage in a health-risk behavior in a risk conducive situation, compared to behavioral expectations, provides a better prediction of subsequent behavior as it reflects the social reactive nature of many of the health-risk behaviors performed by young people.

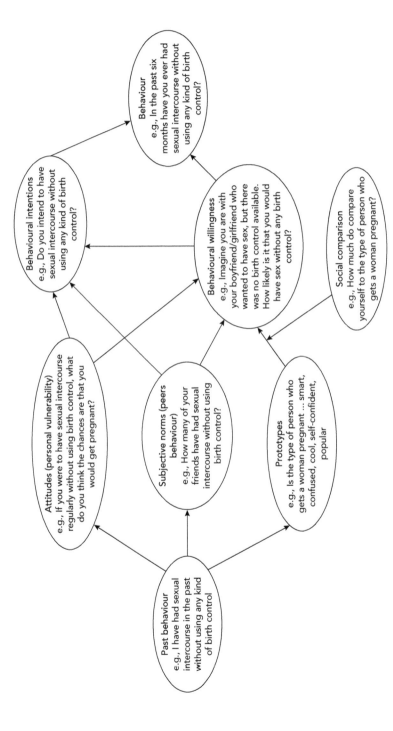

FIGURE 2.12 Prototype Willingness Model (from Gibbons et al., 2015). Applied to sexual intercourse without birth control.

THEORY CRITIQUE BOX 2.11

ADVANTAGES AND DISADVANTAGES OF THE PROTOTYPE-WILLINGNESS MODEL (PWM)

Advantages

1. One of the few models focused on risk behaviors.
2. As a dual process model, it takes into account both reasoned/ reflective and more reflexive routes to behavior.
3. There is empirical support for various components of the model (see Todd et al., 2016, for a meta-analysis of the PWM).
4. The model points to an important but often overlooked distinction between different types of motivation: willingness and expectations.
5. The PWM adds to our understanding of health risk behaviors by highlighting that many health risk behaviors are not intentional or planned. Instead, people may be reacting to risk-conducive situations in which they are willing to perform the behavior.
6. The PWM highlights the importance of prototype perceptions as an additional source of normative influence on health behavior.

Disadvantages

1. The model seems to work better for some behaviors (e.g., alcohol intake) and some age groups (adolescents) than others (Todd et al., 2016).
2. There have been calls for more research identifying differences in predicting health risk vs. health protective behaviors (Todd et al., 2016).
3. Relatively few studies have tested the model as a whole (Elliott et al., 2017).
4. Tests of the model sometimes combine measures of expectations and intentions (Elliott et al., 2017).
5. Evidence for the model is typically considered in the context of imaginary scenarios (e.g., "Imagine being in a night club with friends and they offered you ecstasy. How willing would you be to take it?") rather than real-life situations (see Lewis et al., 2020, for an exception using ecological momentary assessment (EMA) methods to track PWM cognitions over time).

THEORIES OF MAINTENANCE OF BEHAVIOR CHANGE

While health benefits can be achieved by changing some health behaviors once (e.g., promoting attendance at a sexual health clinic), for many health behaviors such as healthy eating, physical activity and smoking cessation, initial changes do not lead to significant or indeed any benefit unless these changes are maintained over an extended period of time. A review by Kwasnicka et al. (2016) identified 100 theories that included hypotheses about behavior change maintenance. Of these, 43 theories suggested distinctions in the processes underlying initiation and maintenance. In reviewing these 43 theories, Kwasnicka et al. identified five themes that appear pivotal for maintenance.

1. Specific *motives* including undertaking the behavior because (a) they enjoy the behavior or are satisfied with the outcomes arising from initial behavior changes; (b) the behavior is consistent with their identity and how they see themselves; (c) they are self-determined (an individual doing something because they feel pressured either by others or by themselves (extrinsic motivation) may be useful for initial change but doing it because they want to do it (intrinsic motivation) is critical for maintenance);
2. Self-regulation which involves controlling behavior by replacing unwanted behaviors triggered through more automatic processes with goal-directed behaviors;
3. Habits (see description of habits earlier in the chapter);
4. Resources. Both physical and psychological resources need to remain high for maintenance;
5. Environment and social influences which can provide incentives or cues which derail initial changes in health behaviors.

Based on responses from 40 experts in theory who were consulted by Kwasnicka et al., the most commonly identified theories relevant to maintenance were the TTM, HAPA, SCT (all described earlier in this chapter), plus the Relapse Prevention Model and Self-Determination Theory which we briefly overview next.

RELAPSE PREVENTION MODEL (MARLATT & GEORGE, 1984; MARLATT & GORDON, 1985)

This model has been typically applied to the maintenance of abstinence from unhealthy or addictive behaviors but could, in principle, also be applied to the maintenance of healthy behaviors. According to the Relapse

Prevention Model, an individual is at risk of relapse when they have weak self-efficacy (whereby the individual feels they have an inability to cope) combined with positive expectancies about engaging in the unhealthy behavior (e.g., thinking that having a cigarette will make them feel better). Relapse is most likely when an individual experiences negative emotions (such as feeling depressed, stressed or anxious), interpersonal conflict (such as difficulties with one's partner or friends) or social pressure from others to engage in the unhealthy behavior.

To encourage maintenance, an individual should view a "relapse" as a transitional process rather than an all-or-nothing process. As such, a smoker who has quit cigarettes who smokes a cigarette again, should view this instance as a lapse or a slip that has been triggered in a high-risk situation rather than a full-blown relapse. To maintain change, an individual should (1) undergo skills training to identify and cope with triggers for lapse (e.g., by using coping plans, along the lines of implementation intentions (see Chapters 3 and 7), to identify triggers and plan how to deal with them); (2) use cognitive re-framing to deal with lapse (e.g., framing lapses as attributable to external, environmental factors that are avoidable rather than internal factors to do with the individual, in order to boost their self-efficacy in maintaining behavior change); (3) develop broader lifestyle changes in order to enhance an individual's general coping capacity. Adopting such techniques strengthens their ability/perceived ability to maintain positive changes in health behavior.

SELF-DETERMINATION THEORY (SDT; DECI & RYAN, 1985)

SDT distinguishes between different types of motivation that can influence behavior. According to this theory, there are three main types of motivation: intrinsic motivation (whereby an individual performs the behavior for its own sake: e.g., Dave exercises because he finds it enjoyable), extrinsic motivation (whereby an individual performs the behavior because of more external reasons: e.g., Maeve exercises to please Dave) and amotivation (whereby an individual has no motivation to do the behavior). Extrinsic motivation can be sub-divided into integrated regulation (whereby an individual does the behavior because it aligns with their values or identity), identified (the individual does the behavior because it leads to outcomes that they value), introjected (the individual does the behavior to avoid negative emotions such as guilt or to obtain approval) and external (to avoid punishment or to get a reward). These types of motivation lie on a continuum from the most autonomous or internalized forms of motivation, where the reasons for performing the behavior originate from oneself, to the least autonomous forms, where the reasons for performing the behavior

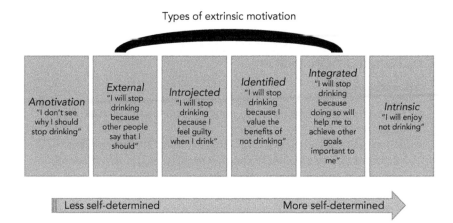

FIGURE 2.13 Self-Determination Theory: The continuum of motivation types. Applied to stopping drinking.

are more pressured by external forces (see Figure 2.13). The more autonomous, or internalized, the motivation underlying the behavior, the greater effort and persistence the individual will put in to drive behavior change and maintenance.

The process of internalization can be facilitated by fulfilling three basic psychological needs: autonomy (when the person feels like they have a sense of choice and undertakes a behavior under their own volition or freewill), competence (when the person feels capable of being able to perform the behavior) and relatedness (when the person feels connected to and understood by important others). The basic needs can be boosted by various behavior change techniques. For example, autonomy can be boosted by exploring values and offering choice; competence can be enhanced by skills-building and problem-solving; relatedness can be improved via techniques such as developing empathy and interpersonal relationships. When these three needs are met in a particular context (e.g., in an exercise class) then the behaviors relevant to that context (i.e., exercising within the class) will be more likely to be autonomously driven and thus more likely to be maintained in the future. In support of the model, a recent review of experimental studies indicated that SDT-based health behavior change interventions positively change SDT constructs and health behaviors and physical/psychological health outcomes, and that changes in autonomous motivation (but not controlled motivation or amotivation) were associated with changes in health behavior (Ntoumanis et al., 2021).

THEORY CRITIQUE BOX 2.12

ADVANTAGES AND DISADVANTAGES OF SELF-DETERMINATION THEORY

Advantages

1. Has a good evidence base including meta-analyses of experimental evidence (e.g., Ntoumanis et al., 2021).
2. As well as positively impacting behavior, there is evidence that interventions based on SDT can also have small, positive benefits for physical and psychological health.
3. Unlike many other models, it differentiates between different types of motivation and thus provides greater depth to this fundamental driver of human behavior.
4. Gives greater emphasis to the role of the social environment than other models by highlighting its role in influencing the basic psychological needs of autonomy, competence and relatedness.
5. Given calls for patients to have more autonomy in their decision-making, SDT has sound potential as it incorporates autonomy as a key basic psychological need.
6. Has various validated measures (e.g., Intrinsic Motivation Inventory; BREQ-2).
7. Benefits from the publication of its own behavior change techniques taxonomy (Teixeira et al., 2020).

Disadvantages

1. Relatively more complex than other models, comprising of several mini theories (e.g., Basic Psychological Needs Theory), meaning that it can be misunderstood and utilized inconsistently.
2. There could be more than three basic psychological needs. For example, Sheldon et al. (2001) present evidence that self-esteem could be an important fourth need related to, but distinct from, competence, plus relatedness and autonomy.
3. Although portrayed as a continuum from more intrinsically to extrinsically-driven motivation, it is possible that an individual could score highly on different types of motivation (e.g., intrinsic, external).
4. Linked to this point, relative measures of motivation (e.g., The Relative Autonomy Index) are problematic because they can score individuals with different motivational profiles in the same way (e.g., individuals who score highly across the board are grouped with those who score low across the board).

5. Similarities between SDT and motivational interviewing can cause some confusion.
6. Ntoumanis et al. (2021) have identified gaps: more work is needed on how to reduce controlled motivation and amotivation, to increase relatedness and to test for long-term effects on motivation and health outcomes.
7. Many experimental tests of the model have not blinded key study personnel to condition and tend to have other methodological limitations (Ntoumanis et al., 2021).

BURNING ISSUE BOX 2.2

CAN WORRY AND RUMINATION INFLUENCE HEALTH OUTCOMES BECAUSE OF THEIR RELATIONS WITH HEALTH BEHAVIORS?

Worry and rumination have been argued to increase, prolong and/or activate stress-related activity linked to a stressor, and this can lead to poorer health. This Perseverative Cognition Hypothesis (PCH; Brosschot et al., 2006) has been extended with Clancy et al. (2016) proposing that worry and rumination can cause poorer health, in part, because worry and rumination can discourage healthy behaviors and encourage unhealthy behaviors.

In support, various studies have indicated (albeit typically small) associations between worry and rumination with unhealthy snacking (e.g., Clancy et al., 2022), more sitting time and less walking (Clancy et al., 2020b) with generally stronger associations with sleep (e.g., Clancy et al., 2020a; McCarrick et al., in press a). Similar relations have also emerged in experimental studies that test interventions to reduce worry/rumination producing changes in these constructs that were associated with changes in health behaviors (see McCarrick et al., 2021, for a review).

Health behavior models such as the Theory of Planned Behavior suggest that variables such as worry and rumination would be distal predictors with their effects on behavior mediated by more proximal constructs. There is some evidence to support this with McCarrick et al. (in press b) reporting greater worry/rumination being associated with less perceived control and, in turn, less sleep. Trying to reduce worry and rumination, constructs not traditionally captured in social cognition models, could be part of novel interventions to change health behaviors.

SUMMARY

In this chapter we covered a range of different theories that have been influential in the field of health behavior change from the traditional to more modern theories. As well as having their own strengths and weaknesses (a number of which have been highlighted in the theory critique sections of this chapter), many of these theories overlap, and researchers have used this as a basis to form more integrative theories. Many of the theories covered in this chapter focus primarily on fairly slow, reflective processes and on the initiation of health behaviors. However, dual process models take into account automatic processes and other modern theories are useful when explaining maintenance of health behaviors. These types of theories include constructs that play important roles in behavior maintenance including habits, satisfaction with the outcomes of behavior and supportive environments.

FURTHER READING

Brandstätter, V., & Bernecker, K. (2022). Persistence and disengagement in personal goal pursuit. *Annual Review of Psychology, 73*, 271–299. This review covers traditional and newer theories relating to persistence (continuing to strive for a goal) and disengagement (moving away from a goal so that one does not feel, think or behave in line with the goal).

Hagger, M.S., & Hamilton, K. (2022). Social cognition theories and behavior change in COVID-19: A conceptual review. *Behaviour Research & Therapy, 154*, 104095. Considers and critiques the application of social cognition models to COVID-19 cognitions and behaviors. In particular, it highlights the preponderance of cross-sectional evidence and general lack of longitudinal and/or experimental tests of theory and a focus on intentions over behavior.

Sniehotta, F.F., Presseau, J., & Araújo-Soares, V. (2014). Time to retire the theory of planned behaviour. *Health Psychology Review, 8*, 1–7. An editorial providing strong criticism against the Theory of Planned Behavior and the need to identify better theories.

GLOSSARY

Autonomy: The extent to which an individual sees they have control over the behavior (whether they do the behavior is up to them).

Behavior change technique: A systematic strategy used in an attempt to change behavior (e.g., providing information on consequences; prompting specific goal setting; modelling the behavior).

Behavioral willingness: An openness to engage in a specific behavior when encountering situations that could make the behavior more likely.

Capacity: Like self-efficacy, the extent to which a person believes they are capable of performing the behavior.

Descriptive norms: Beliefs that important others do/don't do the behavior.

Experiential attitudes: Feelings relating to doing the behavior (e.g., My doing exercise is exciting/boring).

Injunctive norms: Beliefs that important others would approve/not approve of the individual doing the behavior.

Instrumental attitudes: Perceived outcomes of doing the behavior (e.g., My doing exercise is harmful-beneficial).

Intentions: The degree to which an individual is ready and willing to try to perform the behavior.

Perceived norms: Perceived social pressure to do/not do the behavior.

Theories, theory (or model): "a set of interrelated concepts, definitions and propositions that present a *systematic* view of events or situations by specifying relations among variables, in order to *explain* or *predict* the events or situations' (Glanz, Rimer, & Viswanath, 2015, p. 26).

Theory-relevant construct: A key concept or building block within a theory/model upon which the intervention is based. Example constructs in the Theory of Planned Behavior are "attitudes towards the behavior, perceived behavioral control, subjective norms, etc. Constructs can be further broken down into **determinants** (the predictors such as attitudes, subjective norms, PBC) or **outcomes** (such as behavior)."

REFERENCES

Abraham, C. & Sheeran, P. (2015). The health belief model. In Conner, M. and Norman, P. (Eds.). *Predicting and Changing Health Behaviour: Research and Practice with Social Cognition Models. 3rd ed.* Buckingham, UK: Open University Press, 30–69.

Ajzen, I. (1991). The theory of planned behavior. *Organizational Behavior and Human Decision Processes, 50,* 179–211.

Ajzen, I., & Fishbein, M. (1980). *Understanding attitudes and predicting social behavior.* Englewood Cliff, NJ: Prentice-Hall.

Albarracin, D., Gillette, J.C., Earl, A.N. et al. (2005). A test of major assumptions about behavior change: a comprehensive look at the effects of passive and active HIV-prevention interventions since the beginning of the epidemic. *Psychological Bulletin, 131,* 856–897.

Armitage, C.J. (2006). Evidence that implementation intentions promote transitions through the stages of change. *Journal of Consulting and Clinical Psychology, 74,* 141–151.

Armitage, C.J., & Conner, M. (2001). Efficacy of the theory of planned behaviour: A meta-analytic review. *British Journal of Social Psychology, 40,* 471–499.

Armitage, C.J., Sheeran, P., Conner, M., & Arden, M.A. (2004). Stages of change or changes of stage? Predicting transitions in transtheoretical model stages in relation to healthy food choice. *Journal of Consulting and Clinical Psychology, 72,* 491–499.

Ashford, S., Edmunds, J., & French, D.P. (2010). What is the best way to change self-efficacy to promote lifestyle and recreational physical activity? A systematic review with meta-analysis. *British Journal of Health Psychology, 15,* 265–288.

Aulbach, M.B., Knittle, K., & Haukkala, A. (2019). Implicit process interventions in eating behaviour: a meta-analysis examining mediators and moderators. *Health Psychology Review, 13,* 179–208.

Bandura, A. (1971). *Social learning theory.* New York: General Learning Press.

Bandura, A. (1977). Self-efficacy: Toward a unifying theory of behavioral change. *Psychological Review, 84,* 191–215.

Bandura, A. (1997). *Self-efficacy: The exercise of control.* New York: W.H. Freeman and Company.

Bashirian, S., Jenabi, E., Khazaei, S. et al. (2020). Factors associated with preventive behaviours of COVID-19 among hospital staff in Iran in 2020: an application of the Protection Motivation Theory. *Journal of Hospital Infection, 105,* 430–433.

Bassili, J.N. (1996). Meta-judgmental versus operative indexes of psychological attributes: The case of measures of attitude strength. *Journal of Personality and Social Psychology, 71,* 637–653.

Bentler, P.M., & Speckart, G. (1979). Model of attitude-behavior relations. *Psychological Review, 86,* 452–464.

Blanton, H., Van den Eijnden, R.J.J.M., Buunk, B.P. et al. (2001). Accentuate the negative: Social images in the prediction and promotion of condom use. *Journal of Applied Social Psychology, 31,* 274–295.

Bridle, C., Riemsma, R.P., Pattenden, J. et al. (2005). Systematic review of the effectiveness of health behavior interventions based on the transtheoretical model. *Psychology & Health, 20,* 283–301.

Brosschot, J.F., Gerin, W., & Thayer, J.F. (2006). The perseverative cognition hypothesis: a review of worry, prolonged stress-related physiological activation, and health. *Journal of Psychosomatic Research, 60,* 113–124.

Cane, J., O'Connor, D., & Michie, S. (2012). Validation of the theoretical domains framework for use in behaviour change and implementation research. *Implementation Science, 7,* 37.

Champion, V.L., & Skinner, C.S. (2008). The Health Belief Model. In K. Glanz & B. K. Rimer (Eds.), *Health behavior and health education research: Theory, research, and practice* (4th ed., pp. 45–65). Jossey-Bass.

Cialdini, R.B., Reno, R.R., & Kallgren, C.A. (1990). A focus theory of normative conduct: Recycling the concept of norms to reduce littering in public places. *Journal of Personality and Social Psychology, 58,* 1015–1026.

Clancy, F., O'Connor, D.B., & Prestwich, A. (2020b). Do worry and brooding predict health behaviors? A daily diary investigation. *International Journal of Behavioral Medicine, 27,* 591–601.

Clancy, F., Prestwich, A., Caperon, L., & O'Connor, D.B. (2016). Perseverative cognition and health behaviors: A systematic review and meta-analysis. *Frontiers in Human Neuroscience*, *10*, 534.

Clancy, F., Prestwich, A., Caperon, L., Tsipa, A., & O'Connor, D.B. (2020a). The association between worry and rumination with sleep in non-clinical populations: A systematic review and meta-analysis. *Health Psychology Review*, *14*, 427–448.

Clancy, F., Prestwich, A., Ferguson, E., & O'Connor, D.B. (2022). Cross-sectional and prospective associations between stress, perseverative cognition and health behaviours. *Psychology & Health*, *37*, 87–104.

Conn, V.S., Hafdahl, A.R., Brown, S.A., & Brown, L.M. (2008). Meta-analysis of patient education interventions to increase physical activity among chronically ill adults. *Patient Education and Counseling*, *70*, 157–172.

Conner, M., Abraham, C., Prestwich, A. et al. (2016). Impact of goal priority and goal conflict on the intention-health-behavior relationship: Tests on physical activity and other health behaviors. *Health Psychology*, *35*, 1017–1026.

Conner, M., & Norman, P. (2022). Understanding the intention-behavior gap: The role of intention strength. *Frontiers in Psychology*, *13*, 923464.

Conner, M., Sheeran, P., Norman, P., & Armitage, C. J. (2000). Temporal stability as a moderator of relationships in the theory of planned behaviour. *British Journal of Social Psychology*, *39*, 469–493.

Conner, M., Wilding, S., Prestwich, A. et al. (2022). Goal prioritization and behavior change: Evaluation of an intervention for multiple health behaviors. *Health Psychology*, *41*, 356–365.

Cooke, R., & Sheeran, P. (2004). Moderation of cognition-intention and cognition-behaviour relations: A meta-analysis of properties of variables from the theory of planned behaviour. *British Journal of Social Psychology*, *43*, 159–186.

Elliott, M.A., McCartan, R., Brewster, S.E. et al. (2017). An application of the prototype willingness model to drivers' speeding behaviour. *European Journal of Social Psychology*, *47*, 735–747.

Fishbein, M., & Ajzen, I. (2009). *Predicting and changing behavior: The reasoned action approach*. New York, NY: Psychology Press.

Fishbein, M., Triandis, H.C., Kanfer, F.H. et al. (2001). Factors influencing behaviour and behaviour change. In A. Baum, T.A. Revenson, & J.E. Singer (Eds.), *Handbook of health psychology* (pp. 3–17). Mahwah, NJ: Lawrence Erlbaum Associates.

Fogg, B.J. (2009). A behavior model for persuasive design. In *Proceedings of the 4th international Conference on Persuasive Technology* (pp. 1–7).

Forscher, P.S., Lai, C.K., Axt, J.R. et al. (2019). A meta-analysis of procedures to change implicit measures. *Journal of Personality and Social Psychology*, *117*, 522–559.

Friese, M., Wänke, M., & Plessner, H. (2006). Implicit consumer preferences and their influence on product choice. *Psychology and Marketing*, *23*, 727–740.

Gerrard, M., Gibbons, F.X., Bentin, A.C., & Hessling, R.M. (1996). The reciprocal nature of risk behaviors and cognitions: What you think shapes what you do and vice versa. *Health Psychology*, *15*, 344–354.

Gibbons, F.X., & Gerrard, M. (1995). Predicting young adults' health risk behaviour. *Journal of Personality and Social Psychology*, *69*, 505–517.

Gibbons, F.X., Gerrard, M., Blanton, H., & Russell, D.W. (1998). Reasoned action and social reaction: Willingness and intention as independent predictors of health risk. *Journal of Personality and Social Psychology, 74*, 1164–1181.

Gibson, B. (2008). Can evaluative conditioning change attitudes toward mature brands? New evidence from the implicit association test. *Journal of Consumer Research, 35*, 178–188.

Glanz, K., & Rimer, B.K. (2005). *Theory at a Glance: A Guide for Health Promotion Practice* (Second edition). National Cancer Institute, NIH, Public Health Service. U.S. Government Printing Office.

Glanz, K., Rimer, B.K., & Viswanath, K. (2015). Theory, research and practice in health behavior. In K. Glanz, B.K. Rimer, & K. Viswanath (Eds.), *Health Behavior: Theory Research & Practice, 5th Edition*. San Francisco: Jossey-Bass.

Hagger, M.S., Cheung, M.W.L., Ajzen, I., & Hamilton, K. (2022). Perceived behavioural control moderating effects in the Theory of Planned Behavior: A meta-analysis. *Health Psychology, 41*, 155–167.

Hofmann, W., Friese, M., & Wiers, R. (2008). Impulsive versus reflective influences on behavior: a theoretical framework and empirical review. *Health Psychology Review, 2*, 111–137.

Hollands, G.J., Prestwich, A., & Marteau, T.M. (2011). Using aversive images to enhance healthy food choices and implicit attitudes: an experimental test of evaluative conditioning. *Health Psychology, 30*, 195–203.

Janz, N.K., & Becker, M.H. (1984). The health belief model: A decade later. *Health Education Quarterly, 11*, 1–47.

Jones, C.J., Smith, H., & Llewellyn, C. (2014). Evaluating the effectiveness of health belief model interventions in improving adherence: a systematic review. *Health Psychology Review, 8*, 253–269.

Kleis, R.R., Hoch, M.C., Hogg-Graham, R., & Hoch, J.M. (2021). The effectiveness of the transtheoretical model to improve physical activity in healthy adults: A systematic review. *Journal of Physical Activity and Health, 18*, 94–108.

Kothe, E.J., Ling, M., North, M. et al. (2019). Protection motivation theory and pro-environmental behaviour: A systematic mapping review. *Australian Journal of Psychology, 71*, 411–432.

Krejany, C., Kanjo, E., Dadich, A., & Jiwa, M. (2020). Why don't promising innovations always change healthcare behaviours? *The Journal of Health Design, 5*, 250–258.

Kwasnicka, D., Dombrowski, S.U., White, M., & Sniehotta, F. (2016). Theoretical explanations for maintenance of behaviour change: a systematic review of behaviour theories. *Health Psychology Review, 10*, 277–296.

Latham, G.P., Erez, M., & Locke, E.A. (1988). Resolving scientific disputes by the joint design of crucial experiments by the antagonists: Application to the Erez-Latham dispute regarding participation in goal setting. *Journal of Applied Psychology, 73*, 753–772.

Lewis, M.A., Litt, D. M., King, K.M., Fairlie, A.M., Waldron, K.A., Garcia, T.A., … Lee, C. M. (2020). Examining the ecological validity of the Prototype Willingness Model for adolescent and young adult alcohol use. *Psychology of Addictive Behaviors, 34*, 293–302.

Lippke, S., Ziegelmann, J.P., & Schwarzer, R. (2005). Stage specific adoption and maintenance of physical activity: Testing a three-stage model. *Psychology of Sport & Exercise, 6*, 585–603.

Locke, E.A., & Latham, G. P. (2019). The development of goal-setting theory: A half-century retrospective. *Motivation Science*, *5*, 93–105.

Locke, E.A., & Latham, G. P. (2020). Building a theory by induction: The example of goal setting theory. *Organizational Psychology Review*, *10*, 223–239.

Luszczynska, A., & Schwarzer, R. (2015). Social cognitive theory. In Conner, M and Norman, P (Eds.). *Predicting and Changing Health Behaviour: Research and Practice with Social Cognition Models. 3rd ed.* Buckingham, UK: Open University Press, 225–251.

Mace, C.A. (1935). Incentives: Some experimental studies (Report No. 72). Industrial Health Research Board (Great Britain).

Marlatt, G.A. & George, W.H. (1984). Relapse prevention: introduction and overview of the model. *British Journal of Addiction*, *79*, 261–273.

Marlatt, G.A. & Gordon, J.R. (1985). Relapse prevention: Maintenance strategies in the treatment of addictive behaviors. New York, Guildford Press.

McCarrick, D., Prestwich, A., & O'Connor, D.B. (n.d.-a. The role of perseverative cognition in the job strain-health outcome relationship. *Psychology & Health*.

McCarrick, D., Prestwich, A., & O'Connor, D.B. (n.d.-b Perseverative cognition and health behaviours: exploring the role of intentions and perceived behavioural control. *Psychology & Health*.

McCarrick, D., Prestwich, A., Prudenzi, A., & O'Connor, D.B. (2021). Health effects of psychological interventions for worry and rumination: A meta-analysis. *Health Psychology*, *40*, 617–630.

McEachan, R., Taylor, N., Harrison, R. et al. (2016). Meta-analysis of the reasoned action approach (RAA) to understanding health behaviors. *Annals of Behavioral Medicine*, *50*, 592–612.

Michie, S., Abraham, C., Whittington, C., McAteer, J., & Gupta, S. (2009). Effective techniques in healthy eating and physical activity interventions: A meta-regression. *Health Psychology*, *28*, 690–701.

Michie, S., Atkins, L., & West, R. (2014). *The Behaviour Change Wheel: A guide to designing interventions*. Silverback Publishing.

Michie, S., Johnston, M., Abraham, C. et al. (2005). "Psychological theory" group. Making psychological theory useful for implementing evidence based practice: A consensus approach. *Quality and Safety in Health Care*, *14*, 26–33.

Michie, S., van Stralen, M.M., & West, R. (2011). The Behaviour Change Wheel: a new method for characterising and designing behaviour change interventions. *Implementation Science*, *6*, 42.

Milne, S., Sheeran, P., & Orbell, S. (2000). Prediction and intervention in health-related behaviour: A meta-analytic review of protection motivation theory. *Journal of Applied Social Psychology*, *30*, 106–143.

Noar, S.M. & Zimmerman, R.S. (2005). Health behavior theory and cumulative knowledge regarding health behaviors: are we moving in the right direction? *Health Education Research*, *20*, 275–290.

Norman, P., Boer, H., Seydel, E.R., & Mullan, B. (2015). Protection motivation theory. In Conner, M and Norman, P (Eds.). *Predicting and Changing Health Behaviour: Research and Practice with Social Cognition Models. 3rd ed.* Buckingham, UK: Open University Press, 70–106.

Ntoumanis, N., Ng, J.Y.Y., Prestwich, A. et al. (2021). A meta-analysis of self-determination theory-informed intervention studies on the health domain:

effects on motivation, heath behavior, physical and psychological health. *Health Psychology Review, 15,* 214–244.

Orbell, S., & Sheeran, P. (1998). "Inclined abstainers": A problem for predicting health-related behaviour. *British Journal of Social Psychology, 37,* 151–165.

Ouellette, J.A., & Wood, W. (1998). Habit and intention in everyday life: The multiple processes by which past behavior predicts future behavior. *Psychological Bulletin, 124,* 54–74.

Perugini, M. (2005). Predictive models of implicit and explicit attitudes. *British Journal of Social Psychology, 44,* 29–45.

Plak, S., van Klaveren, C., & Cornelisz, I. (in press). Raising student engagement using digital nudges tailored to students' motivation and perceived ability levels. *British Journal of Educational Technology.*

Plotnikoff, R.C., & Trinh, L. (2010). Protection motivation theory: is this a worthwhile theory for physical activity promotion? *Exercise and Sport Sciences Reviews, 38,* 91–98.

Prestwich, A., Ayres, K., & Lawton, R. (2008). Crossing two types of implementation intentions with a protection motivation intervention for the reduction of saturated fat intake: A randomized trial. *Social Science & Medicine, 67,* 1550–1558.

Prestwich, A., & Kellar, I. (2014). How can the impact of implementation intentions as a behaviour change intervention be improved? *European Review of Applied Psychology, 64,* 35–41.

Prestwich, A.J., Lawton, R.J., & Conner, M.T. (2003). The use of implementation intentions and the decision balance sheet in promoting exercise behaviour. *Psychology & Health, 18,* 707–721.

Prestwich, A., Sniehotta, F.F., Whittington, C., Dombrowski, S.U., Rogers, L., & Michie, S. (2014). Does theory influence the effectiveness of health behavior interventions? Meta-analysis. *Health Psychology, 33,* 465–474.

Prochaska, J.O., & DiClemente, C.C. (1983). Stages and processes of self-change smoking: Toward an integrative model of change. *Journal of Consulting and Clinical Psychology, 51,* 390–395.

Quine, L., Rutter, D.R., & Arnold, L. (1998). Predicting and understanding safety helmet use among schoolboy cyclists: a comparison of the theory of planned behaviour and the **health belief model**. *Psychology & Health, 13,* 251–269.

Richetin, J., Perugini, M., Prestwich, A., & O'Gorman, R. (2007). The IAT as a predictor of spontaneous food choice: The case of fruits versus snacks. *International Journal of Psychology, 42,* 166–173.

Rogers, R.W. (1983). Cognitive and physiological processes in fear appeals and attitude change: A revised theory of protection motivation. In J. Cacioppo & R. Petty (Eds.), *Social Psychophysiology.* New York: Guilford Press.

Romain, A.J., Caudroit, J., Hokayem, M., & Bernard, P. (2018). Is there something beyond stages of change in the transtheoretical model? The state of art for physical activity. *Canadian Journal of Behavioural Science, 50,* 42–53.

Rosenstock, I.M., Strecher, V.J., & Becker, M.H. (1988). Social learning theory and the Health Belief Model. *Health Education Quarterly, 15,* 175–183.

Scarabis, M., Florack, A., & Gosejohann, S. (2006). When consumers follow their feelings: The impact of affective or cognitive focus on the basis of consumers' choice. *Psychology & Marketing, 23,* 1005–1036.

Scholz, U., Sniehotta, F. F., & Schwarzer, R. (2005). Predicting Physical Exercise in Cardiac Rehabilitation: The Role of Phase-Specific Self-Efficacy Beliefs. *Journal of Sport and Exercise Psychology, 27,* 135–151.

Schunk, D.H., & DiBenedetto, M.K. (2020). Motivation and social cognitive theory. *Contemporary Educational Psychology, 60,* 101832.

Schwarzer, R. (1992). Self-efficacy in the adoption and maintenance of health behaviors: Theoretical approaches and a new model. In R. Schwarzer (Ed.), *Self-efficacy: Thought control of action* (pp. 217–242). Washington, DC: Hemisphere.

Sheeran, P., Klein, W.M.P., & Rothman, A.J. (2017). Health behavior change: Moving from observation to intervention. *Annual Review of Psychology, 68,* 573–600.

Sheeran, P., Milne, S., Webb, T.L., & Gollwitzer, P.M. (2005). Implementation intentions and health behaviour. In M. Conner & P. Norman (Eds.), *Predicting Health Behaviour, 2nd Edition,* Maidenhead: Open University Press.

Sheeran, P., & Orbell, S. (1999). Augmenting the theory of planned behavior: Roles for anticipated regret and descriptive norms. *Journal of Applied Social Psychology, 29,* 2107–2142.

Sheeran, P., & Webb, T. (2016). The intention-behavior gap. *Social and Personality Psychology Compass, 10,* 503–518.

Sheldon, K.M., Elliot, A.J., Kim, Y., & Kasser, T. (2001). What is satisfying about satisfying events? Testing 10 candidate psychological needs. *Journal of Personality and Social Psychology, 80,* 325–339.

Sheppard, B.H., Hartwick, J., & Warshaw, P.R. (1988). The theory of reasoned action: a meta-analysis of past research with recommendations for modifications and future research. *Journal of Consumer Research, 15,* 325–339.

Skinner, B.F. (1953). *Science and Human Behavior.* New York: Macmillan.

Smith, E.R., & DeCoster, J. (2000). Dual process models in social and cognitive psychology: Conceptual integration and links to underlying memory systems. *Personality and Social Psychology Review, 4,* 108–131.

Sniehotta, F.F., Presseau, J., & Araújo-Soares, V. (2014). Time to retire the theory of planned behaviour. *Health Psychology Review, 8,* 1–7.

Steinmetz, H., Knappstein, M., Ajzen, I., Schmidt, P., & Kabst, R. (2016). How effective are behavior change interventions based on the Theory of Planned Behavior? A three-level meta-analysis. *Zeitschrift für Psychologie, 224,* 216–233.

Strack, F., & Deutsch, R. (2004). Reflective and impulsive determinants of social behavior. *Personality and Social Psychology Review, 8,* 220–247.

Strick, M., van Baaren, R.B., Holland, R.W., & van Knippenberg, A. (2009). *Journal of Experimental Psychology: Applied, 15,* 35–45.

Swann, C., Rosenbaum, S., Lawrence, A. et al. (2021). Updating goal-setting theory in physical activity promotion: a critical conceptual review. *Health Psychology Review, 15,* 34–50.

Teixeira, P., Marques, M.M., Silva, M.N. et al. (2020). A classification of motivation and behavior change techniques used in self-determination theory-based interventions in health contexts. *Motivation Science, 6,* 438–455.

Todd, J., Kothe, E., Mullan, B., & Monds, L. (2016). Reasoned versus reactive prediction of behaviour: a meta-analysis of the prototype willingness model. *Health Psychology Review, 10,* 1–24.

Vancouver, J.B., Ballard, T., & Neal, A. (2022). Goal-setting: Revisiting Locke and Latham's goal-setting studies. In N. K. Steffens, F. Rink, & M. K. Ryan (Eds.) *Organisational Psychology: Revisiting the Classic Studies.* Sage Publications.

Verplanken, B., Aarts, H., Knippenberg, A., & Moonen, A. (1998). Habit versus planned behavior: A field experiment. *British Journal of Social Psychology, 37,* 111–128.

West, R. (2005). Time for a change: putting the Transtheoretical (Stages of Change) Model to rest. *Addiction, 100*, 1036–1039.

West, R. (2006). The Transtheoretical Model of behaviour change and the scientific method. *Addiction, 101*, 774–778.

West, R., & Brown, J. (2013). *Theory of Addiction.* John Wiley & Sons.

Williams, D.M., & Rhodes, R.E. (2016). The confounded self-efficacy construct: conceptual analysis and recommendations for future research. *Health Psychology Review, 10*, 113–128.

Williams, T., & Williams, K. (2010). Self-efficacy and performance in mathematics: Reciprocal determinism in 33 nations. *Journal of Educational Psychology, 102*, 453–466.

Young, M.D., Plotnikoff, R.C., Collins, C.E., Callister, R., & Morgan, P. J. (2014). Social cognitive theory and physical activity: a systematic review and meta-analysis. *Obesity Reviews, 15*, 983–995.

Zhang, C-Q., Zhang, R., Schwarzer, R., & Hagger, M. S. (2019). A meta-analysis of the Health Action Process Approach. *Health Psychology, 38*, 623–637.

3

CHAPTER 3
BEHAVIOR CHANGE TECHNIQUES

OVERVIEW

Behavior change techniques are methods employed by behavioral scientists, psychologists, medical staff and others to try to change the behavior of individuals or groups of people and/or the motivations or other factors/constructs that influence behavior. We first look at how behavior change techniques have been classified within taxonomies. We then consider a number of behavior change techniques, all of which have received extensive examination in the literature. Many of these have a good level of evidence to support their use and have been applied across a wide range of health behaviors. A number of these have links with some of the theories considered in Chapter 2 such as the use of rewards which are closely aligned with operant learning theory. We then look at behavior change techniques in a variety of settings including the workplace and in healthcare. Different contexts bring with them unique challenge, and here we give you a flavor of these as well as an illustration of attempts to change important health behaviors across these varied contexts.

_____

BEHAVIOR CHANGE TECHNIQUE TAXONOMIES

One major goal for the Science of Health Behavior Change is to identify which behavior change techniques are the most effective in changing specific health behaviors. Aside from issues concerning what these specific behaviors might be, an important challenge is to ensure that individuals apply the same definitions of these techniques. Without clearly understood and widely applied definitions, there is a risk that different individuals apply

DOI: 10.4324/9781003302414-4

different labels to the same techniques or the same labels to different techniques. The impact of this would be to delay the development of a clear evidence base either supporting or refuting the effectiveness of specific techniques because it is more difficult to identify and synthesize the evidence from studies testing the same behavior change techniques. In recent years, there have been attempts to identify and categorize behavior change techniques and to clearly define them within behavior change taxonomies.

A key feature of science is replication. Findings demonstrated in one study should be replicated if the method (what was done and to whom) is repeated. To do this, what was done within an experiment needs to be clearly reported. With this in mind, Abraham and Michie (2008) developed a taxonomy of 26 behavior change techniques that provides a common language to describe the techniques that make up an intervention. In addition to increasing the likelihood of replicating studies, using a common language to describe techniques making up an intervention can be helpful in determining what caused any changes in behavior as well as their determinants such as perceived behavioral control and motivation. If techniques were used within interventions but they are not clearly described then potentially important, but "hidden" (as they are not clearly conveyed), techniques might have caused changes in behavior. In this situation, it is not possible to accurately identify which technique caused the change in behavior or determinant (see also: Critical Skills Toolkit 3.1).

Abraham and Michie's (2008) taxonomy of 26 different techniques is presented in *Burning Issue Box 3.1* to give you an indication of the type of strategies that have often been employed as a means to change the actions of individuals or groups of people. Since 2008, this list has been expanded to incorporate a wider range of techniques (Michie et al., 2011) with the latest version incorporating 93 distinct behavior change techniques (Michie et al., 2013). In addition, lists defining behavior change techniques focused on specific behaviors including alcohol intake (Michie et al., 2012) and smoking (Michie, Hyder, Walia, & West, 2011) have been developed. More recently, taxonomies have evolved in different forms including to classify techniques aligned with specific theory (Self-Determination Theory; Teixeira et al., 2020) and to focus on techniques that individuals can use themselves to boost their motivation and change their behavior (Knittle et al., 2020).

Behavior change technique taxonomies have been used to systematically review the evidence to determine the most effective techniques for a variety of behaviors across various contexts using **meta-analyses** (see Table 3.1) or less formal, statistical approaches where meta-analyses were not possible (e.g., Bird et al., 2013; Lyzwinski, 2014).

BURNING ISSUE BOX 3.1

HOW CAN WE CHANGE BEHAVIOR? OVERVIEW OF BEHAVIOR CHANGE TECHNIQUES (ABRAHAM & MICHIE, 2008)

According to Abraham and Michie (2008) there are 26 common methods that individuals can use to try to change the behavior of other people. The 26 techniques overviewed within Abraham and Michie's taxonomy were:

1-3. *Provide information.* These techniques rest on the assumption that educating individuals is a vital component of behavior change. Presenting information is likely to be most effective when the behavior (e.g., buying a particular product) or issue (e.g., climate change) is novel or not well understood. Moreover, while providing basic information about a disease may not have much impact on behavior, other types of information (e.g., providing information on the consequences of behavior) may be more useful (see Fishbein, 1995). Abraham and Michie (2008) categorized providing information into three different techniques:

   1. *On behavior-health link.* This can include factual information concerning the risks one has of developing illness or educational materials concerning the health benefits or problems concerned with health behaviors.
   2. *On consequences.* This educational technique concerns what happens if one performs/does not perform the behavior and the benefits and costs associated with these.
   3. *About others' approval.* Provides information relating to whether others would approve/disapprove of the behavior.

4. *Prompt* intention *formation.* Encourages people to come to a decision to act (e.g., I will exercise) or to achieve a goal (e.g., I will be healthy). This is distinct from technique 10 (specific goal setting) as the decision is not accompanied with a plan regarding how to act (e.g., when and where to act).
5. *Prompt barrier identification.* An individual is asked to think about the factors (e.g., competing goals/demands/situations) that might disrupt one's plans and ways to overcome then.
6. *Provide general encouragement.* This can involve praise or rewards for effort. It can also include attempts to increase one's confidence in their ability through persuasion. It is distinct from technique 14 (contingent rewards) as the rewards do not depend

on achieving one's goal/sub-goal. *See Incentives section in this chapter for further details.*

7. *Set graded tasks.* This involves setting the individual a series of tasks to work towards one's goals. The tasks in the sequence gradually become more demanding, challenging or difficult.

8. *Provide instruction.* Involves *telling* the person individually or in groups, or by tips, *how* to perform the behavior or preparatory behaviors.

9. *Model/demonstrate the behavior. Showing* the individual (e.g., in classes, videos, etc.) how to perform the behavior.

10. *Specific goal setting.* Prompts an individual to plan to perform a specific behavior (e.g., with reference to frequency, intensity or duration of the behavior) in a specific context (e.g., with reference to at least one of the following: where, when, how or with whom the behavior will be performed). *See Implementation Intentions section in this chapter for further details.*

11. *Review of behavioral goals.* An individual is asked to review previous goals or plans. Typically this will follow goal setting (technique 10) and an attempt to act on these goals.

12. *Self-monitoring.* An individual keeps a record (e.g., diary) of their target behaviors. *See Self-Monitoring section in this chapter for further details.*

13. *Feedback.* Receiving information about how the performance of the individual compares to their set goals (building on technique 10) or the behavior of others.

14. *Contingent rewards.* Praise, encouragement or other rewards (e.g., money) are given to reward achievement of one's goal or sub-goals. *See Incentives section in this chapter for further details.*

15. *Teach to use prompts/cues.* Teaches the individual to identify cues in the environment (e.g., time of day, places) which can remind an individual to perform a behavior.

16. *Agree behavioral contract.* Typically involves signing a contract/statement, witnessed by another, which specifies the behavior that the individual will perform.

17. *Prompt practice.* This involves encouraging practice of the behavior.

18. *Use of follow-up prompts.* This technique follows other components of an intervention and often involves sending letters, making telephone calls or visits.

19. *Provide opportunity for social comparison.* This technique places participants in situations in which they can compare their behaviors against those of others (e.g., in group sessions, through video, etc.)

20. *Plan social support/social change.* Provides an individual with support from another (e.g., a buddy system) or encourages the individual to think about how others can help them change behavior.
21. *Prompt identification as a role model/position advocate.* Gives an opportunity to the individual to be a good example to others (e.g., giving talks, persuading others).
22. *Prompt self-talk.* Encourages individuals to talk to themselves (silently or out loud) before and during behavior performance to motivate and support action.
23. *Relapse prevention.* Similar to technique 5 (identify barriers) but occurs after initial behavior change has taken place. An individual is asked to identify situations that put them at risk of relapse and/or situations that can help them maintain the initial change in behavior.
24. *Stress management.* Can comprise a range of techniques (e.g., slow breathing) which attempt to reduce anxiety/stress rather than change the behavior directly.
25. *Motivational interviewing. See Motivational Interviewing section in this chapter for details.*
26. *Time management.* Any technique that helps the individual be able to fit the behavior into their schedule.

Taxonomies of behavior change techniques are useful for accumulating evidence from different studies within **systematic reviews**/meta-analyses, in that they help to group together studies that have employed the same behavior change techniques. Such studies are then compared against studies that have not used the specific behavior change technique in question. However, a common criticism of this approach is that interventions can comprise multiple behavior change techniques, and so it is difficult to identify which specific behavior change techniques help change behavior and which do not (see Critical Skills Toolkit 3.1).

The most detailed taxonomy (i.e., the taxonomy comprising the most behavior change techniques) was produced by Michie et al. (2013). Although it comprises 93 techniques, to help individuals in their coding or use of behavior change techniques, the techniques are grouped into 19 clusters. For instance, a cluster labeled "social support" comprises three behavior change techniques relating to social support (social support-unspecified; social support-practical; social support-emotional), while another cluster labeled "self-belief" comprises of four techniques designed to increase an individual's belief that they can perform a particular behavior (verbal persuasion about capability, mental rehearsal of successful

CRITICAL SKILLS TOOLKIT 3.1

HOW TO IDENTIFY EFFECTIVE COMPONENTS OF AN INTERVENTION

Interventions often comprise of a number of different behavior change techniques. Take this example. Milne et al. (2002) conducted a study testing which techniques can increase the likelihood of engaging in at least one 20-minute session of exercise over a week. They randomly allocated their participants to one of three groups:

Group 1 (control group) did not receive any active behavior change techniques (they were simply asked to read three paragraphs of a novel).

Group 2 (experimental group 1) were asked to read a motivational message.

Group 3 (experimental group 2) were asked to read a motivational message and form an implementation intention regarding when and where they would exercise over the following week.

They demonstrated that at follow-up, 38% of participants in group 1 (control group) and 35% of participants in group 2 (experimental group 1) reported exercising. However, in group 3 (experimental group 2) the percentage of participants reporting exercising increased dramatically to 91%.

Based on the above, it is not clear whether forming an implementation intention *by itself* was responsible for increasing exercise or whether it was the *combination* of forming an implementation intention and reading the motivational message that increased exercise (the motivational message *by itself* was not effective in increasing exercise as the percentage of participants reporting exercise in experimental group 1 and the control group were similar).

In summary, when an intervention comprises a number of different behavior change techniques, it is not clear which specific behavior change technique was responsible for specific changes in constructs or behavior unless a **fully crossed (full-factorial) design** is used.

When an intervention comprises two behavior change techniques, it could use a 2×2 (4 groups) fully-crossed factorial design; when it comprises three behavior change techniques, it could use a $2 \times 2 \times 2$ (8 groups) design; four behavior change techniques could use a 2 × 2 × 2 × 2 (16 groups) design, and so on. For the most basic of these (the 2 × 2 design), there will be 4 groups (group 1 receives technique A and technique B, group 2 receives technique A but not technique B, group 3 receives technique B but not technique A and group 4 receives neither technique A or B). This design is illustrated below In Figure 3.2:

| | | Technique B:
MOTIVATIONAL MESSAGE? | |
		YES	NO
Technique A: IMPLEMENTATION INTENTION?	YES	Implementation intention + motivational message	Implementation intention only
	NO	Motivational message only	No intervention control group

FIGURE 3.2 2 × 2 full-factorial design that could have been incorporated by Milne et al. (2002) to help identify the active component(s) of their interventions.

In the example above, for Milne et al. (2002) to conclude which techniques or combination of techniques caused the differences in exercise across conditions, they should have used a 2 × 2 design (implementation intention + motivational message; implementation intention only; motivational message only; no intervention control). By omitting the implementation intention only condition, Milne et al. could not determine whether it was the combination of implementation intentions plus the motivational message that caused the increase in exercise or whether implementation intentions (without the motivational message) would have increased exercise behavior by itself.

Employing these fully-crossed designs (along with statistical procedures such as ANOVA, see Chapter 6) allows you to identify which specific behavior change technique is responsible for the effects of your intervention and also which behavior change techniques interact (i.e., lead to bigger effects when used in combination rather than using each technique alone). Alternatively, test an intervention that comprises of only one behavior change technique!

TABLE 3.1 Overview of meta-analyses identifying the most effective behavior change techniques to change specific health behaviors

Authors	Year	Behavior(s)	Sample	Taxonomy*	Number of studies (k)	Most effective behavior change techniques
Abraham & Graham Rowe	2009	Physical activity	Healthy Employees	1 (sub-set only)	37	Review of goals; set graded tasks
Avery et al.	2012	Glucose control	Type-2 diabetics	2	17	Prompting generalization of a target behavior; use of follow-up prompts; prompt review of behavioral goals; provide information on where and when to perform PA; plan social support/social change; goal setting (behavior); time management; prompting focus on past success; barrier identification/problem-solving; and providing information on the consequences specific to the individual
Bartlett et al.	2014	Smoking	Smokers with COPD	6	17	Facilitate action planning/develop treatment plan; prompt self-recording; advise on methods of weight control; advise on/facilitate use of social support
Black et al.	2016	Alcohol	Individuals without mental health conditions	4	81	Providing normative information; review of goals; prompting commitment; options for additional support

Brannon & Cushing	2015	Physical activity/diet	Children & Adolescents	1	74	PA: modeling; providing consequences for behavior; providing information on others' approval; intention formation; self-mon toring; behavioral contract Diet: modeling; practice; social support
Bull et al.	2018	Healthy eating/ physical activity/ smoking	Low-income adults	3	35	Healthy eating: self-monitoring; PA: practice; instruction on how to do; smoking: none
Carraça et al.	2021	Physical activity	Overweight adults	3, 7	62	Digital interventions: goal-setting; graded tasks; social incentive In-person: behavioral practice/rehearsal
Dombrowski et al.	2012	Weight-related	Obese adults with comorbidities	1	44	Provide instruction; self-monitoring; relapse prevention; prompt practice
Eckerstorfer et al.	2018	Physical activity	No restrictions	2	50	Behavioral goals; self-monitoring
Finne et al.	2019	Physical activity	Cancer survivors	3	30	Prompts/cues; reduce prompts/cues; non-specific rewards; social reward; graded tasks

(Continued)

TABLE 3.1 (Continued)

Authors	Year	Behavior(s)	Sample	Taxonomy*	Number of studies (k)	Most effective behavior change techniques
French et al.	2014	Physical activity	Older adults	2	16	Barrier identification/problem solving; provide rewards contingent on successful behavior; model/demonstrate the behavior
Garnett et al.	2018	Alcohol intake	Hazardous/ harmful drinkers	3	41	Goal-setting; problem-solving; information about antecedents; behavior substitution; credible source
Henrich et al.	2015	IBS symptoms & well-being	Adult patients with IBS	2 (modified)	48	General empathic support; self-monitoring of symptoms; self-monitoring of cognitions; drawing an explicit link between self-monitored symptoms and cognitions; providing feedback; relapse prevention or coping planning; assertiveness training; prompt practice of new behaviors
Hill et al.	2013	Gestational weight gain	Pregnant women	2	19	Providing information on the consequences of behavior to the individual; provide rewards contingent on successful behavior; prompt self-monitoring of behavior; motivational interviewing

	Year	Behavior	Population			Description
Howlett et al.	2019	Physical activity	Inactive adults	3	16	Postintervention: biofeedback; behavior practice/rehearsal; demonstration of behavior; graded tasks.
Kassavou & Sutton	2018	Medication adherence	Adults prescribed medication related to cardio-metabolic conditions	3	17	Information about health consequences; whether or not participants were asked during the study (e.g., via text) whether they had taken the medication (new BCT not included in the BCTTv1 taxonomy).
Lara et al.	2014	Healthy eating	Older adults	2	22	Barrier identification/problem solving; plan social support/ social change; use of follow-up prompts; goal-setting
McDermott et al.	2016	Healthy eating/ physical activity	No restriction	2	25	None led to larger effects on behavior
Michie et al.	2009	Healthy eating/ physical activity	Adults without chronic illness	1	101	None were significant (but self- monitoring was the best)
Michie et al.	2012	Alcohol	Primary care pop.	4	18	Prompt self-recording; prompt commit-ment from the client there and then

(Continued)

TABLE 3.1 (Continued)

Authors	Year	Behavior(s)	Sample	Taxonomy*	Number of studies (k)	Most effective behavior change techniques
Murray et al.	2017	Physical activity maintenance	Adults	2	62	6–9 months: self-monitoring; follow-up prompts
Olander et al.	2013	Physical activity	Obese adults	2	42	Various but especially: teach to prompts/cues; prompt practice; prompt rewards contingent on effort or progress towards behavior; goal setting (behavior); action planning; provide feedback on performance; barrier identification/problem solving; provide instruction; provide normative information about others' behavior; plan social support/social change; provide Rewards for behavior; self-monitoring of behavior; provide information on the consequences in general; provide information on the consequences for individual
Patterson et al.	2022	Physical activity via apps	People with cardio vascular disease	3	19	Action planning; graded tasks

Samdal et al.	2017	Physical activity/diet	Overweight adults	3	48	Goal-setting and self-monitoring
Taylor et al.	2011	Physical activity	Healthy employees	1	26	None
Taylor et al.	2022	Physical activity	Hospitalized patients	2	18	Goal-setting
Vargas-Garcia	2017	Sugar-sweetened beverage intake	Children, adolescents adults	1	40	adults: no particular technique children model/demonstrate behavior
Webb et al.	2010	Physical activity	General	1 (modified)	85	Several, especially: stress management; general communication skills training; relapse prevention/coping planning; gcal setting; action planning; provide feedback on performance; barrier identification; provide instruction

(Continued)

TABLE 3.1 (Continued)

Authors	Year	Behavior(s)	Sample	Taxonomy*	Number of studies (k)	Most effective behavior change techniques
West et al.	2010	Smoking	Stop Smoking Service attendees	5	43 Stop Smoking Services	Strengthen ex-smoker identity; Elicit client views; measure CO; give options for additional/later support; provide rewards contingent on stopping smoking; advise on changing routine; facilitate relapse prevention and coping; ask about experiences of stop smoking medication; advise on stop smoking medication
Williams & French	2011	Physical activity	Healthy, non-student adults	2	27	Provide information on consequences of the behavior in general; action planning; reinforcing effort or progress towards behavior; provide instruction; facilitate social comparison; time management

* Taxonomy used: 1. Abraham & Michie (2008); 2. Michie et al. (2011) CALO-RE taxonomy; 3. Michie et al. (2013); 4. Michie et al. (2012); 5. Michie et al. (2011a); 7. Teixeira et al. (2020).

performance, focus on past success, self-talk). Despite the behavior change techniques being grouped into hierarchies to make the task of identifying the behavior change techniques within study reports easier, there is evidence suggesting that users fail to code many behavior change techniques reliably, even after training (Wood et al., 2015).

Another limitation of taxonomies is that there are instances where the techniques described actually consist of multiple behavior change techniques. Even in Michie et al.'s (2013) taxonomy, which covers 93 behavior change techniques, there are instances in which certain techniques can be broken down into lower-order techniques. For example, the technique of "restructuring the physical environment" does not account for the various ways in which aspects of the physical environment can be altered to change behavior. Hollands et al. (2017) later developed TIPPME (Typology of Interventions in Proximal Physical Micro-Environments) as a framework to reliably describe and accumulate evidence regarding the impact of different ways of altering the physical environment on the selection, purchase or consumption of food, alcohol or tobacco. TIPPME incorporates two classes of strategies relating to placement or properties that subdivide into six intervention types across three levels of focus (*product* including its packaging or tableware needed to consume the product; *related objects* that typically accompany the product and is typically part of its proximal surroundings and *wider environment* such as temperature or lighting. More discussion, including a critique, of behavior change technique taxonomies is presented in Chapter 10.

POPULAR BEHAVIOR CHANGE TECHNIQUES

There are many reasons for attempting to change health behaviors across many sectors of society such as business, health services, education and general living as well as a number of important questions to address. For example, how might marketing companies encourage consumers to select their healthier product? How might doctors help patients to take the correct amount of medication and continue to do so throughout their treatment period (or even better, how might doctors help the patient to avoid illness in the first place)? How can governments build healthier societies? In an attempt to address these questions, we could employ a range of different behavior change techniques aimed at educating people (see Burning Issue Box 3.1, techniques 1–3); try to encourage individuals to play closer attention to their actions (see Burning Issue Box 3.1, technique 12); provide opportunities for different groups of people to find out more information about one another (see Burning Issue Box 3.1, technique 19) or manipulate aspects of the environment or wider policy (see Chapter 8).

A broad range of behavior change techniques is outlined in Burning Issue Box 3.1. The relative impact of these techniques on behavior, according to Michie et al.'s (2009) review of healthy eating and physical activity interventions, is shown in Figure 3.1. On the basis of this review, **self-monitoring** appears to be the most useful behavior change technique for promoting healthy eating/physical activity, while prompting self-talk appears to be the least useful. Even when we consider a broader range of systematic reviews that attempt to identify the most effective behavior change techniques across various behaviors (see Table 3.1), self-monitoring is often identified as an effective technique. Specifically, self-monitoring has been shown to be particularly effective for smoking reduction (Bartlett et al., 2014), alcohol reduction (Michie et al., 2012), improving Irritable Bowel Syndrome symptoms and well-being (Henrich et al., 2015), as well as promoting

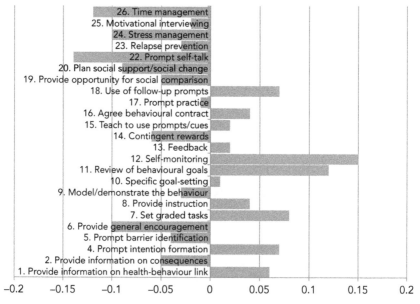

FIGURE 3.1 Relative benefit of including a particular behavior change technique vs. not including the behavior change technique in an intervention (effect of intervention including the specific behavior change technique minus effect of intervention not including the specific behavior change technique) on physical activity and dietary behaviors. Positive scores indicate that the technique is beneficial. Negative scores indicate the technique is less beneficial.

Based on Michie et al. (2009).

physical activity and/or healthy diets (Bull et al., 2018; Brannon & Cushing, 2015; Dombrowski et al., 2012; Eckerstorfer et al., 2018; Hill et al., 2013; Murray et al., 2017; Olander et al., 2013; Samdal et al., 2017).

These reviews are useful when we wish to have a general picture of which techniques are most effective for changing different types of behavior. Reviews that focus on specific behavior change techniques, however, have the potential to more clearly establish the overall effect of a specific behavior change technique because they typically comprise studies that compare interventions that differ only in the presence or absence of that specific behavior change technique (e.g., self-monitoring). We consider this type of review in the following section. Of particular use in identifying whether a specific behavior change technique is effective or not is the use of full factorial designs (see Critical Skills Toolkit 3.1).

Throughout the book we will cover a variety of behavior change techniques. For example, message framing is considered in Chapter 7 and choice architecture or "nudge"-type interventions in Chapter 8. However, as there is a wide range of techniques available to change behavior (see for example, Michie et al., 2013, who identify 93 techniques), we address some techniques in more depth than others. In the following section we outline a number of techniques commonly used to change health behaviors: **self-monitoring**, **motivational interviewing**, **implementation intentions**, **incentives** and **gamification**. In addition, we consider how effective these techniques appear to be and look at *how* they are thought to change behavior. We focus on these techniques due to the large amount of literature devoted to them as well as their potential application to various health behaviors. Furthermore, these techniques appeal to healthcare professionals (particularly motivational interviewing) and policymakers (particularly incentives), can easily be integrated into online platforms and have the potential to change behavior at low cost across large populations. Given the suggestion from the broad reviews (that look at the effectiveness of a wide range of behavior change techniques) that self-monitoring is a particularly effective strategy to promote numerous health behaviors, we consider this strategy next.

SELF-MONITORING

What is it?

Self-monitoring involves an individual keeping a record of their target behaviors. This could take many different forms including an individual keeping a diary, completing a wall-chart, or filling in a self-report questionnaire each day or week. For example, in a weight loss study, participants may be required to write down, in a diary, everything they eat and drink each day, perhaps noting down the fat content of each food. In the domain of physical activity, pedometers (i.e., step counters) and accelerometers (i.e., movement measures) can provide an objective measure that an individual can use to self-monitor their level of activity. Typically, an individual will monitor their behavior (e.g., steps walked) but they can alternatively monitor the consequences/outcomes of behavior (e.g., weight).

How does it work?

The majority of self-monitoring studies have focused on the effects of the technique on behavior change rather than trying to identify how or why this technique changes behavior. There are a number of possible mechanisms: increased awareness of one's level of activity which may, or may not, compare favorably with one's targets or goals; serve as a cue to action; be motivational in nature. Further evidence suggests one potential mechanism is that self-monitoring boosts self-efficacy so that an individual is more confident in their ability to perform the target behavior (Prestwich et al., 2014).

Sometimes, within diaries, participants may record their mood, or other barriers to behavior change (such as poor weather). As such, they could use this additional information to identify the impact of different factors or barriers on their behavior and to cue the individual to consider how these barriers may be overcome. As such, they could provide a useful tool to enhance one's knowledge and understanding of behavior and to aid problem-solving.

Is it effective?

On the basis of the set of general reviews of behavior change techniques presented earlier in this chapter (see Table 3.1), self-monitoring generally appears to be effective. For instance, in a comparison of 26 behavior change techniques and their ability in changing physical activity and healthy eating, across a total of 122 tests, Michie et al. (2009) concluded that self-monitoring was the most effective behavior change technique for both behaviors. This conclusion was based on comparing across studies, in other words, the studies that incorporated self-monitoring within their intervention were compared against studies that did not include self-monitoring as part of their intervention.

However, in other reviews that make comparisons across studies, self-monitoring was found to be less effective than other techniques (Carraça et al., 2021; Patterson et al., 2022). Patterson's review related to digital interventions where perhaps monitoring is expected to occur automatically rather than an individual actively doing it themselves. More active versus passive (automatic) monitoring could be more effective. Some support for this idea can be built on the findings of a review by Harkin et al. (2016) that suggested larger improvements were achieved when the information being monitored was physically recorded than when it was not recorded. Moreover, the negative effect of self-monitoring in Patterson et al.'s review related to monitoring outcomes rather than behavior. It may be that the outcomes that were being monitored were those that can take a long-period of time to achieve (such as weight loss) and/or are difficult to achieve via changes in physical activity and thus fails to positively reinforce physical activity. The findings from Carraça et al.'s (2021) review would also be in keeping with this idea given they found weaker effects for self-monitoring in the context of promoting physical activity in overweight/obese individuals.

These reviews typically involve making comparisons across studies. Comparing across studies may be okay when there are a large number of studies upon which to base the analysis. However, as inevitably different studies will pair self-monitoring with various techniques and the studies draw on different samples and test in different contexts there will be some "noise" (i.e., less precision in your conclusions). However, support for self-monitoring can be drawn from reviews that are less affected by this issue. For example, in a review that focused on the effect of self-monitoring on goal attainment (and thus comprised studies that typically compared two conditions that mainly differed only in the presence or absence of self-monitoring), Harkin et al. (2016) found that self-monitoring had an effect on goal attainment that was nearly medium in size ($d = .40$). The effects were slightly stronger for certain behaviors/outcomes (e.g., physical activity, asthma management, blood pressure) than for others (e.g., diet, weight). It should be noted, however, that self-monitoring invariably involves some element of feedback (people can see their own levels of behavior as they record it) so it can be difficult to disentangle the effects of these two techniques. Attempts have been made by comparing standard self-monitoring conditions against augmented self-monitoring plus feedback conditions with some indications that the augmented conditions can provide an additional small-sized benefit in behavior change (e.g., Prestwich et al., 2016).

A key factor in the success of self-monitoring, in general, is likely to be whether the individual continues to self-monitor by filling in self-report diaries or adhering to other self-monitoring methods. In the long term, this can be a time-consuming behavior change method.

MOTIVATIONAL INTERVIEWING (MILLER & ROLLNICK, 2002)

What is it?

Motivational interviewing is a collaborative person-centered approach that attempts to replace ambivalence (feeling both positive and negative towards behavior change) with stronger intrinsic motivation to change. In other words, rather than feeling indifferent to change, the individual becomes really keen to change their behavior. Moreover, they are keen to change their behavior because it is really important to them rather than simply wanting to change because of some external source (e.g., somebody else wants them to change or there are financial rewards on offer for behavior change). In this way, motivational interviewing has connections with Self-Determination Theory (see, for example, Markland, Ryan, Tobin, & Rollnick, 2005) covered in Chapter 2.

How does it work?

Motivational interviewing (MI) can lead to changes in behavior by either the therapist doing something in MI that is not done within the control treatment or by causing particular changes within the client, or both. There are many possible mechanisms that explain how or why MI can cause behavior change and these have been reviewed by Apodaca and Longabaugh (2009) with respect to problem drinking and the use of illegal substances. These include the therapist:

1. showing empathy, acceptance, warmth and genuineness [MI-spirit];
2. being affirming and reflective listeners [MI-consistent behaviors];
3. *not* confronting, directing or warning [MI-inconsistent behaviors];
4. using specific techniques (e.g., decisional balance and personalized feedback) [specific therapist techniques].

Any of these factors can drive changes in the clients' behavior and these changes might occur via change in clients':

5. intention, commitment or plans to change [change talk/intention];
6. readiness to change (e.g., stage of change);
7. cooperation, engagement or disclosure [client engagement/ involvement];
8. resistance to change [client resistance];
9. self-confidence;
10. sense of discrepancy leading to discomfort at how the current behavior fits in with their general values or life goals [experience of discrepancy].

Of these 10 categories, Apodaca and Longabaugh (2009) concluded that MI-inconsistent behaviors had the strongest evidence as a mediator of change (see Chapter 6, Mediation), in other words, by *not confronting, directing or warning the client* (potential features of minimal interventions, standard care and other treatments such as CBT), therapists evoke less resistance to change within the client, engage them more and achieve better outcomes. There was some evidence that *specific therapist techniques* (particularly *decisional balance*) were associated with better outcomes. *Client change talk* was viewed by Apodaca and Longabaugh (2009) as a consistent and promising mediator of change and MI groups compared to standard care control groups tended to have more positive *intentions* to change substance use. MI was more engaging than other methods and greater *engagement* was associated with better outcomes, although this was based on only one test. *Experience of discrepancy* appears an important, promising but understudied potential mechanism of the relationship between MI and positive substance abuse outcomes.

MI-spirit and client confidence did *not* appear to explain the positive effects of MI. Most studies did *not* support the role of readiness to change in explaining the effects of motivational interviewing on changing substance use. There were insufficient tests of MI-consistent behaviors and client resistance.

A more recent review of mechanisms, this time focused on using MI to promote health behaviors (Copeland et al., 2015), consistent with Apodaca and Longabaugh's earlier review, found motivation (intention) to be a promising mediator with "change talk" also having some support. However, unlike Apodaca and Longabaugh (2009), they concluded that MI-sprit was, alongside motivation, one of the most promising mediators. Relatively recently, Miller and Rollnick (2013) added to their theory by highlighting the role of both compassion (putting clients' needs above their own) and evocation (accepting that the client has what is needed to make a change and it is the therapists' role to draw these capabilities out) as well as adding planning as a later step in which commitment to change is reinforced and patients are facilitated in making their plans to change.

Generally speaking, at this time, there is an insufficient evidence base to either strongly support or refute Miller and Rollnick's (2002, 2013) Motivational Interviewing theory. For instance, Apodaca and Longabaugh (2009) and Copeland et al. (2015) bemoaned the lack of studies that have actually presented some test of the mechanisms of MI (i.e., tested how motivational interviewing changes behavior) and the general low quality of the studies reviewed. More recent reviews have also come to similar conclusions regarding the mixed evidence for the mechanisms of motivational interviewing in behavior change (e.g., Pace et al., 2017).

Is it effective?

The evidence is not wholly consistent (i.e., motivational interviewing is not always effective). For example, a review by Morton et al. (2015) found that MI produced positive changes in health behaviors (diet, physical activity, alcohol intake) in only about half of the studies (18 out of 33). Moreover, according to Vasilaki et al. (2006), MI appears to be more useful in the short-term (less than three months) than long term (greater than three months). Hettema et al. (2005) reached similar conclusions: MI produce large behavior change in the short term ($d = .77$) which become small, around one year ($d = .30$). This concurs with the results of a separate review by Cummings et al. (2009) who reported conflicting evidence for MI effectiveness for long-term improvements in lifestyle and health behaviors. They argue that this might be due to differences in the intensity and/or length of treatment (dosage) and the specific type of MI delivered. This general pattern is also apparent in a review of reviews of motivational interviewing on adult behavior change. Specifically, Frost et al. (2018) found in comparisons that provided moderate quality evidence (the other comparisons in their review of reviews provided less quality evidence) MI was somewhat effective for short-term alcohol intake (8 out of 13 comparisons suggested MI benefits up to four months but evidence was weaker after four months) and smoking cessation (1 out of 1 comparison found a benefit for MI). Evidence for physical activity (one out of four comparisons suggested benefits) and drug use (one out of five comparisons suggested benefits) was less compelling and MI was not effective in reducing risky sexual behaviors (0 out of four comparisons suggested benefits). Additional reviews focused on specific health behaviors have indicated that MI is beneficial for promoting medication adherence (Palacio et al., 2016) but for other behaviors such as drug use, the evidence remains mixed (Calomarde-Gómez et al., 2021; Li et al., 2016). Motivational interviewing tends to have modest to no effect on improving distal outcomes like weight loss compared to standard treatments (e.g., Michalopoulou et al., 2022).

IMPLEMENTATION INTENTIONS (GOLLWITZER, 1993)

What are they?

Implementation intention (Gollwitzer, 1993) manipulations often request an individual to think about good (or critical) situations to act and appropriate responses within those situations, then write them down in an IF–THEN form (e.g., to increase exercise levels: IF it's Monday morning at 9am THEN I will go for a run from my house around the park) and commit oneself to act at this time. For example, if John was subjected to an implementation intention manipulation concerning exercise, then he might be asked to consider when and where would be a good time and place for him to exercise and to also think about specific exercises (e.g., playing football, going for a run) that he would be able to do in that situation. Forming such plans have been shown to be useful in promoting desired (e.g., healthy) behaviors and reducing undesired behaviors (e.g., buying unhealthy foods). Individuals can also use "volitional help sheets" that list potential situations or cues to act on one side of a page or screen and responses to achieve the particular goal are listed on the other. In this way, individuals exposed to the manipulation are provided with a list of potential situations and responses that they can consider. After that, individuals need to decide which responses to make in which situations and to indicate this, typically, by drawing a line between the situations and responses that they wish to link together. Implementation intentions (sometimes referred to as action plans) play important roles in bridging the intention-behavior gap that was highlighted as an issue for many theories of behavior in Chapter 2.

How do they work?

Implementation intentions have been argued to be effective through two processes. First, by planning in advance the situation in which one will act, the planned situation (and the cues within it) become particularly accessible such that an individual is less likely to miss (when encountering the situation) a good opportunity to act (see Aarts, Dijksterhuis, & Midden, 1999). Beyond this, by mentally linking together a good situation to act with a suitable action, the association between the situation and response is strengthened meaning the behavior is more likely to be enacted when the planned situation is encountered. In other words, when the planned situation is encountered, the individual does not need to then decide what to do and how. Instead, the planned behavior can occur quickly. Some have argued that, following the formation of an implementation intention, the initiation of behavior in a planned situation is more likely to be automatic, i.e., occurring immediately, more efficiently and can be cued outside of conscious awareness (see Webb & Sheeran, 2007).

Are they effective?

Based on a review that incorporated 94 independent tests of implementation intentions, Gollwitzer and Sheeran (2006) concluded that implementation intentions have a moderate-to-large effect on behavior. Beneficial effects of implementation intentions were demonstrated across a range of behavioral domains including pro-social, environmental-related, health and academic behaviors as well as in prejudice reduction. Further support has been provided in more recent reviews. For example, they can reduce smoking cessation rates versus comparison groups (10.7% vs. 4.9%; McWilliams et al., 2019) and weekly alcohol consumption (Cooke et al., 2022). They can also be used to address COVID-19-related behaviors such as increasing social distancing (Ahn et al., 2021).

A review by Prestwich and Kellar (2014) suggests that a key factor that determines whether implementation intentions are likely to change behavior is whether an individual is actually motivated to perform the behavior in the first place. If an individual is motivated they will benefit more from forming an implementation intention than somebody who is not motivated.

Take somebody who has no intention to try to save money. Forming an implementation intention regarding when, where and how they will save money is unlikely to help them. However, somebody who is keen to become more frugal with their cash should benefit much more from forming a relevant implementation intention. Furthermore, the type of behavior may influence effectiveness. For example, in the domain of healthy eating, Adriaanse et al. (2011) noted stronger effects of implementation intentions for the promotion of healthy eating than for the reduction of unhealthy eating. How implementation intentions are delivered might also impact their effects on behavior. For example, in their review of the effect of implementation intentions on reducing alcohol intake, Cooke et al. (2022) reported they worked better when delivered in a volitional help sheet format (versus standard implementation intention format where participants write their plans down) and on paper (versus online).

INCENTIVES AND REWARDS

What are they?

Michie et al. (2013) distinguish between **incentives** (making individuals *aware* that they will be rewarded contingent on them performing specific behaviors such as exercise or achieving particular outcomes like losing a set amount of weight) and **rewards** (actually *giving* the reward contingent on their actions or achievements). In practice, these two things typically co-occur within the same intervention. Also referred to as contingency management in the mental health or substance abuse fields (e.g., Pilling, Strang, & Gerada, 2007), or as reinforcement therapy, the basic idea is that desired behaviors (e.g., abstinence from cocaine use) are rewarded to reinforce the change. Over time, these reinforcements are removed when the behavior change can be sustained without such reinforcement. The idea of rewarding desired changes in behavior is most consistent with Operant Learning Theory (see Chapter 2). Incentives can be contrasted with disincentives with the latter making the target behavior or outcome less appealing such as increasing taxes on cigarettes and alcohol.

How do they work?

The approach rests on basic behaviorist principles; if behavior is positively reinforced (rewarded) then it will be repeated, and if behavior is punished then it is less likely to be repeated. There are basic variants of this treatment which use different incentives. For example, in voucher-based reinforcement patients earn vouchers that can be exchanged for retail items. There was uproar in the media when the UK National Health Service (NHS) announced plans to trial this treatment in Fife, Scotland. In their scheme, smokers who gave up smoking for three months were entered into a prize draw for a helicopter trip or an overnight stay in a luxury hotel and other prizes included iPods. Similar schemes have operated in other parts of the UK. Camden Primary Care Trust has offered Nintendo Wiis and iPods to those who attend chlamydia testing.

Are they effective?

They have been argued to be cost-effective in that such schemes raise awareness but also have some evidence for their ability to change health and clinical behaviors and thus preventing disease and reducing the costs associated with such disease. Pilling et al. (2007) pointed to over 25 studies that consistently show the effectiveness of these positive reinforcers to shape behavior change in the area of illicit drug use. Despite tending to involve monetary-based rewards, Pilling et al. highlight their cost-effectiveness. Voucher-based incentive therapy has been shown to be particularly effective in treating substance abuse (Lussier et al., 2006) though evidence from Cahill and Perara (2011) generally questions the long-term effectiveness of such schemes (see also Giles et al., 2014; Mantzari et al., 2015). Interestingly, the positive effects on illicit substance use did not initially appear to translate to licit drug use (smoking; Cahill & Perara, 2011; Johnston et al., 2012) though since then a review by Mantzari et al. (2015) noted small, significant benefits of personal financial incentives for three health behaviors that included smoking (physical activity and diet were also represented). Moreover, in this review, a group of six studies with follow-ups between 12 and 18 months, indicated financial incentives have a moderate effect on smoking outcomes. Effects after 18 months post-base-line, or more than three months after the incentives had been withdrawn, were non-significant.

The issue of whether financial incentives can be effective in the longer term is complex and may depend on the nature of the outcome, whether the behavior has become habitualized and the length of follow up. On the one hand, and in keeping with previous thought and some of the evidence presented earlier (e.g., Mantzari et al., 2015), a study comprising over 400 overweight or obese individuals found that while a financial incentive scheme boosted initial weight loss at six months and this was sustained at 12 months, these benefits disappeared after the incentive ended (West et al., 2021). This could be a reflection of the tendency for people who lose weight to put the weight on again further down the line. There are other instances, however, suggesting that incentives can be effective in the longer term, even after the incentive is no longer available. For example, Notley et al. (2019) conducted a review and reported, with high certainty, that incentives have positive benefits on smoking abstinence rates at six months even after incentives had been removed. In addition, a large-scale quasi-experiment comprising nearly 600,000 individuals across three provinces in Canada (Spilsbury et al., 2022) tested the impact of stopping a government-backed physical activity financial incentive scheme (called Carrot) that provided small daily financial rewards for achieving daily physical activity goals (about $0.04 CAD/day in loyalty points that could be redeemed for certain consumer goods like movies) in one province (Ontario, ironically for financial reasons/lack of government funding!) compared to two provinces (British Columbia; Newfoundland and Labrador) where this daily incentive remained. While there was a reduction in steps, this was smaller than expected (198 and 274 fewer steps per day in Ontario compared to the two other provinces across a period 6–13 weeks after the daily incentive was removed). The findings might suggest that removing financial incentives after they have been used over a period time may have limited impact on behavior. However, this is difficult to conclude on the basis of this study alone because while the most popular element of the reward scheme (accounting for about 80% of the financial reward distributed to users) was removed from Ontario, other (less popular, more challenging rewards) based on daily activities of an individual and their friend over the course of a week remained available across all three provinces.

Incentives/rewards can also be presented in different forms. Aside from direct rewards or entry into a lottery, monetary contingency (deposit) contracts represent a quite different alternative. In monetary contingency contracts, individuals deposit their own money which they lose if they do not achieve the set goal or win back if they do achieve the goal. A review of different types of incentives for physical activity and diet–weight control behaviors provided some evidence that standard financial incentives, lotteries and deposit contracts have some modest benefit (at least when the reward was still available) and that deposit contracts may be more useful than standard financial incentives for physical activity at follow-up (Boonmanunt et al., in press). Budworth et al. (2019) have suggested that combining monetary contingency contracts with more standard financial incentives could be a feasible means to promote physical activity. More research directly comparing different forms of incentives/rewards are needed.

Across reviews of this technique, the evidence is quite mixed though there are some positive findings. It is not especially clear which rewards work best, though there is some evidence that cash incentives may be better than other incentives for longer-term smoking reduction (Giles et al., 2014); it is likely, however, the incentive must be perceived as desirable and rewarding to the user.

CRITICAL SKILLS TOOLKIT 3.2

DON'T TAKE MY WORD FOR IT: HOW TO QUICKLY LOCATE USEFUL LITERATURE

One of the best ways of effectively critiquing research is to ensure that your topic-related knowledge is up-to-date. However, in this day and age, where papers can often be readily accessed online through your library or search engines such as Google Scholar https://scholar.google.co.uk/, you can be over-faced with too many potentially relevant health behavior change papers to look for. Often text books (hopefully like this one) can be a good place to start. They should provide a clear summary of the literature. However, there are no guarantees that the studies highlighted in any particular text book are going to be the best, most interesting or relevant for your needs. Importantly, the science of health behavior change is fast moving so what might appear ground-breaking today might appear "old-hat" or irrelevant tomorrow. Here are some tips to help you keep ahead without drowning in a sea of information.

Google Scholar

Google scholar is a search engine through which you can access health behavior change and other academic journal articles. Clearly this is a good thing; you can often, at the very least, access an abstract of any particular article which summarizes the key findings. Sometimes you can access the full-text paper (even better!). However, the website has another benefit. It gives you an indication of the number of times that the article has been cited by other articles. In other words, you can use this to quickly identify the key papers in any particular area; the key papers will be more likely to have been cited more often.

When looking at the citation count of an article keep in mind that a paper published in 2023 would have had less time to have been cited by others than an article published in 2013. As a general rule of thumb, multiply the number of years that an article has been published by 10 as a benchmark for a good impact on any particular field. This is a rough estimate. Citations of key papers will usually grow exponentially, so a paper that has been cited five times within its first year might be cited 10 times the next year, 20 times the year after that and so on.

Let somebody else do the hard work

Along with text books, a good place to start to identify the most important literature is a review paper or meta-analysis. In other words, instead of trying to summarize the relevant material yourself, try to find review papers (and, if you're keen, update them).

To identify relevant reviews quickly you can use Google Scholar. To update the review, use Google Scholar to see which other papers have cited the review (click the "Cited by" tab) and then take a look at those papers.

Articles can often take years to be published in traditional journals but they can be found quicker

From the time that a study is conducted to the time that it is published in traditional journals, a few years might have passed by and so, in some instances, papers might be out-of-date by the time that they are published! So how can you find even more timely research? One option is to "google" the top people in any particular area. Academics often have their articles or working papers online, even before they are published. Look for the phrase "in press" (or "accepted for publication"). This tells you that the manuscript will definitely be published but it hasn't been published yet. Often academics will let you know which projects they are working on now (which is helpful to see where the field could move to in the future). They might even provide additional resources such as online experiments so that you can get a feeling for the sort of experiments that they conduct. For example, Ralf Schwarzer, a Professor at Freie University, Berlin, who has made important contributions to the science of behavior change including the development of theory (particularly the Health Action Process (HAPA) Model), measures and interventions, provides academic papers and resources, including, for the adventurous, access to a free meta-analysis program at http://userpage.fu-berlin.de/health/author.htm. The rise of online journals provides access to papers more quickly, as do preprint servers. Take a look at medRxiv (https://www.medrxiv.org/ for health sciences), PsyArXiv (https://psyarxiv.com/ for psychology) and the Open Science Framework (OSF) for accessing papers pre-publication too. Trial registries (e.g., https://www.isrctn.com/) and review registries (e.g., https://www.crd.york.ac.uk/prospero/) and the OSF can also give you an idea about what type of work is ongoing.

> **Some journals are viewed as more prestigious than others**
>
> Journals are ranked based on the number of times that papers appearing in their journal are cited by others. A proxy measure of the likely importance of an article is to take a look at the impact factor rating of the journal within which it is published. Impact factors are usually published on the website of the journal and change from year to year. The higher the score, the more times the average paper has been cited within a specific period of time. Look for the following journals as they are often ranked as the top journals in the field: *Health Psychology*, *Annals of Behavioral Medicine*, *Health Psychology Review*, *Nature Human Behaviour*. Some high-ranking general journals (within which health behavior change articles can appear) are: *Psychological Bulletin*, *Psychological Review*, *The Lancet*, *Nature*, *Cochrane Database of Systematic Reviews*, *BMJ* and *PLoS Medicine*.

GAMIFICATION

What is it?

Gamification is a collection of strategies that take game-based features and elements, such as leaderboards, avatars, virtual trophies and points, and applies them in non-game contexts. These principles have been used extensively in education often in the form of serious games (full-featured games intended for serious purposes such as training). In Chapter 2, you'll have encountered Milla and Sonny's use of *Times Tables Rock Stars* which uses game-based elements such as points, levels (such as Rock Hero, Rock Legend, etc.) and leaderboards to encourage users to practice their times tables. Similar types of strategies have been applied to change health behaviors too. Although we consider gamification here as a set of behavior change techniques, it should be noted that others may consider it to be a form of mode of delivery. For example, in their classification of different ways of delivering interventions, Marques et al. (2021) consider gamification a mode of delivery.

How does it work?

A variety of mechanisms have been highlighted particularly around increasing motivation (Krath et al., 2021). By and large, gamification has been shown to increase intrinsic motivation (a key form of motivation from Self-Determination Theory) although there has been some conflicting evidence here. Other mechanisms include increased satisfaction and self-efficacy, more positive attitudes to the gamified subject, social collaboration/support and increased engagement. According to Krath et al. (2021) over 100 theories have been applied in some way to explaining the effects of gamification on outcomes. That's a lot! The most popular theory used has been Self-Determination Theory; a theory you will be familiar with from this book (see Chapter 2). Fortunately, Krath et al. have drawn on the 100+ theories to propose ten theoretical principles that help explain how gamification can achieve its effects. These principles broadly fall into one of three categories relating to helping the individual to their intended behavior, making the material more relevant to them and social benefits. As you can see in the descriptions that follow, which of these principles are relevant for any particular gamification-based intervention will depend on which components of gamification they utilize (e.g., leaderboards; rewards/badges) and how the intervention is set up (e.g., the amount of choice offered):

To help goal-striving

1. Providing clear and relevant goals. These can be broken down to smaller achievable goals (e.g., through different levels in the game);
2. Provide immediate feedback (e.g., through points, level changes in the game, indications of whether they are right or wrong) which can build feelings of competence and self-efficacy;
3. Positive reinforcement (e.g., through points, badges, positive messages from other users);
4. Guided paths. Guidance and tips from within the game can help users to achieve their goals and boost self-efficacy and knowledge;
5. Simplified user experience. As the system becomes easier to use, the less users will get distracted, the more capable they will feel about using it, and the more the technology will be accepted;

To increase relevance

6. Users can set their own goals which can boost their autonomy. Leaderboards are noted as an example here as they allow users to choose where in the leaderboard they wish to strive for;
7. Adaptive content. The content can be modified so that it fits the abilities, knowledge or interests of the user;
8. Enables choice with users completing the game via various different routes which can increase engagement and motivation;

Social benefits

9. Social comparison. Users can view the performance of others, learn from these observations and potentially compare their performance against these benchmarks;

10. Social support/norms. Gamification can help connect users to one another to help each other to achieve their goals and to provide norms.

Is it effective?

A lot of the evidence regarding the effectiveness of gamification is based on studies testing its utility in the context of education. However, evidence-based effectiveness is emerging for health behavior change. For example, Patel et al. (2017) randomized participants to a control group (who received daily feedback on whether they had achieved their step goal) or an intervention group. In the intervention, the participants entered a game with their family in which, after signing a pre-study commitment to try their best, received 70 points every Monday. Each day, a family member would be chosen by the game to try to achieve a steps total. If they failed, they would lose 10 points but would keep the points if they succeeded. At the end of the week, families with at least 50 points would move up a level (they started at "bronze"). Those at gold or platinum levels at the end of the study would receive, wait for it…a mug with the study logo! Participants in the intervention condition, compared to the control group, achieved their step goals on a greater percentage of days (during the intervention period: 53% vs. 32%; at follow-up: 44% vs. 33%). Mazeas et al. (2022) have since reported that, on the basis of a meta-analysis of 16 randomized controlled trials, gamification can be used to increase physical activity with a small-to-medium sized effect. Interestingly, Mazeas et al. also reported that they can have small, positive effects when compared to groups who receive active, but non-gamified, content. However, they also reported that the positive effects reduce over time.

A CAUTIONARY NOTE

When you read the overviews of the effectiveness of each of the techniques, you may wonder why, for example, a relatively simple technique such as implementation intentions produce, on average, larger effects than more complex interventions such as motivational interviewing. Remember that it is often difficult to compare across studies, and this is particularly true when you do this to make comparisons of different techniques. In implementation intention studies, comparison groups are often no-intervention controls. For other techniques, such as motivational interviewing, this is much less likely (e.g., usual care or alternative treatments are more likely for motivational interviewing). A size of an effect is dependent not only on what participants in the intervention condition do but also those in the control group. Less change can be expected for those in no-intervention conditions versus those in usual care or alternative treatments. There are likely other confounds too, such as the type of person targeted by each behavior change technique. It might be that those in the average motivational interviewing study are individuals with harder to change behaviors.

APPLYING BEHAVIOR CHANGE TECHNIQUES IN VARIOUS CONTEXTS

Behavior can be changed across a variety of different contexts. In this section, we highlight various reviews and empirical studies demonstrating effective strategies to change a range of health behaviors across a number of contexts: schools, the workplace, sports clubs and in healthcare settings.

SCHOOL-BASED INTERVENTIONS

Why?

The school, given the role of compulsory physical education classes, can be a useful way to increase physical activity and fitness. There are a number of ways in which changes to school-based physical education classes can increase physical activity. For example, the number of classes can be increased, the duration of classes can be increased or the type of exercises/sports conducted in class can be altered. Through classes, educational and other behavior change techniques can also be applied directly to pupils to tackle a range of different health behaviors.

Examples

In a systematic review of physical activity interventions, Kahn et al. (2002) concluded there was strong evidence that modifications to physical activity classes can increase aerobic capacity, flexibility and muscular endurance. These improvements seemed to be achieved without adverse consequences to other school work.

As well as promoting physical activity directly, school-based interventions have been used to reduce sedentary behavior. Television and video-game use are important contributors to sedentary lifestyles which, in turn, have been associated with negative health outcomes. On the basis that American children, outside of sleep, spend most of their time watching television and playing video-games, Robinson (1999) designed an intervention aimed at reducing the time spent doing these activities. It was anticipated that, by changing this activity, children's body mass index could be reduced because replacement activities would use more energy. One group received lessons from their teachers (who were trained first by the experimenters) concerning self-monitoring of television and video game use; students were then challenged to go "cold turkey" by not watching television or playing video games for 10 days before being given a seven-hour per week budget of time they could spend on these activities. This intervention was supported by materials designed to motivate parents to enforce these rules and an electronic monitor that could ration the number of hours the television could be switched on per week. Finally, students were asked to be advocates for reduced media use. Compared to a control group of students who simply reported on their behavior, the students exposed to the school-based intervention appeared to watch significantly less television and play video games less than the control group. The intervention group, relative to the control group, also had significant reductions in body mass index over the course of the study plus additional benefits (e.g., improved waist-to-hip ratios). Consequently, school-based interventions can be used to change health behaviors which may help in the battle against childhood obesity (but see Kahn et al., 2002).

WORKSITE INTERVENTIONS

Why?

The workplace is another important context in which to change health behaviors given many employed adults spend around half of the time that they are awake at work. Improving the health of one's workforce can have important and tangible benefits for companies. In a meta-analysis by Conn, Hafdahl, Cooper, Brown and Lusk (2009), worksite-based interventions, designed to increase physical activity, increased physical activity and had small effects on increasing attendance and reducing job-related stress (see Effect Sizes in Chapter 6). In addition, obesity in the workplace is linked with absenteeism, sick leave, disability, injuries and healthcare claims (Anderson et al., 2009). Reducing obesity through effective behavior change strategies may be one way, therefore, of reducing staff-related costs. Interventions designed to change health behaviors in the workplace can also benefit the economy more widely by reducing the demands on doctors/ GPs and medical costs. The workplace, therefore, can be seen as a convenient and economically viable environment within which to try to change important health behaviors.

Interestingly, the size of the workplace has been shown *not* to influence the success of behavior change interventions linked to health (Conn et al., 2009). Effective interventions can, in principle therefore, be delivered with similar outcomes in small, medium and large-sized companies.

Examples

In a review of worksite-based interventions to promote physical activity, Taylor et al. (2012) concluded that such interventions yield small increases in physical activity, on average. However, the review did not detect any behavior change techniques to be especially effective in this context. Similarly, based on the results of the higher quality studies included in a review of worksite interventions on health outcomes, Heaney and Goetzel (1997) concluded that it is unlikely that simply raising health awareness across the workforce will create substantial change. According to Heaney and Goetzel (1997), a more targeted approach to high-risk individuals involving risk-reduction counselling is likely to be more useful in effecting change.

Anderson et al. (2009) presented an explanatory model highlighting how the worksite can be used to deliver changes in dietary and physical activity-related behaviors and, thus, changes in body size and composition of their employees. According to Anderson et al. (2009), there are three main ways in which an organization can promote exercise and diet. First, an organization can make changes to its policy and environment by, for example, providing free worksite gyms to encourage employees to participate in regular exercise. This would help counter barriers of cost and the inconvenience of finding opportunities to exercise. Second, organizations can raise awareness about the benefits of exercise through, for example, presenting health-related information on the intranet or through posters and leaflets distributed in the workplace. Third, organizations could offer social support or skills training aimed at increasing employees' confidence in their ability to improve diet or increase physical activity.

INTERVENTIONS BY SPORTS CLUBS

Why?

Intervening within sports clubs can be an attractive route to health behavior change for individuals who may be less inclined to utilize standard health services such as men. They can bring individuals together who have shared interests and that, in turn, can increase **relatedness** which can contribute to **intrinsic motivation**. By engaging closely with a sports club they can become involved with an intervention that matches their identity.

Examples

Working with 13 professional football clubs in Scotland, the Football Fans in Training scheme was shown to help individuals lose, on average, nearly 5 kilograms more at one-year follow-up than those allocated to a control group (Hunt et al., 2014). This intervention, which involved 12 weekly sessions each with an educational component and group-based physical activity sessions run by club coaches and follow-up emails and a reunion event, also positively benefited a range of biological (e.g., waist size, body fat, blood pressure), psychological (e.g., self-esteem) and behavioral (self-reported physical activity, diet and alcohol intake) outcomes. This approach has inspired similar interventions using the same or different sports across Europe, Australia, Canada and New Zealand (Hunt et al., 2020).

INTERVENTIONS IN PRIMARY CARE/HEALTHCARE

Why?

In the past, doctors, nurses and other healthcare professionals have focused on treating the sick. In the UK, Lord Darzi's report *NHS Next Stage Review* (Department of Health, 2008) which sets out a strong vision for innovation, quality and personalized care, informed the strategies of many organizations within the National Health Service (NHS). According to this review, a key focus and challenge here is to prevent ill health as well as treating sickness within healthcare settings.

Relative to interventions conducted in the workplace or school-based settings, behavior change in healthcare faces the challenge of lack of time in contact with the person who is the target for behavior change. Previous research has, therefore, focused on screening of people at risk (e.g., using the alcohol use disorders test, AUDIT, Bohn, Barbor, & Kranzler, 1995) within primary care (e.g., at the General Practice). There is a need, therefore, to develop effective brief-interventions to change key health behaviors.

There are other challenges to developing and delivering effective behavior change interventions in healthcare settings. The interventions need to be seen as feasible and acceptable to the users (those delivering it and those receiving it). For example, there has been concern that doctors (general practitioners, GPs) may not be able to deliver brief interventions designed to change health behaviors due to factors such as worries about damaging the GP-patient relationship (e.g., being advised to quit smoking after attending an appointment with a smoking-related illness may make the patient feel like they are being blamed for their illness), lack of incentive for GPs and lack of training (e.g., O'Donnell et al., 2014). Strong evidence for the efficacy (i.e., the ability of the intervention to cause changes in behavior) and how quickly they can be delivered will be key factors in how acceptable the intervention is to the users and whether it will be adopted and used over a sustained period of time, even when intervention studies cease. Fortunately, there is some evidence supporting the use of brief interventions designed to change health behaviors within healthcare settings.

Examples

In a meta-analysis comprising 17 tests, Stead, Bergson and Lancaster (2008) concluded that doctors giving brief advice concerning smoking cessation could increase quit rates significantly compared to groups receiving no advice, raising quit rates to 4–6% compared to 2–3% without assistance. There is a risk, however, that doctors might not view this as a sufficient rise in success rates to warrant the additional time spent within a consultation. Brief advice, however, has also been shown to be useful for other health and drug-related behaviors including alcohol use (Bien, Miller & Tonigan, 1993; O'Donnell, Wallace & Kaner, 2014).

Providing advice to quit smoking might be effective but there are ways to yield larger improvements. In their review, Aveyard et al. (2012) reported that providing advice to quit on medical grounds increased smoking quit attempts but not as much as providing assistance. However, only one study in this review tested the effectiveness of assistance versus advice to quit on medical grounds and while this increased quit attempts, it did not increase quit success (Slama et al., 1990).

A promising brief approach developed by Aveyard et al. (2016) involved a physician offering referral to an effective weight loss program and, if it was accepted by the patient, the physician would both ensure that they signed up there and then and offered a follow-up appointment. Compared to patients who were randomized to a condition provided only with advice to change behavior on health grounds, those randomized to the intervention lost more than double the weight (nearly 2.5kgs versus just over 1kg) at 12 months. The intervention was designed to take the physician less than 30 seconds though it should be acknowledged that the weight loss service, to which the patients would have been directed, is not a brief intervention.

Miller and Sanchez (1993) have also advocated the use of a FRAMES approach to change health behaviors in healthcare settings. The FRAMES approach is a brief intervention comprising Feedback (providing information on behavior relative to goals or others), Responsibility (emphasizing the individual themselves are ultimately responsible for their health), Advice (providing verbal or written advice to change behavior), Menu (providing a range of self-help strategies), Empathy (the healthcare practitioner adopting a warm, understanding approach) and Self-Efficacy (enhancing confidence in one's ability to change through persuasion).

An alternative approach that can be used effectively in healthcare settings involves showing patients pictorial information regarding their risks. For example, Naslund et al. (2019) randomized participants to either a condition that they were provided with images representing a carotid ultrasound and the amount of plaque buildup within an individual (see Figure 3.3) or

Your vascular wall thickness is presented as vascular age
The green sector corresponds to wall thickness in patients being at least 10 years younger than your actual age, and the red sector at least 10 years older

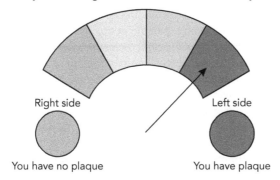

Right side   Left side

You have no plaque   You have plaque

Your picture that shows IMT and plaque

Right side   Left side

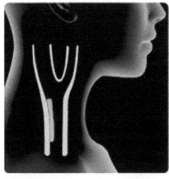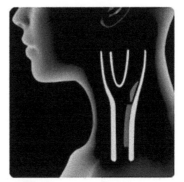

IMT shown with a coloured line   Plaque shown with a marking

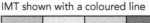

FIGURE 3.3 Health risk visuals used by Naslund et al. (2019) to try to reduce risk of atherosclerotic disease in asymptomatic adults.

Näslund U, Ng N, Lundgren A, Fhärm E, Grönlund C, Johansson H, Lindahl B, Lindahl B, Lindvall K, Nilsson SK, Nordin M, Nordin S, Nyman E, Rocklöv J, Vanoli D, Weinehall L, Wennberg P, Wester P, Norberg M; VIPVIZA trial group. Visualization of asymptomatic atherosclerotic disease for optimum cardiovascular prevention (VIPVIZA): a pragmatic, open-label, randomized controlled trial. *Lancet*. 2019, Jan 12;393(10167):133–142. doi: 10.1016/S0140-6736(18)32818-6. Epub 2018 Dec 3. Erratum in: *Lancet*. 2019 Jun 15;393(10189):2394. PMID: 30522919.

to a comparison group not receiving this visual information. At one-year follow-up, those allocated to the intervention group reduced risk scores relative to the control group. Hollands et al. (2022) have reviewed the effects of interventions that visualize health risk with medical imaging and concluded that they can be useful to help reduce smoking, improve diet, increase physical activity and behaviors related to oral hygiene.

One final point is that the health sector provides services related to behavior change that utilize behavior change techniques. For example, in a review of the Stop Smoking Services treatment manuals used in England, West et al. (2010) coded the behavior change techniques specified in each manual using a smoking specific taxonomy (Michie et al., 2011). They then tested the associations between the use of specific behavior change techniques and treatment success. They found that the manuals contained 22 behavior change techniques, on average. The most common behavior change techniques used were providing advice on stop smoking medication, helping to identify lapse triggers and formulating plans to deal with them, goal-setting (each present in 98% of the manuals) and measuring carbon monoxide levels (95% of manuals). They reported that nine techniques were associated with both four-week self-reported and carbon monoxide verified abstinence rates including measuring carbon monoxide levels, advice on changing routine and relapse prevention. In similar ways, healthcare services are sent recommendations based on psychological literature on behavior change techniques. An example of this is Public Health England's recommendations regarding what techniques to use to aid weight loss and its maintenance (Public Health England, 2017). Moreover, motivational interviewing and relapse prevention are key elements in exercise referral schemes that enable those referred on health grounds to access exercise classes or individual sessions at heavily discounted rates. These schemes have been shown to be effective for those with coronary heart disease (Murphy et al., 2012).

BURNING ISSUE BOX 3.2

QUESTION & ANSWERS ON BEHAVIOR CHANGE

Question 1: Which behavior change technique is the most effective?

At a general level, it has been demonstrated within a review on HIV intervention strategies (Albarracín et al., 2005) that passive interventions (simply presenting arguments) are less effective than more active interventions (such as behavioral skills training).

At the level of specific techniques, self-monitoring appears to be a particularly effective strategy. In a meta-analysis of patient education to increase physical activity, Conn et al. (2008) reported that interventions that incorporated self-monitoring (.56) were more effective than those that did not (.40) while other techniques (barriers management,

contracting, consequences, contracting, exercise prescription, feed
back, fitness testing, goal setting, problem solving and stimulus/cues)
were unrelated to effect sizes. This is consistent with results of a review
by Michie et al. (2009) that also concluded self-monitoring was the
most effective behavior change technique for healthy eating and
physical activity, as well as a review examining the impact of self-monitoring across several types of behavior (Harkin et al., 2016).
While different techniques might be more effective for different
behaviors, and there is a degree of imprecision in the approach
adopted by Conn et al. and Michie et al. (given they consider multiple
behavior change techniques), self-monitoring clearly appears to be a
powerful behavior change technique. This is supported also by the
number of times it emerges as an effective behavior change technique
relative to other techniques in other reviews (see Table 3.1).

Question 2: Is it better to change multiple behaviors at the same
time?

By changing one behavior successfully, this might increase one's
confidence in one's ability to change other behaviors. However, Bull,
Dombrowski, McCleary and Johnston (2014), in a review of health
behavior interventions for low income groups, reported interventions
targeting only physical activity produced larger effects than studies
targeting multiple behaviors including physical activity. This finding
was consistent with Conn et al.'s (2008) meta-analysis which reported
that interventions targeting only physical activity (.57) yielded larger
effects on physical activity than those targeting physical activity and
other behaviors (e.g., diet) together (.38). Attempting to change two
behaviors at the same time has been argued to lead to less than twice
the change of an intervention targeting one behavior (i.e. sub-additivity), as the more complex intervention is more difficult for the participant to adhere to (e.g., The Trials of Hypertension Collaborative
Research Group, 1997). However, even in studies where adherence is
high, sub-additivity still occurs (e.g., Sacks et al., 2001). More recently,
a review by Wilson et al. (2015) suggested that making 2–3 recommendations led to stronger behavioral improvements than making 0, 1 or
4/+ recommendations. In sum, targeting multiple behaviors at the
same time may lead to greater overall change but sub-additivity is one
drawback of this approach along with putting greater demands on
participants, those delivering the intervention, and total costs.

Question 3: Are interventions that comprise more behavior change techniques more effective?

In their review of internet-based interventions to promote physical activity, Webb et al. (2010) reported interventions with more techniques tended to produce greater increases in physical activity. In a review of workplace-based interventions designed to reduce stress, Murphy (1996) concluded studies that used a combination of techniques reported larger effects on outcome measures than studies that incorporated interventions comprising single techniques. More recent reviews have provided equivocal support with more techniques leading to larger effects on some outcomes but not others (e.g., Bishop et al., 2015). When assessing the impact of self-regulatory techniques on exercise and dietary behaviors (prompting intention formation; providing feedback on performance; self-monitoring; prompting specific goal-setting; prompting review of behavioral goals), Michie et al. (2009) reported that combining three self-regulatory techniques generated a moderate effect on behavior; using 2, 4 or 5 self-regulatory techniques resulted in small-to-moderate effects; while 0 or 1 self-regulatory techniques generated the smallest effects. Thus, it appears that moderately complex interventions (that combine a small number of techniques) might be the most useful for behavior change.

Question 4: Does tailoring educational materials to the needs of the individual rather than presenting everybody with the same information yield larger changes in behavior?

Tailoring involves individualizing interventions based on information specific to that individual (such as their characteristics, circumstances, needs and preferences) rather than using a one-size-fits-all approach, which gives the same intervention to everybody. Advances in technology can enable complex tailoring with relative ease. Tailoring interventions via computers, for example, allows those delivering interventions to provide personalized self-assessment and feedback and respond to the specific beliefs and cognitions of individuals. By providing only information that is relevant to the individual, the amount of irrelevant information is reduced and this may explain why this approach could increase the likelihood that the educational materials are read and the key points recalled (Brug, Campbell, & van Assema, 1999). Personalized feedback should seek to compare the individual's behavior against peer averages which highlights to the individual the need to change (e.g., Brug et al., 1996). In a review of 57 studies, however, tailoring was found to have a small benefit on the effectiveness of behavioral interventions (Noar, Benac & Harris, 2007).

Engagement, or involvement in the message, is likely to be a key factor in the influence of tailoring as with any form of educational materials (see Petty & Cacioppo, 1986). Presenting tailored information in an interactive format might be one way to maximize user engagement and subsequent behavior change. For example, Hurling, Fairley and Dias (2006) demonstrated that an interactive version of an internet website was rated as more engaging as indexed by higher user retention, it enhanced exercise expectations, and it increased self-reported exercise more than a less interactive version and no intervention.

Brug et al. (1999) tentatively concluded that computer-tailored information may be more motivating, especially in reducing fat intake, than general information. However, Conn et al. (2008) reported that individually tailored interventions were no more effective than presenting the same content to everybody within their meta-analysis of educational physical activity interventions for patients.

Ma et al. (2021) has argued that there is a need to establish which factors should be taken into account in tailoring, what to tailor (e.g., behavior change techniques, intensity of intervention, mode of delivery, etc.) and how best to develop tailored interventions. They recommend input from a range of stakeholders and co-design/co-production methods (see Chapter 5) to improve tailored interventions.

BURNING ISSUE BOX 3.3

HOW CAN WE DEVELOP HEALTHY HABITS AND BREAK UNHEALTHY HABITS?

Forming healthy habits feels like the holy grail; if we can achieve them, healthy behaviors are much more likely to be maintained over time. Part of the reason is that once habits are formed, fluctuating motivation levels are less likely to derail healthy behaviors with behavior propelled forward by impulse (Gardner, 2015). So, how can these be developed? Part of the solution involves understanding how habits develop in the first place.

Wood and Neal (2016) explain that habits develop when sufficiently rewarding or rewarded behaviors are consistently repeated in the same place, time or other context. For example, it is quite easy to see how, at the first signs of mild hunger in the evening (context), one of the authors of this book (Andrew) reaching for, and subsequently consuming, a packet of chips (behavioral response) which he enjoys (rewarding) becomes habitual and hard to stop if repeated over successive nights (repeated actions in the same context). As a result, over time, through these learned associations between the context and the behavior, when an individual encounters that context, these cue behavior more automatically in a way that it can happen quickly, without deliberation or mental effort.

Based around their definition of habits, Wood and Neal (2016) suggest three categories of interventions to promote healthy habits: repetition of the behavior, having stable contextual cues and the behavior being rewarded. As such, if you want to develop a healthy habit, try to:

1. Choose a goal for yourself and select a behavior that you'll likely enjoy in order to achieve that goal, in this sense, the behavior will become rewarding in itself (behavior → enjoyment).
2. There's no harm in ensuring the behaviors themselves are relatively simple (complex behaviors may be harder to habitualize) and are behaviors that you're reasonably confident in performing (this may not always be possible and you may want to build up confidence a little first!).
3. Next, identify a stable context (same time, place, etc.) in which to perform the behavior. You could even piggyback on an existing habit. You regularly watch TV but want to do more exercise; no problem, choose a TV show that you watch regularly and do floor exercises (if that's your thing) while watching the TV show.
4. Aim to repeat the behavior regularly in response to your stable contextual cue. It'll get easier over time. Studies have shown, for example, that regularly attending the gym for around five weeks can lead to new exercise habits (Armitage, 2005). Context dependent repetition has also been reported to be an effective means to promote medication adherence (Robinson et al., in press).
5. Reward the behavior. As noted above, the behavior itself could be rewarding or you can do it alongside other activities that you enjoy. Alternatively, doing the behavior can be rewarded in different ways. It has been argued that if behavior is rewarded through extrinsic rewards (e.g., buying a new clothing item), it is best done at the beginning (when the habit is developing, possibly to offset any short-term negative effects of starting a new healthy behavior). Further, rewards work best when they are

uncertain (rather than guaranteed rewards every time) and promote behavior repetition.

Gardner (2015) argues that, once stimulus-response associations are learned, habits represent a process in which a context automatically cues an *impulse* towards the behavior. These impulses can be overridden, though this can be difficult even when they have not been acted on for a while, as traces of the old habits can remain dormant in memory, ready to be re-enacted upon encountering old cues or when motivation or willpower is lacking (Bouton et al., 2011; Gardner et al., 2021). Thus, how these impulses can be overridden or avoided in the first place serve as useful pointers for how to break unhealthy habits such as smoking.

Again, Wood and Neal (2016) highlight three categories of interventions to break habits involving disrupting the cue (e.g., avoiding exposure to cues which can sometimes occur around major life events like moving house), environmental restructuring (adding friction to unhealthy choices like banning smoking in public places or heavily taxing junk foods and/or removing friction for healthy choices such as discounting healthy foods; ensuring there's always fresh fruit in the house, etc.) and strategies to aid monitoring (e.g., red traffic lights on unhealthy foods; signs to promote stair use over lift use etc.).

There are additional strategies that may also help to break unwanted habits. Gardner et al. (2021) suggest trying to replace old habitual behaviors by practicing new alternative behaviors repeatedly in the same context. These alternative behaviors should serve the same goal as the old behavior and/or when this is not appropriate (i.e., if the goal is unhealthy) the replacement behavior should be at least as appealing as the original behavior. In addition, implementation intentions (see elsewhere in this chapter and Chapter 7) can be used to link the cue to a new behavior rather than the old unhealthy behavior, and conserving mental resources to focus on engaging in the new behavior and not performing the old undesired behavior can also be helpful. If the cues to the undesired behaviors are not known, Gardner et al. (2021) recommend a period of self-monitoring to identify potential cues that occur prior to performing the unwanted behaviors.

In sum, there are recommended strategies to form new habits and break old ones. Neither of these are necessarily easy to do but the rewards can be great.

SUMMARY

Many behavior change techniques are available and represent different ways to change behavior. These techniques have been defined and categorized within taxonomies enabling consistent use and descriptions of interventions. As these taxonomies become refined over time, and effective training methods developed to ensure such taxonomies can be used reliably, they will become an increasingly important means to organize the evidence base. Of the techniques available, self-monitoring appears to have a lot of promise. The techniques that we have focused on within this chapter tend to produce medium to large effects in the short term but their effects become smaller in the longer term.

FURTHER READING

Adams, J., Giles, E.L., McColl, E., & Sniehotta, F.F. (2014). Carrots, sticks and health behaviours: a framework for documenting the complexity of financial incentive interventions to change health behaviours. *Health Psychology Review*, *8*, 286–295. Identifies nine different domains across which to describe financial incentive interventions: direction, form, magnitude, certainty, target, frequency, immediacy, schedule and recipient.

BCT Taxonomy v1 Online Training website provides online training in how to use Michie et al.'s (2013) classification of 93 behavior change techniques. See: http://www.bct-taxonomy.com/ The National Centre for Smoking Cessation and Training (NCSCT) website provides access to a variety of resources relevant to behavior change techniques. These include videos and other training resources concerning very brief advice on smoking, as well as a variety of documents designed for smoking cessation practitioners. See: http://www.ncsct.co.uk/

Verplanken, B., & Orbell, S. (2022). Attitudes, habits, and behavior change. *Annual Review of Psychology*, *73*, 327–352.

Comprehensive overview of how habits develop, how they enable long-term behavior change and how they can be disrupted.

GLOSSARY

Behavior change technique: A systematic strategy used in an attempt to change behavior (e.g., providing information on consequences; prompting specific goal setting; modelling the behavior).

Fully-crossed (full factorial) design: A methodological approach in which each behavior change technique used in a study is delivered individually and in combination with all other behavior change techniques. Useful for identifying which behavior change techniques change behavior and which do not.

Gamification: An approach to behavior change that utilizes game-like features like scoring points and moving up or down ranking ladders in non-game contexts (e.g., to promote walking steps).

Implementation intention: A specific plan an individual makes, in advance, regarding the context (e.g., when/where) one will perform a specific action.

Incentives/rewards: Typically reflects informing (incentives)/ giving (rewards) a reward to encourage behavior change (though a broader definition may also encompass the removal of punishment or related threat).

Intrinsic motivation: A type of motivation which reflects an individual doing a behavior for its own sake because it is enjoyable and satisfying or personally interesting.

Meta-analysis: A statistical procedure used to combine, compare and contrast the findings of studies on a related topic.

Motivational interviewing: "Prompting the person to provide self-motivating statements and evaluations of their own behavior to minimize resistance to change" (Abraham & Michie, 2008, p. 382).

Relatedness: A sense of belonging or connectedness which, according to Self-Determination Theory, is an important need or component underlying intrinsic motivation.

Self-monitoring: "The person is asked to keep a record of specified behavior(s) (e.g., in a diary)" (Abraham & Michie, 2008, p. 382).

Systematic review: a rigorous and replicable approach to identify, and synthesize evidence from, studies tackling a specific issue.

REFERENCES

Aarts, H., Dijksterhuis, A., & Midden, C. (1999). To plan or not to plan? Goal achievement or interrupting the performance of a mundane behaviours. *European Journal of Social Psychology, 29*, 971–979.

Abraham, C., & Graham-Rowe, E. (2009). Are worksite interventions effective in increasing physical activity? A systematic review and meta-analysis. *Health Psychology Review, 3*, 108–144.

Abraham, C., & Michie, S. (2008). A taxonomy of behavior change techniques used in interventions. *Health Psychology, 27*, 379–387.

Adriaanse, M.A., Vinkers, C.D., De Ridder, D.T., Hox, J.J., & De Wit, J.B. (2011). Do implementation intentions help to eat a healthy diet? A systematic review and meta-analysis of the empirical evidence. *Appetite, 56*, 183–193.

Ahn, J.N., Hu, D., & Vega, M. (2021). Changing pace: using implementation intentions to enhance social distancing behavior during the COVID-19 pandemic. *Journal of Experimental Psychology, 27*, 762–772.

Albarracín, D., Gillette, J.C., Earl, A.N. et al. (2005). A test of major assumptions about behavior change: A comprehensive look at the effects of passive and active HIV-prevention interventions since the beginning of the epidemic. *Psychological Bulletin, 131*, 856–897.

Anderson, L.M., Quinn, T.A., Glanz, K. et al. (2009). The effectiveness of worksite nutrition and physical activity interventions for controlling employee overweight and obesity. *American Journal of Preventive Medicine, 37*, 340–357.

Apodaca, T.R. & Longabaugh, R. (2009). Mechanisms of change in motivational interviewing: a review and preliminary evaluation of evidence. *Addiction, 104*, 705–715.

Armitage, C.J. (2005). Can the theory of planned behavior predict the maintenance of physical activity? *Health Psychology, 24*, 235–245.

Avery, L., Flynn, D., van Wersch, A., Sniehotta, F.F., & Trenell, M.I. (2012). Changing physical activity behavior in type 2 diabetes: A systematic review and meta-analysis of behavioral interventions. *Diabetes Care*, 35, 2681–2689.

Aveyard, P., Begh, R., Parsons, A., & West, R. (2012). Brief opportunistic smoking cessation interventions: a systematic review and meta-analysis to compare advice to quit and offer of assistance. *Addiction, 107*, 1066–1073.

Bartlett, Y.K., Sheeran, P., & Hawley, M.S. (2014). Effective behaviour change techniques in smoking cessation interventions for people with chronic obstructive pulmonary disease: A meta-analysis. *British Journal of Health Psychology, 19*, 181–203.

Bien, T.H., Miller, W.R., & Tonigan, J.S. (1993). Brief interventions for alcohol problems: A review. *Addiction, 88*, 315–336.

Bird, E.L., Baker, G., Mutrie, N., et al. (2013). Behaviour change techniques used to promote walking and cycling: A systematic review. *Health Psychology, 32*, 829–838.

Bishop, F.L., Fenge-Davies, A.L., Kirby, S., & Geraghty, A.W.A. (2015). Context effects and behaviour change techniques in randomized trials: A systematic review using the example of trials to increase adherence to physical activity in musculoskeletal pain. *Psychology & Health, 30*, 104–121.

Black, N., Mullan, B., & Sharpe, L. (2016). Computer-delivered interventions for reducing alcohol consumption: meta-analysis and meta-regression using behaviour change techniques and theory. *Health Psychology Review, 10*, 341–357.

Bohn, M.J., Barbor, T.F., & Kranzler, H.R. (1995). The alcohol use identification test (AUDIT): Validation of a screening instrument for use in medical settings, *Journal of Studies on Alcohol, 56*, 423–432.

Boonmanunt, S., Pattanaprateep, O., Ongphiphadhanakul, B. et al. (in press). Evaluation of the effectiveness of behavioral economic incentive programs for goal achievement on healthy diet, weight control and physical activity: A systematic review and network meta-analysis. *Annals of Behavioral Medicine.*

Bouton, M.E., Todd, T.P., Vurbic, D., & Winterbauer, N.E. (2011). Renewal after the extinction of free operant behavior. *Learning & Behavior, 39*, 57–67.

Brannon, E.E., & Cushing, C.C. (2015). Is there an app for that? Translational science of pediatric behavior change for physical activity and dietary interventions: A systematic review. *Journal of Pediatric Psychology, 40*, 373–384.

Brug, J., Campbell, M., & van Assema, P. (1999). The application and impact of computer-generated personalized nutrition education: A review of the literature. *Patient Education and Counseling, 36,* 145–156.

Brug, J., Steenhuis, I.H.M., Van Assema, P., & De Vries, H. (1996). The impact of a computer-tailored nutrition intervention. *Preventive Medicine, 25,* 236–42.

Budworth, L., Prestwich, A., Sykes-Muskett, B. et al. (2019). A feasibility study to assess the individual and combined effects of financial incentives and monetary contingency contracts on physical activity. *Psychology of Sport & Exercise, 44,* 42–50.

Bull, E.R., Dombrowski, S.U., McCleary, N., & Johnston, M. (2014). Are interventions for low-income groups effective in changing healthy eating, physical activity and smoking behaviours? A systematic review and meta-analysis. *BMJ Open, 4,* e006046.

Burke, B.L., Arkowitz, H. & Menchola, M. (2003). The efficacy of motivational interviewing: a meta-analysis of controlled clinical trials. *Journal of Consulting and Clinical Psychology, 71,* 843–861.

Cahill, K. & Perara, R. (2011). Competitions and incentives for smoking cessation. *Cochrane Database of Systematic Reviews,* Issue 4. Art. No.: CD004307.

Calomarde-Gómez, C., Jimenez-Fernandez, B., Balcells-Olivero, M., Gaul, A., & Lopez-Pelayo, H. (2021). Motivational interviewing for cannabis use disorders: a systematic review and meta-analysis. *European Addiction Research, 27,* 413–427.

Carraça, E., Encantado, J., Battista, F. et al. (2021). Effective behavior change techniques to promote physical activity in adults with overweight or obesity: A systematic review and meta-analysis. *Obesity Reviews, 22,* e13258.

Conn, V.S., Hafdahl, S.R., Cooper, P.S., Brown, L.M., & Lusk, S.L. (2009). Meta-analysis of workplace physical activity interventions. *American Journal of Preventive Medicine, 37,* 330–339.

Cooke, R., McEwan, H., & Norman, P. (2022). The effect of forming implementation intentions on alcohol consumption: a systematic review and meta-analysis. *Drug and Alcohol Review, 42,* 68–80.

Copeland, L., McNamara, R., Kelson, M., & Simpson, S. (2015). Mechanisms of change within motivational interviewing in relation to health behaviour outcomes: A systematic review. *Patient Education & Counseling, 98,* 401–411.

Coster, S., Gulliford, M.C., Seed, P.T., Powrie, R.K., & Swaminathan, R. (2000). Self-monitoring in Type 2 diabetes mellitus: a meta-analysis. *Diabetic Medicine, 17,* 755–761.

Cummings, S.M., Cooper, R.L., & Cassie, K.M. (2009). Motivational interviewing to affect behavioral change in older adults. *Research on Social Work Practice, 19,* 195–204.

Department of Health (2008). High quality care for all: NHS next stage review final report.

Dombrowski, S.U., Sniehotta, F.F., Avenell, A. et al. (2012). Identifying active ingredients in complex behavioural interventions for obese adults with obesity-related co-morbidities or additional risk factors for comorbidities: A systematic review. *Health Psychology Review, 6,* 7–32.

Eckerstorfer, L.V., Tanzer, N.K., Vogrincic-Haselbacher, C. et al. (2018). Key elements of mHealth interventions to successfully increase physical activity: Meta-regression. *JMIR mHealth uHealth, 6,* e10076.

Finne, E., Glausch, M., Exner, A. et al. (2018). Behavior change techniques for increasing physical activity in cancer survivors: a systematic review and meta-analysis of randomized controlled trials. *Cancer Management and Research, 10,* 5125–5143.

Fishbein, M. (1995). Developing effective behavior change interventions: Some lessons learned from behavioral research. In T.E. Becker, S.L. David, & G. Saucey (Eds.) *National Institute on Drug Research Monograph Series 155* (pp. 246–261). Rockville, MD: National Institute on Drug Research.

French, D.P., Olander, E.K., Chisholm, A., & McSharry, J. (2014). Which behaviour change techniques are the most effective at increasing older adults' self-efficacy and physical activity behaviour? A systematic review. *Annals of Behavioral Medicine, 48,* 225–234.

Frost, H., Campbell, P., Maxwell, M. et al. (2018). Effectiveness of motivational interviewing on adult behaviour change in health and social care settings: A systematic review of reviews. *PLoS ONE, 13,* e0204890.

Gardner, B. (2015). A review and analysis of the use of "habit" in understanding, predicting and influencing health-related behaviour. *Health Psychology Review, 9,* 277–295.

Gardner, B., Richards, R., Lally, P. et al. (2021). Breaking habits or breaking habitual behaviours? Old habits as a neglected factor in weight loss maintenance. *Appetite, 162,* 105183.

Garnett, C.V., Crane, D., Brown, J. et al. (2018). Behavior change techniques used in digital behavior change interventions to reduce excessive alcohol consumption: A meta-regression. *Annals of Behavioral Medicine, 52,* 530–543.

Giles, E.L., Robalino, S., McColl, E., Sniehotta, F.F., & Adams, J. (2014). The effectiveness of financial incentives for health behaviour change: systematic review and meta-analysis. PLoS ONE, *9,* e90347.

Gollwitzer, P.M. (1993). Goal achievement: The role of intentions. In W. Stroebe & M. Hewstone (Eds.), *European Review of Social Psychology, 4,* 141–185. Chichester, England: Wiley.

Gollwitzer, P.M., & Sheeran, P. (2006). Implementation intentions and goal achievement: A meta-analysis of effects and processes. *Advances in Experimental Social Psychology, 38,* 249–268.

Harkin, B., Webb, T.L., Chang, B.P.I. et al. (2016). Does monitoring goal progress promote goal attainment? A meta-analysis of the experimental evidence. *Psychological Bulletin, 142*(2), 198–229.

Hartmann-Boyce, J., Johns, D.J., Jebb, S., & Aveyard, P. (2014). Effect of behavioural techniques and delivery mode on effectiveness of weight management: systematic review, meta-analysis and meta-regression. *Obesity Reviews, 15,* 598–609.

Heaney, C.A., & Goetzel, R.Z. (1997). A review of health-related outcomes of multi-component worksite health promotion programs. *American Journal of Health Promotion, 11,* 290–307.

Henrich, J.F., Knittle, K., De Gucht, V. et al. (2015). Identifying effective techniques within psychological treatments for irritable bowel syndrome: A meta-analysis. *Journal of Psychosomatic Research, 78,* 205–222.

Hettema, J., Steele, J., & Miller, W.R. (2005). Motivational Interviewing. *Annual Review of Clinical Psychology, 1,* 91–111.

Hill, B., Skouteris, H., & Fuller-Tyszkiewicz, M. (2013). Interventions designed to limit gestational weight gain: a systematic review of theory and meta-analysis of intervention components. *Obesity Reviews, 14,* 435–450.

Hilton, C.E. & Johnston, L.H. (2017). Health psychology: It's not what you do, it's the way that you do it. *Health Psychology Open, 4*(2).

Hollands, G.J., Bignardi, G., Johnston, M. et al. (2017). The TIPPME intervention typology for changing environments to change behaviour. *Nature Human Behaviour, 1,* 140.

Hollands, G.J., Usher-Smith, J.A., Hasan, R. et al. (2022). Visualising health risks with medical imaging for changing recipients' health behaviours and risk factors: Systematic review with meta-analysis. *PLoS Medicine, 19,* e1003920.

Howlett, N., Trivedi, D., Troop, N.A., & Chater, A.M. (2019). Are physical activity interventions for healthy inactive adults effective in promoting behavior change and maintenance, and which behaviour change techniques are effective? A systematic review and meta-analysis. *Translational Behavioral Medicine, 9,* 147–157.

Hunt, K., Wyke, S., Bunn, C. et al. (2020). Scale-up and scale-out of a gender sensitized weight management and healthy living program delivered to overweight men via professional sports clubs: The wider implementation of Football Fans in Training (FFIT). *International Journal of Environmental Research and Public Health, 17,* 584.

Hunt, K., Wyke, S., Gray, C.M. et al. (2014). A gender-sensitised weight loss and healthy living programme for overweight and obese men delivered by Scottish Premier League football clubs (FFIT): a pragmatic randomised controlled trial. *Lancet, 383,* 1211–1221.

Hurling, R., Fairley, B.W., & Dias, M.B. (2006). Internet-based exercise intervention systems: Are more interactive designs better? *Psychology & Health, 21,* 757–772.

Johnston, V., Liberato, S., & Thomas, D. (2012). Incentives for preventing smoking in children and adolescents. *Cochrane Database of Systematic Reviews,* Issue 10. Art. No.: CD008645.

Kahn, E.B., Ramsey, L.T., Brownson, R.C. et al. (2002). The effectiveness of interventions to increase physical activity. A systematic review. *American Journal of Preventive Medicine, 22,* 73–107.

Kassavou, A., & Sutton, S. (2018). Automated telecommunication interventions to promote adherence to cardio-metabolic medications: meta-analysis of effectiveness and meta-regression of behaviour change techniques. *Health Psychology Review, 12,* 25–42.

Knittle, K., Heino, M., Marques, M.M. et al. (2020). The compendium of self-enactable techniques to change and self-manage motivation and behaviour v. 1.0. *Nature Human Behaviour, 4,* 215–223.

Lara, J., Evans, E.H., O'Brien, N. et al. (2014). Association of behaviour change techniques with effectiveness of dietary interventions among adults of retirement age: a systematic review and meta-analysis of randomised controlled trials. *BMC Medicine, 12,* 177.

Li, L., Zhu, S., Tse, N., Tse, S., & Wong, P. (2016). Effectiveness of motivational interviewing to reduce illicit drug use in adolescents: a systematic review and meta-analysis. *Addiction, 111,* 795–805.

Lussier, J.P., Heil, S.H., Mongeon, J.A., Badger, G.J., & Higgins, S.T. (2006). A meta-analysis of voucher-based reinforcement therapy for substance use disorders. *Addiction, 101*, 192–203.

Lyzwinski, L.N. (2014). A systematic review and meta-analysis of mobile devices and weight loss with an intervention content analysis. *Journal of Personalized Medicine, 4*, 311–385.

Mantzari, E., Vogt, F., Shemilt, I. et al. (2015). Personal financial incentives for changing habitual health-related behaviors: A systematic review and meta-analysis. *Preventive Medicine, 75*, 75–85.

Markland, D., Ryan, R.M., Tobin, V.J., & Rollnick, S. (2005). Motivational interviewing and self-determination theory. *Journal of Social and Clinical Psychology, 24*, 811–831.

Marques, M.M., Carey, R.N., Norris, E. et al. (2021). Delivering behaviour change interventions: Development of a mode of delivery ontology. *Wellcome Open Research, 5*, 125.

Mazeas, A., Duclos, M., Pereira, B., & Chalabaev, A. (2022). Evaluating the effectiveness of gamification on physical activity: systematic review and meta-analysis of randomized controlled trials. *Journal of Medical Internet Research, 24*, e26779.

McDermott, M.S., Oliver, M., Iverson, D., & Sharma, R. (2016). Effective techniques for changing physical activity and healthy eating intentions and behaviour: A systematic review and meta-analysis. *British Journal of Health Psychology, 21*, 827–841.

McWilliams, L., Bellhouse, S., Yorke, J., Lloyd, K., & Armitage, C.J. (2019). Beyond "planning": A meta-analysis of implementation intentions to support smoking cessation. *Health Psychology, 38*, 1059–1068.

Michalopoulou, M., Ferrey, A.E., Harmer, G. et al. (2022). Effectiveness of motivational interviewing in managing overweight and obesity: a systematic review and meta-analysis. *Annals of Internal Medicine, 175*, 838–850.

Michie, S., Abraham, C., Whittington, C., McAteer, J., & Gupta, S. (2009). Effective techniques in healthy eating and physical activity interventions: A meta-regression. *Health Psychology, 28*, 690–701.

Michie, S., Ashford, S., Sniehotta, F.F. et al. (2011). A refined taxonomy of behaviour change techniques to help people change their physical activity and healthy eating behaviours: The CALO-RE taxonomy. *Psychology & Health, 26*, 1479–1498.

Michie, S., Churchill, S., & West, R. (2011a). Identifying evidence-based competences required to deliver behavioural support for smoking cessation. *Annals of Behavioral Medicine, 41*, 59–70.

Michie, S., Hyder, N., Walia, A., & West, R. (2011b). Development of a taxonomy of behaviour change techniques used in individual behavioural support for smoking cessation. *Addictive Behaviors, 36*, 315–319.

Michie, S., Richardson, M., Johnston, M. et al. (2013). The behavior change technique taxonomy (v1) of 93 hierarchically clustered techniques: Building an international consensus for the reporting of behavior change interventions. *Annals of Behavioral Medicine, 46*, 81–95.

Michie, S., Whittington, C., Hamoudi, Z. et al. (2012). Identification of behaviour change techniques to reduce excessive alcohol consumption. *Addiction, 107*, 1431–1440.

Miller, W. R. & Rollnick, S. (2002). *Motivational Interviewing: Preparing People for Change*, 2nd ed. Guilford Press.

Miller, W.R. & Rollnick, S. (2013). *Motivational Interviewing: Helping People Change*, 3rd ed. Guilford Press.

Miller, W.R., & Sanchez, V. C. (1993). Motivating young adults for treatment and lifestyle change, in: Howard, G. (Ed.) *Issues in Alcohol Use and Misuse by Young Adults*. Notre Dame, IN: University of Notre Dame Press.

Milne, S.E., Orbell, S., & Sheeran, P. (2002). Combining motivational and volitional interventions to promote exercise participation: Protection motivation theory and implementation intentions. *British Journal of Health Psychology*, 7, 163–184.

Morton, K., Beauchamp, M., Prothero, A. et al. (2015). The effectiveness of motivational interviewing for health behaviour change in primary care settings: a systematic review. *Health Psychology Review*, 9, 205–223.

Murphy, L.R. (1996). Stress management in work settings: A critical review of health effects. *American Journal of Health Promotion*, 11, 112–135.

Murphy, S.M., Edwards, R.T., Williams, N. et al. (2012). An evaluation of the effectiveness and cost effectiveness of the National Exercise Referral Scheme in Wales, UK: a randomised controlled trial of a public health policy initiative. *Journal of Epidemiology and Community Health*, 66, 745–753.

Näslund, U., Ng, N., Lundgren, A. et al. (2019). Visualization of asymptomatic atherosclerotic disease for optimum cardiovascular prevention (VIPVIZA): a pragmatic, open-label, randomised controlled trial. *Lancet*, 393, 133–142.

Noar, S.M., Benac, C.N., & Harris, M.S. (2007). Does tailoring matter? Meta-analytic review of tailored print health behaviour change interventions. *Psychological Bulletin*, 133, 673–693.

Notley, C., Gentry, S., Livingstone-Banks, J. et al. (2019). Incentives for smoking cessation. *Cochrane Database of Systematic Reviews*, 7, CD004307.

O'Donnell, A., Wallace, P., & Kaner, E. (2014). From efficacy to effectiveness and beyond: What next for brief interventions in primary care? *Frontiers in Psychiatry*, 5, 113.

Ogden, J. (2016). Celebrating variability and a call to limit systematisation: the example of the Behaviour Change Technique Taxonomy and the Behaviour Change Wheel. *Health Psychology Review*, 10, 245–250.

Olander, E., Fletcher, H., Williams, S. et al. (2013). What are the most effective techniques in changing obese individuals' physical activity self-efficacy and behaviour: A systematic review and meta-analysis. *International Journal of Behavioral Nutrition and Physical Activity*, 10, 29.

Pace, B.T., Dembe, A., Somer, C.S. et al. (2017). A multivariate meta-analysis of motivational interviewing process and outcome. *Psychology of Addictive Behaviors*, 31, 524–533.

Palacio, A., Garay, D., Langer, B. et al. (2016). Motivational interviewing improves medication adherence: a systematic review and meta-analysis. *Journal of General Internal Medicine*, 31, 929–940.

Patel, M.S., Benjamin, E.J., Volpp, K.G. et al. (2017). Effects of a game-based intervention designed to enhance social incentives to increase physical activity among families: The BE FIT randomized clinical trial. *JAMA Internal Medicine*, 177, 1586–1593.

Patterson, K., Davey, R., Keegan, R. et al. (2022). Behaviour change techniques in cardiovascular disease smartphone apps to improve physical activity and sedentary behaviour: Systematic review and meta-regression. *International Journal of Behavioral Nutrition and Physical Activity, 19*, 81.

Petty, R.E., & Cacioppo, J.T. (1986). The elaboration likelihood model of persuasion. *Advances in Experimental Social Psychology, 19*, 123–205.

Pilling, S., Strang, J., & Gerada, C. (2007). Psychosocial interventions and opioid detoxification for drug misuse: summary of NICE guidance. *British Medical Journal, 335*, 203–205.

Prestwich, A., Conner, M., Hurling, R., Ayres, K., & Morris, B. (2016). An experimental test of control theory-based interventions for physical activity. *British Journal of Health Psychology, 21*, 812–826.

Prestwich, A., & Kellar, I. (2014). How can implementation intentions as a behaviour change intervention be improved? *European Review of Applied Psychology, 64*, 35–41.

Prestwich, A., Kellar, I., Parker, R. et al. (2014). How can self-efficacy be increased? Meta-analysis of dietary interventions. *Health Psychology Review, 8*, 270–285.

Public Health England (2017). *Changing behaviour: Techniques for tier 2 adult weight management services.* London: Public Health England.

Robinson, L., Arden, M.A., Dawson, S. et al. (in press). A machine-learning assisted review of the use of habit formation in medication adherence interventions for long-term conditions. *Health Psychology Review.*

Robinson, T.M. (1999). Reducing children's television viewing to prevent obesity: A randomized controlled trial. *Journal of the American Medical Association, 282*, 1561–1567.

Sacks, F.M., Svetkey, L.P., Vollmer, W.M., et al., for the DASH-Sodium Collaborative Research Group (2001). A clinical trial of the effects on blood pressure of reduced dietary sodium and the DASH dietary pattern (the DASH-Sodium Trial). *New England Journal of Medicine, 344*, 3–10.

Samdal, G.B., Eide, G.E., Barth, T., Williams, G., & Meland, E. (2017). Effective behaviour change techniques for physical activity and healthy eating in overweight and obese adults; systematic review and meta-regression analyses. *International Journal of Behavioral Nutrition and Physical Activity, 14*, 42.

Slama, K., Redman, S., Perkins, J., Reid, A.L., & Sanson-Fisher, R.W. (1990). The effectiveness of two smoking cessation programmes for use in general practice: a randomised clinical trial. *BMJ, 300*, 1707–1709.

Spilsbury, S., Wilk, P., Taylor, C., Prapavessis, H., & Mitchell, M. (2022). Paying people to be healthy: Limited time offer. *Research Square*, https://www.research square.com/article/rs-1723426/v1. doi.org/10.21203/rs.3.rs-1723426/v1

Stead, L.F., Bergson, G., & Lancaster, T. (2008). Physician advice for smoking cessation. *Cochrane Database of Systematic Reviews*, Issue 2. Art. No.: CD000165.

Tate, D.F., Lytle, L.A., Sherwood, N.E. et al. (2016). Deconstructing interventions : approaches to studying behavior change techniques across obesity interventions. *Translational Behavioral Medicine, 6*, 236–243.

Taylor, N., Conner, M., & Lawton, R. (2011). The impact of theory on the effectiveness of worksite physical activity interventions: a meta-analysis and meta-regression. *Health Psychology Review, 6*, 33–73.

Taylor, N.F., Harding, K.E., Dennett, A.M. et al. (2022). Behaviour change interventions to increase physical activity in hospitalised patients: a systematic review, meta-analysis and meta-regression. *Age and Ageing, 51*, afab154.

Teixeira, P.J., Marques, M.M., Silva, M.N., et al. (2020). A classification of motivation and behavior change techniques used in self-determination theory based
interventions in health contexts. *Motivation Science, 6*, 438–455.

The Trials of Hypertension Prevention Collaborative Research Group (1997).
Effects of weight loss and sodium reduction intervention on blood pressure and
hypertension incidence in overweight people with high normal blood pressure:
the trials of hypertension prevention, phase II. *Archives of Internal Medicine, 157*,
657–667.

Vargas-Garcia, E.J., Evans, C.E.L., Prestwich, A. et al. (2017). Interventions to
reduce consumption of sugar-sweetened beverages or increase water intake:
evidence from a systematic review and meta-analysis. *Obesity Reviews, 18*,
1350–1363.

Vasilaki, E.I., Hosier, S.G., & Cox, W.M. (2006). The efficacy of motivational
interviewing as a brief intervention for excessive drinking: A meta-analytic
review. *Alcohol & Alcoholism, 41*, 328–335.

Verplanken, B., & Orbell, S. (2022). Attitudes, habits, and behavior change. *Annual
Review of Psychology, 73*, 327–352.

Webb, T.L., Joseph, J., Yardley, L., & Michie, S. (2010). Using the internet to
promote health behavior change: A systematic review and meta-analysis of the
impact of theoretical basis, use of behavior change techniques, and mode of
delivery on efficacy. *Journal of Medical Internet Research, 12*(1), e4.

Webb, T.L., & Sheeran, P. (2007). How do implementation intentions promote goal
attainment? A test of component processes. *Journal of Experimental Social
Psychology, 43*, 295–302.

West, D.S., Krukowski, R.A., Monroe, C.M. et al. (2022). Randomized controlled
trial of financial incentives during weight-loss induction and maintenance in
online group weight control. *Obesity, 30*, 106–116.

West, R., Walia, A., Hyder, N., Shahab, L., & Michie, S. (2010). Behavior change
techniques used by the English Stop Smoking Services and their associations
with short-term quit outcomes. *Nicotine & Tobacco Research, 12*, 742–747.

Williams, S. & French, D. (2011). What are the most effective behaviour change
techniques for changing physical activity self-efficacy and physical activity
behaviour, and are they the same? *Health Education Research, 26*, 308–322.

Wilson, K., Senay, I., Durantini, M. et al. (2015). When it comes to lifestyle
recommendations, more is sometimes less: A meta-analysis of theoretical
assumptions underlying the effectiveness of interventions promoting multiple
behavior domain change. *Psychological Bulletin, 141*, 474–509.

Wood, C. E., Richardson, M., Johnston, M. et al. (2015). Applying the behaviour
change (BCT) taxonomy v1: a study of coder training. *Translational Behavioral
Medicine, 5*, 134–148.

Wood, W., & Neal, D.T. (2016). Healthy through habit: Interventions for initiating
and maintaining health behavior change. *Behavioral Science & Policy, 2*, 71–83.

4

CHAPTER 4
THEORY-BASED INTERVENTIONS

OVERVIEW

In the previous chapters you were introduced to a variety of **theories** and **behavior change techniques** that have been used to understand, predict and change behavior. In this chapter, we deal with more challenging issues: what are theory-based interventions and why is it useful for a health-related intervention to be theory-based? As this chapter extends what you have learned in the opening chapters, it is important that you read these first. The issues covered in Chapter 4 are challenging, but hopefully stimulating, and represent key obstacles for the progression of the science of health behavior change.

A great deal of research has been conducted to identify what factors (**determinants**) predict behavior and you would have come across many of these determinants (expressed as theoretical constructs) in Chapter 2. In the context of behavior change interventions, such determinants (e.g., motivation), when they are targeted by interventions (e.g., providing information on the health consequences of doing or not doing a behavior) to promote health behavior (e.g., taking medication), are sometimes referred to as **mechanisms of action**, or targets in the experimental medicine approach.

Various studies have highlighted the importance of a variety of determinants/constructs/mechanisms of action/targets (we will use these terms interchangeably) including attitudes (whether a person has a positive or negative evaluation of a particular object or behavior or thinks positive outcomes will follow from performing the behavior), self-efficacy (whether an individual feels they have the ability to

DOI: 10.4324/9781003302414-5

perform a particular behavior or are confident they can perform it), threat appraisal (which comprises an individual considering both the likelihood and the severity of the negative consequences (e.g., illness) associated with doing or not doing certain behaviors), intentions (one's willingness to try to perform a particular behavior) and a whole host of other determinants that drive a wide variety of behaviors. By identifying the determinants of health behavior, individuals can then set about changing health behavior by selecting techniques that change the determinant in order to change behavior. This approach of identifying a mechanism, targeting it for change and measuring and assessing to what extent changes in the mechanism account for changes in behavior is in keeping with the science of behavior change/experimental medicine approach that we cover later in this chapter and also in Chapter 7. By assessing not only changes in behavior but also potential changes in determinants, we open the "black box" to help us to figure out why an intervention was effective or not effective. This chapter will also reflect on what constitutes a **theory-based intervention** and highlight the potential benefits, and problems, associated with designing and evaluating a theory-based intervention. We then consider how to develop theory-based interventions using different approaches including the experimental medicine approach, a four-step approach and intervention mapping.

WHAT IS A THEORY-BASED INTERVENTION?

Behavioral scientists within the field of health behavior change research often refer to their interventions as "theory-based." What does this actually mean? In practice, its meaning can vary, and vary a lot! Without wanting to become overly philosophical about theory and theory-based interventions, one could argue that waking up one day and having the thought that an intervention could work because it may change a particular determinant of behavior could constitute a **theory**, regardless of whether this lies or does not lie within an established theory like those covered in Chapter 2. This could simply represent an idea based on common sense. This idea regarding how an intervention might work could, like magic, turn your everyday intervention into a "theory-based" intervention. Sounds seductive, doesn't it? When those interested in changing health behavior design interventions and call them "theory-based," it is likely that they do not have this vision of a theory-based intervention in mind. Instead, theory-based interventions are likely to range from an author loosely referring to their intervention in the context of a particular theory within the introduction of a journal article to using theory systematically at the various steps of the research process.

THE THEORY CODING SCHEME (MICHIE & PRESTWICH, 2010)

To measure the extent to which theory is used to develop and test a behavior change intervention, Michie and Prestwich (2010) developed the **Theory Coding Scheme**. The Theory Coding Scheme comprises 19 items. These items cover whether theory is mentioned; whether the constructs within a particular theory were targeted for change by specific behavior change techniques; whether theory is used to select participants (e.g., only targeting individuals that lack motivation, or hold weak intentions, to stop drunk driving) or tailor interventions to the needs of particular interventions (e.g., delivering different behavior change techniques to those who are not motivated to change their behavior but have the skills to do so and those who are motivated to change their behavior but lack the skills to do so); whether the theory underlying the intervention is tested by a) measuring the appropriate theoretical constructs before and/or after the delivery of the intervention, b) whether changes in the theoretical constructs explain the effectiveness of the intervention on behavior change (see Mediation Analysis, Chapter 6); and finally whether theory is refined on the basis of the results of the study in which the intervention was tested.

The Theory Coding Scheme has a number of potential benefits and applications. First, within **systematic reviews** and **meta-analyses** (see Chapters 5 and 6) it can be used to rigorously and systematically examine the use of theory within intervention research. Such reviews in the past have tended to rely on very basic examination of theory (e.g., Albarracin et al., 2005; Baban & Craciun, 2007; Trifiletti et al., 2005; Webb & Sheeran, 2006) such as comparing those studies which explicitly state that the interventions described are based on theory against those that are not. As stated above, this is problematic as there is great variation in what researchers have termed theory-based interventions. Moreover, the attempts to compare theory-based behavior change interventions against more **atheoretical interventions** have consistently failed to consider exactly how theory has informed the intervention. The Theory Coding Scheme provides a means to test, in a much more rigorous fashion, whether the use of theory can enhance the effects of interventions and *how* these benefits can be accrued. Second, the scheme might influence the design of theory-based interventions by encouraging researchers to systematically consider and examine what constitutes a theory-based intervention and the role of theory in informing and evaluating such interventions. Third, it might encourage a more systematic approach to describe interventions, and the role that theory has played, within journal articles by providing a framework upon which to do so.

Regarding the first point, certainly, systematic reviewers have used the Theory Coding Scheme to describe and evaluate the role of theory in their reviews. Typically, this has been done in three forms either using all 19 items separately (e.g., Meade et al., 2019) or clustering these 19 items into groups (e.g., Arnott et al., 2014) or doing both (e.g., Sediva et al., 2022). Regarding the second point, researchers have described using the coding scheme to guide their intervention design (e.g., Kavussanu et al., 2022) or to evaluate their own intervention (e.g., Gomis-Pastor et al., 2020). Regarding the third point, however, a formal test is needed to show that the coding scheme has led to better reporting.

THE LITMUS TEST OF THEORY (NIGG & PAXTON, 2008)

Alternatives to the Theory Coding Scheme exist. For example, Nigg and Paxton's (2008) Litmus Test of Theory incorporates eight items relating to theory use. There is a reasonably large overlap between the Litmus Test and the Theory Coding Scheme. For instance, both consider whether a theory has been mentioned, the relationship between behavior change techniques and theoretical constructs, and the measurement and change in theoretical mediators following intervention. The key differences are that the Litmus Test, but not the Theory Coding Scheme, considers whether the theory has been described by the authors, the fidelity of the intervention and whether the target of the theory-based intervention is consistent with the measure used to assess the intervention. In relation to the latter, an example in which there is inconsistency is when an intervention targets a specific type of physical activity (e.g., walking) but the measure relates to overall physical activity. On the other hand, the Theory Coding Scheme considers the relationship between behavior change techniques and theoretical constructs in more detail (i.e., using five items), as well as considering other factors not present in the Litmus Test such as how theory has been used to tailor interventions, the implications of the results for theory, whether the intervention is based on a single or multiple theories and the reliability and validity of the measures. In addition, the process of developing the Theory Coding Scheme has been made clear along with its ability to be used reliably across multiple coders.

CRITICAL SKILLS TOOLKIT 4.1

"THEORY-BASED" INTERVENTIONS

In health behavior change research, those who design an intervention might describe their intervention as theory-based. By using the term "theory-based intervention," their intervention is open to a number of potential criticisms as the term "theory-based intervention" can take on multiple different meanings and interpretations:

IS THE INTERVENTION BASED ON ONE THEORY OR A COMBINATION OF THEORIES?

Often an intervention might be based on elements of different theories. As such, basing an intervention on multiple theories means that the theories have been combined and synthesized into a new untested theory. Being untested, and by combining elements of different theories together in a non-systematic, evidence-based way could in effect make their intervention atheoretical (i.e. not theoretical). In Figure 4.1, the underlying constructs specified within the Theory of Planned Behavior (TPB) are targeted by an intervention (comprising three behavior change techniques: BCT1, BCT2, BCT3) but an additional construct (threat) is also targeted. Given this combination of constructs, the rationale would need to be clear (and convincing) why threat was also targeted alongside the constructs within the TPB. That's not to say an appropriate rationale cannot be built. For example, the theories may be complementary, as they cover generally different constructs or a theory helps address limits in

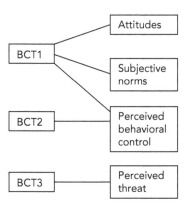

FIGURE 4.1 A diagrammatic representation of an intervention comprising three behavior change techniques (BCT1, BCT2, BCT3) targeting the Theory of Planned Behavior constructs *plus* perceived threat.

another theory (such as the intention-behavior gap); or previous research may have been conducted already suggesting combining particular theories could be beneficial.

ARE ALL CONSTRUCTS SPECIFIED WITHIN A THEORY (EXCLUDING BEHAVIOR) TARGETED BY THE INTERVENTION?

If only some elements are targeted then is the intervention faithful to the theory? Maybe not. If only particular constructs were targeted, do the authors provide a clear rationale why they have targeted these constructs rather than others? Figure 4.2 provides a diagrammatic representation of some, but not all, underlying constructs from the Theory of Planned Behavior being targeted by two behavior change techniques (BCT1, BCT2).

IN ANY INTERVENTION, IT SHOULD BE CLEAR WHY EACH BEHAVIOR CHANGE TECHNIQUE HAS BEEN INCORPORATED WITHIN AN INTERVENTION

In a *theory-based* intervention, it should be clear *which behavior change technique is targeting which specific construct.* Ideally, the authors should present evidence and a reasoned rationale why a specific technique should change a specific construct and how, in turn, changing this construct should change behavior. It is fairly common for an intervention to incorporate multiple behavior change techniques but it is not especially common for the inclusion of each behavior change technique to be clearly justified and linked to a specific theoretical construct (see Prestwich et al., 2014b). Figure 4.3a provides a diagrammatic representation where all three behavior change techniques (BCT1, BCT2, BCT3) used within an intervention are linked to two constructs within a theory (C1, C2). Figure 4.3b

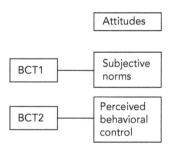

FIGURE 4.2 A diagrammatic representation of an intervention comprising two behavior change techniques (BCT1, BCT2) targeting only two of the Theory of Planned Behavior constructs.

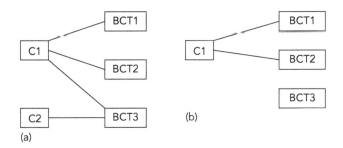

FIGURE 4.3 *a*: A diagrammatic representation where all behavior change techniques (BCT1 BCT2, BCT3) are linked to at least one construct (C1 and/or C2). *b*: A diagrammatic representation where some, but not all, of the behavior change techniques (BCT1, BCT2, but not BCT3) are linked to at least one construct (C1).

provides a diagrammatic representation where only two of the behavior change techniques (BCT1, BCT2 but not BCT3) are linked to a construct within a theory.

IDENTIFYING WHY AN INTERVENTION IS EFFECTIVE OR INEFFECTIVE

The authors might describe their intervention as theory-based but not test its theoretical basis. The theory-based intervention could be appropriately tested by measuring participants' levels on each construct after (and, if they choose, before) the intervention and testing statistically whether these changes mediate (i.e., explain) the effect of the intervention on behavior change (see Mediation analysis, Chapter 6). Sometimes authors do take steps to measure theoretical constructs within their study or randomized controlled trial. However, even when they do this and present evidence that their intervention changes behavior and changes at least one theoretical construct, they might fail to test whether changes in the theoretical construct explain the effect of the intervention on behavior (i.e., conduct mediation analysis). As such, it is not clear why their intervention was effective in changing behavior and it does not provide sufficient evidence to validate and support the theory upon which the intervention was based.

FOR BEHAVIOR CHANGE, DOES THEORY ACTUALLY MATTER?

Many scientists like to label themselves as either "theoretical" or "applied" in perspective. Theoretical scientists develop theories and may look to test them. Applied scientists are more focused on solving problems. However, the two perspectives go hand-in-hand. Applied scientists can use theory to guide and develop their behavior change interventions. In turn, the **outcomes** from theory-based interventions can inform the refinement of current theories and inspire the generation of "better" theories that are more effective in real-life settings. The benefits of using theory to develop and test health behavior interventions are:

i. *Identify key constructs (determinants) to target*
   If there is evidence that a construct (e.g., attitudes; threat; self-efficacy) is associated with (or, even better, *causes*) health behavior, changing these constructs should change health behavior. However, if a particular theory or **model** specifies a number of constructs, which construct is the most important to target? Constructs might be selected by considering the following factors (see also Burning Issue Box 4.1 and Critical Skills Toolkit 4.1 and Critical Skills Toolkit 4.2):
   a) Whether your sample scores high or low on a particular theoretical construct.
   b) The amount of variance in health behavior that is explained by the construct (see Chapter 2, Critical Skills Toolkit 2.1) or, put more simply, the extent to which health behavior is associated with a determinant (see Critical Skills Toolkit 4.1) ideally after ruling out or adjusting for confounders that can co-occur with your variables of interest. In the absence of a measure of health behavior, researchers could focus on targeting constructs which are strongly related to (explain a lot of variance in) behavior such as behavioral intentions.
   c) The variability in the measure assessing a particular construct (see Critical Skills Toolkit 4.2).
   d) The targeted construct must be amenable to sufficient change; if a construct is difficult to change, it might not be a good target for intervention.

ii. *Help to select appropriate intervention techniques*
   Theory can be used as a guide to select the most appropriate combination of behavior change techniques to incorporate within a behavior change intervention (see Step 2 of the "Four-Step Cycle of Theory Based Behavior Change" outlined later in this chapter).

BURNING ISSUE BOX 4.1

IF YOU HAD TO CHOOSE, HOW WOULD YOU DECIDE WHICH THEORETICAL DETERMINANT TO TARGET IN YOUR INTERVENTION?

You're tasked with changing the eating patterns of a group of over-weight people. You may decide to target the theoretical construct which has the highest correlation with unhealthy eating patterns. However, assume for a minute that the theoretical construct that correlates most strongly with unhealthy eating patterns is attitudes towards dieting and that most, or all, of your target sample already have positive attitudes towards dieting. In this sense, there might be better determinants to tackle.

If you are using the Theory of Planned Behavior (see Chapter 2) as a basis for your intervention then the other candidates for behavior change would be to alter subjective norms and/or perceived behavioral control (PBC). Of these constructs, subjective norms might already be positive, many people within the target group might already perceive their friends, family and/or important others to want them to diet. This leaves PBC, the degree to which an individual feels they have the skills to diet. In a sample of overweight people, PBC might be low and thus targeted for intervention.

One further consideration to keep in mind is whether the theoretical construct can be changed and changed enough to lead to behavior change. If a construct is difficult to change, at least sufficiently to change behavior, other constructs may need to be targeted.

CRITICAL SKILLS TOOLKIT 4.2

LACK OF VARIABILITY AND ITS IMPACT ON CORRELATION. SHOULD YOU TARGET ONLY THE CONSTRUCTS THAT EXPLAIN SIGNIFICANT PORTIONS OF VARIANCE IN BEHAVIOR (OR MORE PROXIMAL DETERMINANTS)?

Imagine you've run a pilot study where you've measured Theory of Planned Behavior (TPB) constructs (attitudes, subjective norms, PBC, intentions and behavior) in a sample of students. The study attempts to identify the constructs that most strongly relate to/predict the number of days per week that students exercise for 30 minutes.

After measuring these constructs, you've assessed the correlations (relationships) between them (for more information on correlations, see Chapter 6). The average level of each construct (mean), the spread/variability of the scores in your sample (standard deviation, SD) and the intercorrelations between the variables are presented below.

TABLE 4.1 Descriptives and intercorrelations between variables from a fictitious study

	Scale	Mean	SD Attitude	SN	PBC	Intention	Exercise
Attitudes	1–7	2.25	0.25	.08	.02	.05	-.02
SN	1–7	4.50	1.30	–	.11	.12	.09
PBC	1–7	3.25	1.25		–	.42	.33
Intention	1–7	4.45	1.23			–	.35
Exercise	0–7	1.50	1.50				–

All of the mean scores are comfortably below their maximum possible score (7) and thus there is room for an intervention to try to increase the levels of any of the constructs. On this basis, all of the constructs (attitudes, SN, PBC) could be targeted for intervention as a means to make students' intentions to exercise more positive (and, in turn, to increase their exercise participation). So what else could we use to determine what construct to target with our intervention?

We can look at the size of the correlations between the variables to identify which variables most strongly relate to intentions and/or behavior. In this example, PBC looks like the best candidate as it more strongly correlates with intention ($r = .42$) and exercise behavior ($r = .33$) than the other candidates (SN and Attitudes). As it is the most strongly related, changing PBC (rather than attitudes or SN) should lead to the biggest/most reliable changes in intentions and ultimately behavior. However, this isn't the full story...

Look at the standard deviation of scores for attitudes, it is very low. This means that nearly all of your participants have the same level of attitudes towards exercising. When a construct (in this case, attitudes) has very little variability then it is almost impossible that it will correlate with anything (and looking at the correlations between attitudes and the other variables, the correlations are near zero reflecting very weak relationships). This weak correlation might arise from poor reliability and/or validity of your attitude measure (see Chapter 5). In this instance, attitudes might still be an important determinant of intentions and behavior. Targeting attitudes in an attempt to make them more positive towards exercising might still be an effective method to change behavior.

Looking at subjective norms (SN), although its mean score is rather low (suggesting that there is room for an intervention to make subjective norms more positive), it does not correlate highly with intentions or behavior nor is it hindered by low levels of variability. As such, there would be less benefit in your intervention targeting subjective norms compared to the other constructs. On the basis of the Theory of Planned Behavior (which informs your initial list of candidate target constructs – attitudes, subjective norms, PBC) and the data above, your intervention should target PBC. You should also consider trying to change attitudes.

iii.   *It can be used to refine or tailor intervention techniques and theories.*
   a) Attitudes and perceived behavioral control (PBC), according to certain theories, are two key determinants of behaviors such as exercising. Take Barry and Jeremy, two individuals who have difficulty in exercising frequently. On the basis of the theories highlighting the importance of attitudes and PBC, Barry and Jeremy should complete measures of attitudes and PBC. After completing such measures, it turns out Barry has a positive attitude towards exercising but low PBC and Jeremy who has a negative attitude towards exercising but high PBC. On this basis, Barry should be exposed to an intervention designed to enhance PBC and Jeremy should receive an intervention to make his/her attitudes towards exercising more positive. This example illustrates how theory can be used to tailor interventions to the specific needs of the individual.
   b) By designing and implementing studies that have a theoretical framework, then we can continuously test the theory and identify in which contexts and for which populations and behaviors it is most effective. This can lead to the refinement of theory and helps to build up the generalizability of the theory (by identifying various situations that the theory can be usefully applied; see Step 4 of the "Four-Step Cycle of Theory Based Behavior Change" outlined later).

iv.   *Inform interventions that more effectively change health behavior.*
   There is some evidence that basing an intervention on theory can lead to larger effects on behavior. For example, in a meta-analysis, Albarracin et al. (2005) indicated that studies that reported using theory as a basis for their intervention yielded stronger changes in

HIV-related behaviors than studies that did not do this. However, there are other reviews out there and they do not necessarily show such a clear picture. We consider whether using theory to help develop an intervention really does lead to big changes in health behavior in Burning Issue Box 4.2.

BURNING ISSUE BOX 4.2

DOES BASING AN INTERVENTION ON A THEORY INCREASE HEALTH BEHAVIOR CHANGE?

Theory is good because it helps us to change health behavior better, for longer. This mantra is likely held by the majority of researchers interested in changing (health) behavior. It sounds appealing, not least because this line of thought serves to validate the usefulness of a theory. But is it accurate?

The answer is, probably not. Across 13 different reviews, Prestwich et al. (2015) reported that only three reviews support that theories increase intervention effects on health behaviors or health-related outcomes, seven provided mixed evidence and a further three (cue horrified face) implied that theory-based interventions actually produced smaller changes in health behavior compared to those not based on theory. Dalgetty et al. (2019) in a systematic review of systematic reviews reported likewise with eight out of nine reviews suggesting that using theory did not increase the effectiveness of health behavior interventions.

However, there are various things to keep in mind:

1. *Well, what is being compared?* On the one side, "theory-based" interventions can vary a lot, see the definition at the start of this chapter. At the other side, where studies compare an intervention not based on theory against a comparison condition, even these studies probably draw on the same knowledge and ideas articulated in theories either through (i) common sense, (ii) by drawing on theory without knowledge of the theory and/or (iii) not referencing the theory in the study report/article. In short, the picture is messy; there is variation in theory-based interventions, variation in interventions that are "not theory-based" and there is variation in how this information is reported in articles and subsequently synthesized in the form of a review.

2. *Pick a side.* Most reviews compare studies that have tested "theory-based" interventions against studies that have tested interventions that do not use theory. This splitting of studies into one of two camps creates a comparison that is rather blunt. An alternative question is "Do studies that use theory more generate larger intervention effects than those that use it less?" A further question is "Does using theory in a particular way lead to larger effects?" For instance, do interventions that use theory to tailor or customize an intervention to different groups of people lead to stronger effects than studies that do not use theory to tailor their intervention? Do studies that use theory to select each of their behavior change techniques produce larger changes in health behavior than studies that do not do this? These alternative questions have been considered less and may paint a different picture than the "theory does not help" view.

3. *Interventions based on some theories may be better than others.* Some reviews considering the impact of theory on health behavior intervention effectiveness have presented evidence that may imply some theories may be used to develop interventions that achieve larger changes in health-related behaviors and outcomes than other theories. For instance, Dombrowski et al. (2012) and Michie et al. (2009) present evidence alluding to the potential benefits of Control Theory, while Samdal et al. (2017) suggest interventions based on theories like Self-Determination Theory yield more positive changes in health behaviors in the long-term compared to other types of theories. Interventions based on single rather than multiple theories may yield larger effects (e.g., Prestwich et al., 2014) although specific combinations of theories could be particularly effective, more evidence is needed though to support these assertions more strongly.

4. *It is probably not a fair fight.* Authors who take the time and effort to develop a truly theory-based intervention are also those who probably employ more rigorous methods in their evaluation. Employing more rigorous research methods tends to reduce the size of study effects. As a result, there is likely to be an important confound between the studies that test theory-based interventions and those that test other interventions. This confound (study quality) makes it harder for studies testing theory-based interventions to achieve large effects on health behaviors.

So, all in all, the evidence is mixed regarding whether using theory to develop health behavior interventions leads to stronger changes in behavior. Over time, as more interventions fully based on specific theories are tested, a clearer picture will hopefully emerge to identify the best theories upon which to base interventions, or perhaps even find out which theories work best in which contexts (for which groups of people, settings, behaviors, etc.). When the picture becomes clearer, more and more interventions will likely be developed based on these "better" theories meaning that, in the future, interventions based on theory may be more effective than interventions not based on theory. That's the optimistic, long-term view, anyway.

v.   *Using theory in designing interventions can indicate why an intervention was effective, or ineffective, in changing behavior.*
      By measuring key determinants (constructs) in your participants after they have been exposed to an intervention one can gain an understanding of why an intervention was effective (or ineffective) in changing behavior. By taking this approach, the following outcomes are possible.

      a)   *Successfully change theoretical constructs and behavior.*
           Here, there is a possibility that you can identify why your intervention was effective. Essentially if your intervention changes a determinant (e.g., attitudes) and behavior (e.g., exercise) then you could potentially conclude that your intervention successfully changed exercise by changing attitudes. This conclusion would be stronger on the basis of process evaluations and mediation analysis (see Chapter 6).
      b)   *Does not change theoretical construct but does change behavior.*
           If this outcome is achieved then one might gain an understanding of how the intervention was effective by ruling out (or minimizing) the role of the theoretical constructs not affected by the intervention.
      c)   *Successfully change theoretical constructs but behavior does not change.*
           In this instance either: a) the change in the theoretical constructs was not sufficient to change behavior (e.g., your intervention might have made your sample's attitudes towards exercising more positive, but not positive enough, to promote exercise; or you might have changed attitudes but not other determinants that are necessary to change behavior), or b) the theoretical determinant/construct does not cause behavior. In the latter case, the theory might be refined by removing this "determinant" from the theory. This illustrates an additional benefit of using theory to inform behavior change interventions, using *theory-based intervention can be used to refine and improve theories.* Theory-based

interventions are only as good as the theories upon which the intervention is based. If an intervention is based on a theory which identifies inappropriate determinants then the intervention is unlikely to change behavior and the theory needs to be improved. In this way, there is a "synergistic cycle" where theory informs intervention development and evaluation and this evaluation informs (refines or supports) the theory upon which the intervention was based.

d) *Does not change the theoretical construct and does not change behavior.* Here, the theory might be appropriate but the intervention technique was inappropriate (as it didn't change a key behavioral determinant or behavior). One might conclude here that the intervention was ineffective because it did not change the underlying behavioral determinant (although this is not fully testable, if the intervention had changed the behavioral determinant in question then it might not necessarily have changed behavior).

DEVELOPING & TESTING THEORY-BASED INTERVENTIONS 1: THEORY CODING SCHEME

As noted above, the Theory Coding Scheme can be used to influence the design and testing of theory-based interventions. In particular, it can encourage researchers to systematically target and measure all components of a theory, provide a rationale for each behavior change technique by explicitly linking each to a theory-relevant determinant, caution against combining theories, recruit appropriate participants, consider tailoring and assess/test mechanisms and, on the basis of the results, identify/act on implications for the underlying theory.

DEVELOPING & TESTING THEORY-BASED INTERVENTIONS 2: SCIENCE OF BEHAVIOR CHANGE AND THE EXPERIMENTAL MEDICINE APPROACH

The Science of Behavior Change is an initiative involving a working group of researchers who advocate an experimental approach to identify which interventions and techniques work and which do not in order to change behavior. The focus is very much on understanding what mechanisms change as a result of exposure to a particular intervention and whether changes in these mechanisms cause changes in behavior. They argue it is not enough to identify whether or not something works; it's important also to understand how or why an intervention may work or may not work or even work for some people, or in some contexts, but not others.

It involves three steps: Identify, Measure, Influence. The idea is that if you can identify a potentially modifiable target that relates to behavior, measure it reliably (creating what they call "assays") checking when and how much it relates to behavior, and then influence the target (change it in a meaningful and measurable way), then you can positively influence the associated behaviors. For example, if worry is a key determinant of sleep (Clancy et al., 2020) then creating and detecting reductions in worry (e.g., through mindfulness) should lead to improved sleep. Fuller descriptions of the Experimental Medicine Approach to behavior change (e.g., Riddle, Science of Behavior Change Working Group, 2015), in addition to noting the need to (1) identify a target, (2) measure and (3) influence a target, highlighted a fourth element which is to test the extent to which changing the determinant leads to behavior change.

The determinants the Science of Behavior Change team focus on are grouped into three broad classes: (1) self-regulation (e.g., temporal discounting, the extent to which immediate smaller rewards are favored over later larger rewards), (2) stress resilience and stress reactivity (e.g., heart rate in response to a stressor), (3) interpersonal and social processes (e.g., emotional responses such as anger following interactions with a partner). The Science of Behavior Change website (https://scienceofbehaviorchange.org/) overviews a range of projects that adopt this approach to change behavior as well as a range of measures that can be used to assess the key determinant or mechanism.

DEVELOPING & TESTING THEORY-BASED INTERVENTIONS 3: FOUR-STEP CYCLE

In the first edition of the textbook, we presented a slightly different approach to the science of behavior change approach noted above. This alternative approach involving a four-step cycle is overviewed again here. After identifying the health behavior to change, changing behavior essentially incorporates (up to) four steps (see Figure 4.4). Step 1 involves using the best theories to identify the most likely determinants of behavior from the relevant **theory-relevant constructs**. Step 2 then requires the identification of behavior change techniques that are most likely to change the key determinants of behavior and consequently the behavior of interest. Much behavior change work have incorporated Step 2, focusing on what works, neglecting Step 1. Step 3 requires the adoption of the stringent methods and statistics that we overview in Chapters 5 and 6 to evaluate the effect of the intervention. These include the use of reliable and valid measures of behavior as well as any proposed mechanisms of action plus statistical consideration of the role of changing the mechanism of action on changing behavior. The final step is to use the evaluation to refine the intervention and/or underlying theory. Given the results of the study should be used to refine the underlying theory, the process should be seen as a cycle that continually refines and improves the underlying theory in order to develop better theories that lead to the development of more effective behavior change interventions.

Many individuals and organizations interested in health behavior change such as the UK National Health Service (NHS) or multinational businesses, might argue that Step 1 is unnecessary and that Step 2 simply involves the

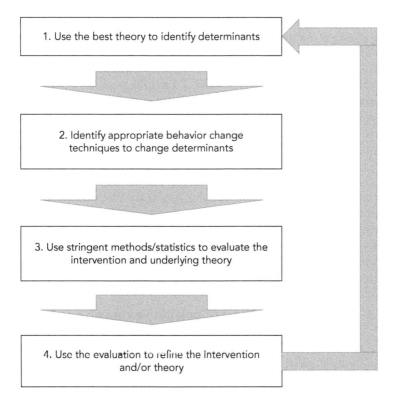

FIGURE 4.4 Basic four-step cycle to theory-based behavior change.

identification of a technique that changes health behavior directly (without changing, necessarily, the determinants specified within any particular theory). They might view the ultimate aim as changing health behavior (e.g., increasing attendance for cervical cancer screenings; increasing physical activity; reducing alcohol intake, etc.) and as long as a particular strategy changes behavior (more women attend cervical cancer screenings; more people increase their physical activity levels and people drink less alcohol), then they are happy (particularly if they meet their targets). However, omitting Step 1 and passing quickly over Step 2 eliminates the role of theory and the potential benefits that it might bring in terms of providing a structured approach to accumulating evidence and potentially selecting the most appropriate approach to behavior change. Not considering how or why a behavior change technique may or may not change behavior in Step 3 would also be a key omission. We now consider the "four steps" in more detail.

STEP 1: USE THE BEST THEORIES TO IDENTIFY DETERMINANTS TO TARGET

At the very least, there should be some evidence to support the theory; this could be correlational evidence showing that determinants within the theory correlate with behavior. Preferably, however, there would be experimental evidence that changes in theoretical determinants cause changes in behavior. Ideally, there will be lots of studies providing consistent experimental evidence demonstrating that the theory is supported and outperforms other theories that could be used as a starting point to develop your intervention. A rigorous systematic review and meta-analysis (an approach that statistically combines the findings from lots of relevant studies, see Chapters 5 and 6) supporting a particular theory would be useful at this first step, should such a review exist.

Over time, it will become clearer which theories are the best theories upon which to base your intervention (see Burning Issues Box 4.4 for more detailed consideration of this issue). Once you've identified an appropriate theory upon which to develop and evaluate your intervention, you can identify the theory-relevant constructs to target as the theory suggests that they determine behavior (see Burning Issues Box 4.1 for further information about which determinants/theory-relevant constructs to target).

STEP 2: IDENTIFY APPROPRIATE BEHAVIOR CHANGE TECHNIQUES TO CHANGE DETERMINANTS

By identifying theoretical constructs (determinants) to target, theory provides a means for selecting one behavior change technique over another.

According to Bandura (1977), for instance, self-efficacy (one's belief that they are capable of performing a particular task or behavior) can be promoted by persuasion, successfully performing the task/behavior yourself or seeing somebody else complete the task. However, most health/social cognition models, highlighted in Chapter 2, only specify which constructs predict behavior and do not specify which intervention techniques change these constructs.

A major development over the past few years has been the creation of a toolkit to help researchers identify the best behavior change techniques to change specific determinants. Part of the Human Behaviour Change Project, the Theory and Techniques Tool maps 74 behavior change techniques to 26 mechanisms of action. This interactive tool (available at: https://theoryandtechniquetool.humanbehaviourchange.org/), identifies whether there is evidence that a particular behavior change technique will likely change a particular mechanism of action, whether it won't change it, whether the evidence is inconclusive or whether there is no evidence for a link. According to this tool, for example, what you believe about your ability to perform a particular behavior (beliefs about capabilities) can be influenced by various techniques including providing instruction, problem solving, watching a demonstration of the behavior, practice or rehearsing the behavior, verbal persuasion, self-talk (telling yourself that you're able to perform a behavior), focusing on past successes or using graded tasks (breaking a task down into easier sub-tasks, accomplishing them, before moving onto increasingly difficult tasks).

The basis for deciding which mechanisms of action should be affected by which behavior change techniques within the interactive tool come from a series of studies. In these studies, the researchers either gathered information from text of published papers in which authors specify what they believe the links to be based on their understanding of the evidence (Carey et al., 2019) or an equivalent in which groups of experts try to agree, using consensus methods (see Chapter 5), which behavior change techniques they believe should change which determinants (Connell et al., 2019). The final decisions regarding whether or not any specific behavior change technique should change any specific determinant was achieved by a study that compared and contrasted the findings of these prior studies and attempted to resolve any disagreements or inconsistencies through another consensus study (Johnston et al., 2020).

There are alternative methods to choose behavior change techniques to tackle specific determinants, and we evaluate these different methods in Burning Issue Box 4.3.

BURNING ISSUE BOX 4.3

HOW DO YOU CHOOSE WHICH BEHAVIOR CHANGE TECHNIQUE(S) TO CHANGE WHICH DETERMINANTS?

Option 1: Use the Theory & Techniques Tool

As noted in the main text, the Theory and Techniques Tool is an interactive, online tool that can be used to identify recommendations regarding which behavior change techniques should be used to change which determinants.

Advantages

1. The easy to use tool provides a straightforward means to draw on expert opinion to inform your choice.
2. The matrix covers a much wider range of combinations of behavior change techniques and determinants than any other approach aside from your own or your research team's educated guesswork.

Disadvantages

1. As the tool is predicated on consensus methods and the opinions of authors, it is not particularly evidence-based as compared to forming decisions on the basis of experimental data.
2. For some combinations, opinions are not consistent.

Option 2: Draw on relevant reviews and meta-analyses

One possibility is to conduct or identify relevant reviews that have attempted to find which techniques are the most useful methods to change the determinant of interest (e.g., Prestwich et al., 2014a). Typically, these reviews involve collating evidence from studies that have tested the effectiveness of different interventions, comprising different behavior change techniques, in changing a specific behavior. To be included in these reviews, the researchers conducting each study will have needed to have also measured a specific determinant such as motivation after some participants have been exposed to an intervention and some participants have not (these individuals forming the control or comparison group). In each study, an effect size will be calculated reflecting the difference in the level of the determinant (e.g., motivation) in the intervention and comparison groups. For each behavior change technique, the average effect size of the studies that have tested a specific behavior change technique will be compared against the average effect size of the studies that have not tested the behavior change technique. If you compare the effect sizes of the studies that have tested the effect of interventions that comprise a specific behavior change technique, such as self-monitoring against the studies that have not tested self-monitoring, and the studies that have tested self-monitoring generate more favorable effect sizes, that would suggest self-monitoring is a useful strategy.

Advantages

1. Where these reviews have been conducted, they can save a lot of time and energy in identifying behavior change techniques that are potentially good candidates to change specific determinants.
2. They can provide information on a range of different behavior change techniques and their ability to change a specific determinant.
3. They generate outcomes and suggestions based on empirical data.

Disadvantages

1. Given the studies lumped together in the reviews will likely differ in many aspects (e.g., their interventions will likely involve different combinations of behavior change techniques; use different outcome measures, etc.), any "signal" implying a benefit of a specific behavior change technique is likely to be noisy. What this means is that the evidence provided from such reviews will be relatively weak. For that reason, these reviews may provide useful pointers regarding which techniques might change which deter-minants, but the answers provided from such reviews will not be definitive.
2. If reviews do not exist and new reviews need to be conducted, you're in trouble, as these reviews can require a lot of time and energy!

Option 3: Small-scale testing or use of adaptive designs

Small-scale tests such as pilot testing and N-of-1 trials (see Chapter 5 and Critical Skills Toolkit 5.8) can enable you to test whether a specific behavior change technique may be useful in changing specific determinants. Adaptive designs (see Chapter 10) enable you to change the design based on prior results with a view to identifying the best outcomes.

Advantages

1. Can be relatively quick to conduct.
2. A more evidence-based approach than some alternative approaches.
3. Can guide larger-scale testing and identify issues early prior to expensive, larger-scale trials.
4. In the context of behavior change techniques, adaptive designs can be used to consider not only whether a behavior change technique might change a particular determinant, but also how much of the technique is needed and/or whether its effects can be enhanced through combining it with other behavior change technique(s).
5. It can enable testing in samples that are representative of your target population. If you rely on previous studies, the findings from these prior studies may not replicate due to a variety of differences including the unique characteristics of your target population.

Disadvantages

1. It is difficult to consider the impact of more than a few behavior change techniques at one time.
2. Requires subsequent, more large-scale testing for more definitive answers.

Option 4: Intervention Mapping

You could apply the techniques theorized within Intervention Mapping (IM) to change specific determinants (see the supplementary materials provided by Kok et al., 2016).

Advantages

1. Like the Theory and Techniques Tool, Intervention Mapping (Kok et al., 2016) provides recommendations for a wide range of determinants and techniques.
2. Comprehensive approach to behavior change.

Disadvantages

1. The Intervention Mapping procedures, if followed in full, can require significant time and cost.
2. The evidence-base required for various linkages (e.g., determinants to techniques) could be lacking.
3. The process of linking determinants to techniques (e.g., by conducting systematic reviews) is often not clearly articulated. More generally, IM does not give detailed guidance regarding *how* to use theory to design interventions, nor how theory can be tested and improved through appropriate modifications (Michie, Sheeran & Rothman, 2007).
4. More broadly, the generation of determinants encourages the integration of various theories within a single intervention. By combining theories, does the intervention remain theory-based?

STEP 3: USE STRINGENT METHODS/STATISTICS TO EVALUATE THE INTERVENTION AND UNDERLYING THEORY

It is important to use an appropriate methodological and statistical approach to evaluate the effect of the intervention on the theoretical constructs and its subsequent impact on health behaviors. We consider appropriate methodological approaches throughout the book including, in particular, this chapter and Chapter 5. A useful statistical analysis, called mediation analysis (see Chapter 6), helps identify whether the changes in behavior can be attributed to changes in the theoretical constructs stipulated in the underlying theory used to inform the intervention. If the changes in behavior can be attributed to changes in the relevant theoretical constructs then there is evidence to support the theory.

STEP 4: USE THE EVALUATION TO REFINE THE INTERVENTION AND/OR THEORY

If the changes in behavior are not explained by changes in the relevant theoretical constructs that the theory stipulates (and assuming the study is sufficiently methodologically strong with a sufficient number of participants) then there is evidence to suggest that the theory is inadequate. While one may not want to change a theory on the basis of one null finding, over time, if such null results accumulate within several studies, then the theory should be refined in line with the evidence. Based on a review by Prestwich et al. (2014b) which explored how theory is used in relation to developing and evaluating physical activity and dietary interventions, there appears to be a real reluctance by authors to do this. In fact, on the basis of this review, fewer than 3% of experimental studies that test theory-based interventions involve the authors suggesting refinements to the theory through the addition or removal of new constructs to the theory or by identifying which relationships between theoretical constructs should be changed. Relatedly only 1 in 10 studies provided adequate support (or refutation) of a theory based on appropriate mediation analyses. These low rates of theory-based inferences and suggested refinements serve to slow down the progress of the science of behavior change as poor theories will continue to be used and newer, better theories will develop more slowly (see Prestwich et al., 2015).

DEVELOPING & TESTING THEORY-BASED INTERVENTIONS 4: INTERVENTION MAPPING

Intervention Mapping (IM) is a process, outlined by Bartholomew et al. (1998) and more recently by Kok et al. (2016), to design, develop and evaluate behavior change interventions. Central to the process is the need for the intervention to be theory-based and evidence-based. IM provides guidance regarding the steps that (IM recommends) should be taken when developing an intervention. In essence it takes a problem (e.g., obesity), identifies the key behaviors (e.g., diet, physical activity) that should be changed to address the problem, attempts to identify the factors that determine these key behaviors (e.g., high availability of energy dense foods; poor self-efficacy), the methods that change these determinants (e.g., changes to the environment; modelling) which are then tweaked so that they can be adopted by the users (the people delivering the intervention and the people that receive it) before the intervention is evaluated in the final step (see Figure 4.5).

The IM procedure is outlined below in more detail. Reference to Kwak et al.'s (2007) development of a worksite intervention to prevent weight gain using IM (The NHF-NRG In Balance-Project) is presented within brackets.

1. *Needs assessment.* The nature of the problem [weight gain], the underlying behaviors [reduction in routine, daily physical activities; eating larger portions of food and energy dense foods], the key associated environmental contexts in which the underlying behaviors take place [workplace] are each identified. The stage culminates in the

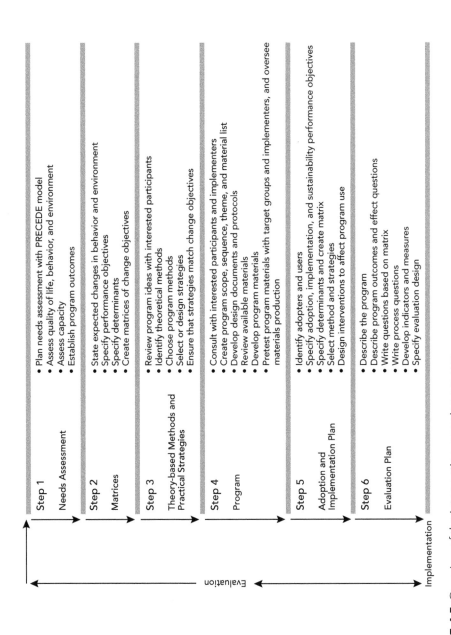

Step 1

Needs Assessment

- Plan needs assessment with PRECEDE model
- Assess quality of life, behavior, and environment
- Assess capacity
- Establish program outcomes

Step 2

Matrices

- State expected changes in behavior and environment
- Specify performance objectives
- Specify determinants
- Create matrices of change objectives

Step 3

Theory-based Methods and Practical Strategies

- Review program ideas with interested participants
- Identify theoretical methods
- Choose program methods
- Select or design strategies
- Ensure that strategies match change objectives

Step 4

Program

- Consult with interested participants and implementers
- Create program scope, sequence, theme, and material list
- Develop design documents and protocols
- Review available materials
- Develop program materials
- Pretest program materials with target groups and implementers, and oversee materials production

Step 5

Adoption and Implementation Plan

- Identify adopters and users
- Specify adoption, implementation, and sustainability performance objectives
- Specify determinants and create matrix
- Select method and strategies
- Design interventions to affect program use

Step 6

Evaluation Plan

- Describe the program
- Describe program outcomes and effect questions
- Write process questions
- Write questions based on matrix
- Develop indicators and measures
- Specify evaluation design

Evaluation

Implementation

FIGURE 4.5 Overview of the intervention mapping process.

Intervention Mapping. http://interventionmapping.com

specification of program objectives [decrease energy intake through diet and/or increase physical activity within 25–40 year olds in the workplace].

2. *Identify performance objectives, determinants and change objectives.* The program objectives identified in the first step are broken down into behaviors that can be targeted for change [increase walking/cycling as mode of transport; increase physical activity at work; decrease food portion sizes; replace high-fat foods with low fat foods; replace low fiber with high fiber foods; replace saturated fats with unsaturated fats]. These are then broken down into *performance objectives* which tends to involve writing down the step-by-step changes that you wish to make [e.g., for replacing low fiber with high fiber foods, the target population: a) need to know what fiber-rich foods are; b) self-assess their fiber-intake; c) have a negative attitude towards foods low in fiber; d) indicate the importance of consuming fiber-rich foods; e) choose to consume fiber rich foods; f) set achievable goals; g) form plans to reach these goals]. These changes can occur at multiple levels (e.g., changes to the individual or environment).

   The performance objectives are then linked to the *key determinants* [at the level of the individual knowledge; awareness; taste preference; attitude; self-efficacy; habit. At the level of the environment: availability; management commitment/support; social support; company policy; cost] often through focus groups and/or systematic literature reviews. A matrix of behavior change objectives is formed by mapping the *performance objectives* to *key determinants*, at various levels (individual, interpersonal, organizational, community, societal).

3. *Theory-based intervention methods and practical strategies.* The general techniques for changing determinants (theory-based methods) are identified (by reviewing empirical evidence and theories) [prompts; social support, etc.] and then translated into practical strategies that can be deployed within the population/environment in question [e.g., placing prompts at elevators = prompts; setting up lunchtime walking groups = support)].

4. *Producing and integrating the intervention program.* The practical strategies identified in Step 3 are then put together in a plan where the sequence of strategies and their scope are determined. The program materials are put together at this stage. It is often useful to check that the materials are pretested and one checks that the materials match the performance objectives [brainstorm with experts to identify useful materials that already exist; tweak existing materials, where necessary; develop new materials where needed].

5. *Adoption and implementation plan.* This step follows the procedures outlined in Step 2 but the end-point is the formation of a detailed plan regarding program adoption and implementation by influencing the

behavior of the people that will use the intervention. This stage needs to take account of the environment in which the intervention will be delivered (and those delivering it) and modified, where necessary, to ensure adoption. Pre-testing of the materials in the environment can be useful to identify, at an early stage, any potential problems regarding adoption and implementation.

6. *Evaluation.* This stage is useful to identify whether the assumed linkages (e.g., between key determinants and performance objectives) were supported. This stage should attempt to assess changes in quality of life and health, behaviors, performance objectives, change determinants and level of implementation. Of course in order to assess these factors, they need to be considered during the earlier stages of IM and reliable and valid measures should be used or developed.

BURNING ISSUE BOX 4.4

Q&A ON THEORY-BASED INTERVENTIONS

Question 1: Which theory should I base my intervention upon?

At the moment, it is unclear which theory is the most useful for basing interventions. It is likely that some theories might be more appropriate in different situations and for different behaviors. For instance, a key factor might be whether the intervention is concerned with the initiation of behavior change or with the maintenance of the behavior (for the former, many of the theories outlined in Chapter 2 would be helpful; for the latter, theories such as the Relapse Prevention Model, Marlatt & George, 1984, might be useful). However, the selection of the most appropriate theory remains a complex issue. This is partly as a result of the variation in what comprises a theory-based intervention (i.e., even with two interventions described as being based on the Theory of Planned Behavior (TPB), there is likely to be some variation in the number of TPB constructs targeted, the selection of different behavior change techniques, variation in measures used to evaluate the effectiveness of the intervention, etc.). Consequently, an adequate answer to this question is some way off, the evidence base is insufficient.

Question 2: Should my intervention always be theory-based?

From a pragmatic viewpoint, where you want to change behavior and you are not interested in why your intervention is effective or ineffective then there is less need for an intervention to be theory-based.

Instead, your intervention should be selected on the criterion that it is *evidence-based* (i.e., previous studies have shown that a particular intervention is effective in changing your target behavior in a population that is representative of your population). If, however, you wish to understand the mechanisms underlying the effects of your intervention (for example, if you want to improve your intervention in the future or you wish to test a particular theory) then your intervention should ideally be theory-based and you should test it accordingly. That's not to say that an intervention *has* to be theory-based in the sense of it has to be built around an established theory like Self-Determination Theory or the Theory of Planned Behavior to test mechanisms. Any variable or construct expected to change as a result of exposure to an intervention could be proposed and tested (assuming it is measurable) to be a variable that explains how your intervention changes health behavior. However, the benefits of testing mechanisms based on an established theory are that you are provided with a framework guiding you around what to measure and how these variables should operate in relation to one another. Furthermore, by measuring the same variables, evidence can accumulate more rapidly in an organized manner to provide support for (or refute) the underlying theory.

Question 3: How should I test my theory-based intervention?

At the most basic level, one might choose to (a) design an intervention which comprises a number of different behavior change techniques that targets each of the constructs within a theory, (b) randomly allocate participants to the intervention group or a no-intervention control group, (c) measure each of the constructs after (and, if you choose, before) the intervention in both groups, and (d) then compare the effectiveness of the intervention relative to a no-intervention control group in changing the theoretical constructs and behavior. This approach would give us an indication of:

a.   whether an intervention based on all constructs of a theory is effective in changing behavior,
b.   which constructs were changed by the intervention and
c.   which construct changes (if any) explained the changes in behavior.

However, there are limitations. If there are multiple behavior change techniques within the intervention then additional experimental conditions are required to identify which components (behavior change techniques within the intervention) were effective in changing a theoretical construct or behavior (see Critical Skills Toolkit 3.1 in Chapter 3). In addition, simply measuring constructs, such as intentions, has been shown to be able to change behavior itself and thus can be viewed as an intervention in itself. This is known as the *meremeasurement or Question-Behavior effect* (see Chapter 7). As well as potentially reducing the size of the benefit of the intervention over the control (or even eliminating it), it is unclear whether the intervention would have been effective over the control condition *without* measuring the constructs. A Solomon four-group design is an approach to combat this problem whereby exposure to the intervention is crossed with exposure to measures of key determinants before completing the follow-up measure (i.e., resulting in four study conditions: intervention+ measures, measures only, intervention only, control (neither intervention or measures).

Question 4: How many constructs should my intervention target?

One viewpoint would be that, if you're basing your intervention on a particular theory, your intervention should target all of the constructs underlying or predicting behavior. However, doing so leads to the problems described in response to Question 3, either you have two groups (one intervention and one control) and consequently you struggle to find one technique that can change each of the theoretical constructs or you use a number of different behavior change techniques and you consequently do not know which behavior change techniques underlies your study effects (to do so, you would need to adopt a fully-crossed design).
An alternative might be to target only certain (key) constructs allowing you to use fewer behavior change techniques and more basic designs (which comprises fewer intervention groups). The drawback here is that you are not being fully faithful to the theory as a whole. To complicate matters, some constructs appear in more than one theory (thus a TPB-based intervention that targets only PBC/self-efficacy could be described as a social cognitive theory-based intervention, for example).

Question 5: Is it okay to target constructs from different theories at the same time?

Yes, you might choose to target constructs that most strongly correlate with behavior regardless of the theory from which it is derived (see Critical Skills Toolkit 4.1). However, a consequence is that by putting together constructs from different theories, you are essentially developing and testing a new theory.

Question 6: Is there anything else I should bear in mind when designing a theory-based intervention?

One thing to keep in mind with theory-based interventions, as with any intervention, is that it should be consistently delivered to your participants in the way it is intended; in other words, it should have high fidelity. For example, you could design a brilliant intervention on paper but if only part of this intervention is delivered then your intervention might be ineffective in changing behavior. It is often useful, particularly when you are relying on others to deliver your intervention (and where time and funds permit), to run a process evaluation (see Chapter 6) where you assess, among other things, whether or not participants receive the intervention as intended.

SUMMARY

In this chapter we considered the degree of variation that exists in claims regarding whether particular health behavior change interventions are theory-based, as well as different approaches that can be used to assess the extent of theory use. In addition, we considered the various benefits of using theory and critically evaluated whether the use of theory leads to stronger effects than interventions not based on theory. We conclude that the evidence is rather mixed but that theory use still has several benefits. We also overview critical issues such as how to select an underlying theory and the best techniques to change specific determinants. We ended the chapter by considering four different ways in which theory-based interventions can be developed and tested: using the Theory Coding Scheme, the experimental medicine approach, intervention mapping and a four-step cycle approach.

FURTHER READING

Hagger, M.S., & Weed, M. (2019). DEBATE: Do interventions based on behavioral theory work in the real world? *International Journal of Behavioral Nutrition and Physical Activity*, *16*, 36. It's not often that academics are given the opportunity to slug it out in a lively debate published in a single article. Hagger argues in favor of interventions based on theory working in the real world to aid population health; Weed argues against.

Kok, G., Gottlieb, N.H., Peters, G.Y., Mullen, P.D., Parcel, G.S., Ruiter, R.A.C., Fernández, M.E., Markham, C., & Bartholomew, L.K. (2016). A taxonomy of behaviour change methods: an Intervention Mapping Approach. *Health*

Psychology Review, *10*, 297–312. A paper highlighting the intervention mapping approach and which provides tables overviewing methods to change different determinants of health behavior.

Michie, S., & Prestwich, A. (2010). Are interventions theory-based? Development of a Theory Coding Scheme. *Health Psychology*, *29*, 1–8. A 19-item coding scheme that can be used to assess how, and to what extent, any particular health behavior intervention is theory-based.

Prestwich, A., Webb, T.L., & Conner, M. (2015). Using theory to develop and test interventions to promote changes in health behaviour: Evidence, issues, and recommendations. *Current Opinion in Psychology*, *5*, 1–5. A paper challenging the assumption that using theory to inform health behavior interventions leads to larger changes in behavior.

GLOSSARY

Atheoretical intervention: An attempt using one or more behavior change techniques to change behavior or related outcomes without reference to, or use of, theory.

Behavior change technique: A systematic strategy used in an attempt to change behavior (e.g., providing information on consequences; prompting specific goal setting; prompting barrier identification; modelling the behavior; planning social support).

Determinant: Construct that is assumed to causally influence another construct (typically behavior). Often used interchangeably with *mechanism of action*.

Mechanism of action: Construct that changes in response to an intervention which, in turn, leads to changes in behavior or other related outcomes. Often used interchangeably with *determinant*.

Meta-analysis: A statistical procedure used to combine, compare and contrast the findings of studies on a related topic.

Systematic review: A rigorous and replicable approach to identify, and synthesize evidence from, studies tackling a specific issue.

Theories, theory (or model): "A set of interrelated concepts, definitions and propositions that present a *systematic* view of events or situations by specifying relations among variables, in order to *explain* or *predict* the events or situations" (Glanz, Rimer, & Viswanath, 2015, p. 26).

Theory-based intervention: An approach to change behavior or other outcomes (such as those related to health) that draws on one or more underlying theories to identify which determinants of behavior/outcomes to target, which behavior change techniques to employ and for whom.

Theory coding scheme: An approach to assess how, and the extent to which, theory has been used to inform the development and evaluation of an intervention.

Theory-relevant construct: A key concept or building block within a theory/model upon which the intervention is based. Example constructs in the Theory of Planned Behavior are attitudes towards the behavior, perceived behavioral control, subjective norms, etc. Constructs can be further broken down into **determinants** (the predictors such as attitudes, subjective norms, PBC) or **outcomes** (such as behavior).

REFERENCES

Ajzen, I. (1991). The theory of planned behavior. *Organizational Behavior and Human Decision Processes, 50*, 179–211.

Albarracin, D., Gillette, J.C., Earl, A.N., Glasman, L.R., Durantini, M.R., & Ho, M.H. (2005). A test of major assumptions about behavior change: a comprehensive look at the effects of passive and active HIV-prevention interventions since the beginning of the epidemic. *Psychological Bulletin, 131*, 856–897.

Baban, A., & Craciun, C. (2007). Changing health-risk behaviors: A review of theory and evidence-based interventions in health psychology. *Journal of Cognitive and Behavioral Psychotherapies, 7*, 45–67.

Bandura, A. (1977). Self-efficacy: Toward a unifying theory of behavioral change. *Psychological Review, 84*, 191–215.

Bartholomew, L.K., Parcel, G. S., & Kok, G. (1998). Intervention Mapping: A Process for Developing Theory- and Evidence-Based Health Education Programs. *Health Education and Behavior, 25*, 545–563.

Carey, R.N., Connell, L.E., Johnston, M., Rothman, A.J., de Bruin, M., Kelly, M.P., & Michie, S. (2019). Behavior change techniques and their mechanisms of action: a synthesis of links described in published intervention literature. *Annals of Behavioral Medicine, 53*, 693–707.

Clancy, F., Prestwich, A., Caperon, L., Tsipa, A., & O'Connor, D. (2020). The association between worry and rumination with sleep in non-clinical populations: A systematic review and meta-analysis. *Health Psychology Review, 14*, 427–448.

Connell, L.E., Carey, R.N., de Bruin, M., Rothman, A.J., Johnston, M., Kelly, M.P., & Michie, S. (2019). Links between behavior change techniques and mechanisms of action: an expert consensus study. *Annals of Behavioral Medicine, 53*, 708–720.

Dalgetty, R., Miller, C.B., Dombrowski, S.U. (2019). Examining the theory-effectiveness hypothesis: A systematic review of reviews. *British Journal of Health Psychology, 24*, 334–356.

Dombrowski, S.U., Sniehotta, F.F., Avenell, A., Johnston, M., MacLennan, G., & Araujo-Soares, V. (2012). Identifying active ingredients in complex behavioural interventions for obese adults with obesity-related co-morbidities or additional risk factors for co-morbidities: A systematic review. *Health Psychology Review, 6*, 7–32.

Glanz, K., Rimer, B.K., & Viswanath, K. (2015). Theory, research and practice in health behavior. In K. Glanz, B.K. Rimer and K. Viswanath (Eds.), *Health Behavior: Theory Research & Practice, 5th Edition*. San Francisco: Jossey-Bass.

Gomis-Pastor, M., Roig, E., Mirabet, S. et al. (2020). A mobile app (mHeart) to detect medication nonadherence in the heart transplant population: Validation study. *JMIR mHealth uHealth*, *8*, e15957.

Johnston, M., Carey, R.N., Connell Bohlen, L.E., Johnston, D. W., Rothman, A.J., de Bruin, M., … Michie, S. (2021). Development of an online tool for linking behavior change techniques and mechanisms of action based on triangulation of findings from literature synthesis and expert consensus. *Translational Behavioral Medicine*, *11*, 1049–1065.

Kavussanu, M., Barkoukis, V., Hurst, P., Yukhymenko-Lescroart, M., Skoufa, L., Chirico, A., … Ring, C. (2022). A psychological intervention reduces doping likelihood in British and Greek athletes: A cluster randomized controlled trial. *Psychology of Sport & Exercise*, *61*, 102099.

Kok, G., Gottlieb, N.H., Peters, G.Y., Mullen, P.D., Parcel, G.S., Ruiter, R.A.C., … Bartholomew, L.K. (2016). A taxonomy of behaviour change methods: an Intervention Mapping Approach. *Health Psychology Review*, *10*, 297–312.

Kwak, L., Kremers, S.P.J., Werkman, A., Visscher, T.L.S., van Baak, M., & Brug, J. (2007). The NHF-NRG in Balance-Project: The Application of Intervention Mapping in the Development, Implementation and Evaluation of Weight Gain Prevention at the Worksite. *Obesity Reviews*, *8*, 347–361.

Marlatt, G.A., & George, W.H. (1984). Relapse prevention – introduction and overview of the model. *British Journal of Addiction*, *79*, 261–273.

Meade, L.B., Bearne, L.M., Sweeney, L.H., Alageel, S.H., & Godfrey, E.L. (2019). Behaviour change techniques associated with adherence to prescribed exercise in patients with persistent musculoskeletal pain: Systematic review. *British Journal of Health Psychology*, *24*, 10–30.

Michie, S., Abraham, C., Whittington, C., McAteer, J., & Gupta, S. (2009). Effective techniques in healthy eating and physical activity interventions: A meta-regression. *Health Psychology*, *28*, 690–701.

Michie, S., Johnston, M., Francis, J., Hardeman, W., & Eccles, M. (2008). From theory to intervention: mapping theoretically derived behavioural determinants to behaviour change techniques. *Applied Psychology: an International Review*, *57*, 660–680.

Michie, S., & Prestwich, A. (2010). Are interventions theory-based? Development of a Theory Coding Scheme. *Health Psychology*, *29*, 1–8.

Michie, S., Sheeran, P., & Rothman, A. (2007). Advancing the Science of Behaviour Change. Invited editorial, *Psychology and Health*, *22*, 249–253.

Nigg, C.R., & Paxton, R.J. (2008). Conceptual perspectives used to understand youth physical activity and inactivity, (pp. 79–113). In Smith, A.L. & Biddle, S.J.H. (Eds.), *Youth Physical Activity and Inactivity: Challenges and Solutions*. Champaign, IL: Human Kinetics.

Prestwich, A., Kellar, I., Parker, R., MacRae, S., Learmonth, M., Sykes, B., … Castle, H. (2014a). How can self-efficacy be increased? Meta-analysis of dietary interventions. *Health Psychology Review*, *8*, 270–285.

Prestwich, A., Sniehotta, F.F., Whittington, C., Dombrowski, S.U., Rogers, L., & Michie, S. (2014b). Does theory influence the effectiveness of health behavior interventions? Meta-analysis. *Health Psychology*, *33*, 465–474.

Prestwich, A., Webb, T.L., & Conner, M. (2015). Using theory to develop and test interventions to promote changes in health behaviour: Evidence, issues, and recommendations. *Current Opinion in Psychology*, *5*, 1–5.

Riddle, M., Science of Behavior Change Working Group (2015). News from the NIH: using an experimental medicine approach to facilitate translational research. *Translational Behavioral Medicine, 5,* 486–88.

Samdal, G. B., Eide, G. E., Barth, T., Williams, G., & Meland, E. (2017). Effective behaviour change techniques for physical activity and healthy eating in over-weight and obese adults; systematic review and meta-regression analyses. *International Journal of Behavioral Nutrition and Physical Activity, 14,* 42.

Sediva, H., Cartwright, T., Robertson, C., & Deb, S.K. (2022). Behavior change techniques in digital health interventions for midlife women: Systematic review. *JMIR mHealth uHealth, 10,* e37234.

Trifiletti, L.B., Gielen, A.C., Sleet, D.A., & Hopkins, K. (2005). Behavioural and social sciences theories and models: are they being used in unintentional injury prevention research? *Health Educational Research, 20,* 298–307.

Webb, T.L., & Sheeran, P. (2006). Does changing behavioral intentions engender behavior change? A meta-analysis of experimental evidence. *Psychological Bulletin, 132,* 249–268.

5

CHAPTER 5
THE METHODOLOGY OF HEALTH BEHAVIOR CHANGE

OVERVIEW

Love it or hate it, research methods (and its best friend, statistics) represent a vital element of health behavior change. What are the most effective behavior change techniques to tackle obesity? How can we prevent medical errors? What are the barriers that prevent people, particularly those from lower socio-economic groups, from eating healthily? While we can try to answer such questions without scientific investigation – for example, in relation to the last question, we could suppose cost is a crucial barrier preventing people from eating healthily – what evidence supports this and how strong is this evidence? In this chapter, as well as introducing various methods of data collection, we highlight their pros and cons, and overview means to evaluate the quality of data. We cover the key, burning issue of replicability too, the extent to which findings from equivalent studies lead to equivalent outcomes. Towards the end of the chapter, we also consider recommendations for developing and evaluating health behavior change interventions and methods related to translating health behavior change intervention into real-world settings over the longer term.

SURVEY/QUESTIONNAIRE METHODS

Within surveys or questionnaires, behavioral scientists can look to identify the relationships between a whole range of different factors including those that are societal (e.g., socio-economic status) and individual (e.g., attitudes towards exercising).

DOI: 10.4324/9781003302414-6

CRITICAL SKILLS TOOLKIT 5.1

ADVANTAGES AND DISADVANTAGES OF SURVEYS/ QUESTIONNAIRES USING RATING SCALES

The following advantages and disadvantages refer specifically to surveys and questionnaires that use rating scales rather than open-ended questions.

To illustrate the advantages and disadvantages of questionnaires/ surveys, the examples below have been applied to assess attitudes towards exercising.

Rating scales assessing attitudes towards exercising could look like this:

	Strongly Disagree		Strongly Agree	
I really like exercising	1	2	3	4
Exercising is fun	1	2	3	4

Or

Exercising is:	Boring	1	2	3	4	5	Exciting
	Harmful	1	2	3	4	5	Beneficial
	Bad	1	2	2	4	5	Good

Advantages

1. Rating scales quickly assess people's attitudes (or other constructs). For example, a random sample of school children could respond to questions like those above to give an indication of the attitudes of school children to exercising.
2. They can be relatively cheap to develop.
3. When applied in correlational studies (see Chapter 6), they can indicate which variables correlate (i.e., are related) with each other. For example, questionnaire measures of attitudes towards exercising may correlate with questionnaire measures of the number of

times that people exercise per week. By identifying which variables correlate with one another, behavioral scientists can generate hypotheses that can be tested using experimental designs. For example, one could hypothesize that exposing school children to an intervention designed to promote more favorable attitudes towards exercising will result in these school children exercising more in the future compared to a second group of school children not exposed to this intervention.

Disadvantages

1. Their potential utility is dependent on their design. To be of use, the questionnaire/survey should have strong evidence of **reliability** (e.g., **internal reliability, test-retest reliability**) and **validity** (e.g., **convergent validity, divergent validity**).
2. If the questionnaire is not reliable then you have an inaccurate representation of whatever it is you're trying to measure (e.g., school children's attitudes towards exercising). In turn, it would have limited use in *predicting* behavior (e.g., how often school children exercise).
3. When used in correlational (rather than experimental) designs they tell us little about causation. For example, measuring attitudes towards exercising and the number of times people exercise per week does not determine whether positive attitudes towards exercising encourages more frequent exercise (attitudes cause behavior), or whether frequently exercising promotes positive attitudes towards exercising (behavior causes attitudes) or neither. Experimental designs provide stronger evidence than correlational designs regarding causation.

To maximize the likelihood that any particular survey or questionnaire provides a good snapshot of current opinions, rather than just a snapshot, and to increase the likelihood that it accurately, rather than inaccurately, predicts future outcomes (such as the number of times people exercise), one must ensure that their survey/questionnaire is well-designed. In other words, it should have good evidence of reliability and validity (see Critical Skills Toolkit 5.2: Designing a reliable and valid questionnaire).

TABLE 5.1 Different types of questionnaire items

Type	Description	Sample items
Categorical	Participants are asked to select a specific category that best fits them or their opinion (the response options may or may not be provided)	"Are you a student?" Yes No "How much money do you earn per year?" Less than £20,000, £20,000 to £40,000, ore than £40,000.
Ranking	Require partici-pants to rank order several response options	"Rank the following food types in order of preference from 1=most preferred to 4= least preferred:" Fruit Confectionary Savory Vegetables snacks
Likert	Require individu-als to rate their level of agree-ment with a statement along a scale	"I enjoy playing football" Strongly Strongly disagree agree 1 2 3 4
Semantic differential	Similar to Likert scales but use opposing adjective pairs as anchors	"I find playing football is:" Fun 1 2 3 4 5 Boring Good 1 2 3 4 5 Bad Healthy 1 2 3 4 5 Unhealthy
Open-ended	Participants are not constrained in their response options (unlike the other types of questionnaire items)	"Why do you exercise as often as you do?" "Tell me about your feelings towards exercising" "What factors influence the foods that you buy?"

CRITICAL SKILLS TOOLKIT 5.2

DESIGNING A RELIABLE AND VALID RATING SCALE QUESTIONNAIRE

Designing a reliable and valid questionnaire can take time and benefits from careful development. When you are evaluating questionnaires, you should look for evidence of scale development plus reliability and validity. A reliable measure produces consistent responses. A valid measure assesses what it claims to measure. If a measure is said to assess attitudes towards exercise but actually assesses emotions concerning food then the measure would be said to be invalid.

Ensuring a measure has reliability and validity helps reduce measurement error (the difference between what the individual responds on the measure and their actual "true" score). If behavioral scientists use measures that do not have evidence of reliability and/or validity, the conclusions that arise from their studies are more likely to be inaccurate and the findings are less likely to be replicated by others in the future.

Developing a reliable/valid scale requires careful development via the following steps:

1. *Generate a large pool of items*
   You might think attitudes, and other psychological constructs, may be accurately measured through a single item within a questionnaire. A single item measure is less likely than a measure with multiple items, however, to accurately represent a person's attitude. Think of a person (Jimmy) who was asked to try to hit the bulls-eye on a dartboard with a single dart. Think of another person (Ted) who was asked to try to hit the bulls-eye on a dartboard with 20 darts. You want to use these scenarios to measure the dart-playing ability of Jimmy and Ted by measuring the distance of the (average) dart from the bulls-eye. Your estimate of Ted's ability is likely to be more accurate (Jimmy may have one particularly good or bad dart which greatly influences your assessment of his darting ability). The same principle applies to developing a reliable questionnaire; more items (questions) on your questionnaire should enhance its reliability.
2. *Take care when writing the specific items*
   a) The set of items should accurately and comprehensively represent the diversity and complexity of the psychological

construct (e.g., attitudes towards healthy eating, self-esteem) that is being assessed. This will help ensure **content validity** of the measure.

b) Some of the items should be reversed to avoid acquiescence bias (the tendency to agree with statements). For example, when measuring attitudes towards exercise, somebody with a very favorable attitude towards exercise would likely respond "5" to item "i" and "1" to item "ii":

i. Doing physical active is fantastic

Strongly disagree	Strongly agree
1 2 3 4 5	

ii. Doing physical activity is dull

Strongly disagree	Strongly agree
1 2 3 4 5	

c) Reliability and validity of the questionnaire can also be enhanced by constructing specific items carefully. Here are common problems that could apply to items within a questionnaire:

i. The items should be answerable on the scale provided. For example, somebody would struggle to answer the question: "How much money do you earn?" on a "strongly agree" to "strongly disagree" rating scale.

ii. Items should avoid acronyms as the participant may not understand them. For example: "The BPS is a worthwhile organization" may be difficult to answer for somebody who doesn't know that the BPS stands for the British Psychological Society.

iii. Ambiguous language should be avoided: "I like rock" could refer to rock music, rocks on the ground or rock candy.

iv. Loaded questions that make assumptions or assess only one part of the issue should be avoided. For example, "Are you still exercising?" assumes the individual used to exercise.

v. It is important that a question helps to differentiate between people and this wouldn't happen when everybody agrees or disagrees with a particular statement. Thus,

statements that everybody would agree (or disagree) with such as "Murder is a bad thing" should not be used.
vi. Leading questions are problematic: "Everybody should exercise, shouldn't they?"
vii. Double-barreled questions or statements should be avoided as people may not feel the same to each element (e.g., "Skin self-examinations are boring and unpleasant"; somebody may find them unpleasant but not boring).
viii. Double negatives can be difficult to understand (e.g., instead of saying "not unpleasant" use "pleasant" as the simpler language is easier to follow).
ix. Items should be brief, jargon-free, simple to understand and not intellectualized.

3. *Pilot the measure*
Once a set of items has been generated, it is useful for the measure to be trialed by handing the questionnaire to participants (representative of those you plan to recruit) and asking them to complete it. This pilot step can be used to identify any weak items.

a) *Remove items that elicit responses that are inconsistent with responses on other related items*
In a scale assessing individuals' intentions to exercise all items should attempt to measure intentions towards exercising. As the items should all be striving to measure the same thing (i.e. intentions towards exercising) then participants should respond to the items in a consistent way. See responses to item set A and responses to item set B. Responses to item set A are consistent, while responses to item set B are inconsistent.

SET A: CONSISTENT RESPONSES INDICATIVE OF A RELIABLE SCALE (RESPONSES SUGGEST STRONG INTENTIONS TO EXERCISE)

		Strongly Disagree			Strongly Agree	
		1	2	3	4	5
1	I intend to exercise	1	2	3	4	**5**
2	I am keen to exercise	1	2	3	4	**5**
3	My desire to exercise is weak	**1**	2	3	4	5
4	I want to exercise	1	2	3	4	**5**

SET B: INCONSISTENT RESPONSES INDICATIVE OF AN UNRELI- ABLE SCALE (IT IS UNCLEAR FROM THE SET OF RESPONSES WHETHER THE INDIVIDUALS HAS STRONG, MODERATE OR WEAK INTENTIONS TO EXERCISE)

		Strongly Disagree			Strongly Agree	
		1	**2**	**3**	**4**	**5**
1	I intend to exercise	1	2	3	4	**5**
2	I am keen to exercise	**1**	2	3	4	5
3	My desire to exercise is weak	1	2	**3**	4	5
4	I want to exercise	**1**	2	3	4	5

A measure that elicits consistent responses across items is said to have high **internal reliability**. Internal reliability is assessed by Cronbach's alpha and should be between 0.7 and 1 in a reliable measure. If it falls below 0.7 then the level of internal reliability is typically judged to be unacceptable (the lower the number, the less internally reliable the measure). In statistical packages (such as SPSS), when requesting Cronbach's alpha, the output will typically also show the impact on the Cronbach's alpha score should any specific item be deleted. This is a helpful way to identify any items that seem to elicit responses that are inconsistent with responses on other items. Another way is to assess the correlation between responses on each specific item with the total (summed) score across all items. To generate a more reliable scale, researchers would remove from their questionnaire any item that has a low item-total correlation.

b) *Remove items that are unlikely to discriminate among individuals* If the measure is to be of use, it should be able to discriminate accurately between different groups of people. Take the measure of intentions to exercise above; one might expect that people who exercise a lot would have stronger intentions to exercise than people who do little exercise. If the measure is trialed on a sample where half of the participants exercise a lot and the other half exercise little or not at all (more sedentary individuals) then one may expect the standard deviation of responses would not be too low and thus has some discriminatory value. One strategy to enhance validity of the scale is to remove items that have very low standard deviations. Alternatively, or in addition, items that do not seem to differentiate between your two groups of participants (high exercisers and more sedentary people) in the expected manner could be removed in the pilot phase of scale development. This strategy will help maximize the **criterion-related validity** of your scale: the extent that your measure is related to distinct criteria in the real world (in this case, the extent that it can differentiate between high exercisers and more sedentary people).

4. *Further test the reliability and validity of your measure*
   The **dimensionality** of the scale should be examined to help make clear whether the scale is measuring one thing (thus making it unidimensional) or several things (thus making it multidimensional). This can be achieved through factor analysis.

   Test-retest reliability should be assessed by giving participants the same questionnaire twice on two separate occasions. If the measure has high test-retest reliability then responses should be very similar across both time-points.

   When looking through the items of a scale, judge the **face validity** – do all of the items look like they assess what they are supposed to assess? This is a pretty straightforward but subjective, non-standardized way of assessing validity. Other types of validity can be assessed more formally.

   The **predictive validity** of a scale can be measured by testing whether responses on the questionnaire predict future events that one would expect it should predict. For example, does the measure of intentions to exercise predict how much exercise people do in the future? If it does then you could argue the measure has predictive validity.

   The **convergent validity** of the measure can be determined by assessing the correlation between the measure and a related measure that has been previously validated. For example, when developing a new measure of intentions to exercise then the responses that participants give on the new measure should be similar to (correlate with) responses on a measure of exercise intentions that has been previously validated.

   The **discriminant (divergent) validity** of the scale can be established by checking that responses on the scale are unrelated to responses on scales that it should be unrelated to. In the example of developing a measure of intentions to exercise, you would expect it would be unrelated to responses on a measure of attitudes towards washing up, for instance.

BURNING ISSUE BOX 5.1

HEALTH RISK BEHAVIORS AND ALTERED STATES

Studies that use models like the Theory of Planned Behavior (TPB) or the Prototype Willingness Model require participants to complete questionnaires reporting their thoughts and feelings about a behavior in a "cold" state (e.g., in a carefully controlled laboratory situation). These self-reports are then used to predict later decisions to perform a behavior taken in a "hot" state (e.g., when under the influence of alcohol or when sexually aroused or when really hungry). The problem is that these cold cognitions measured in the laboratory may not show a good match with the real world hot cognitions that drive behavior in the real world. George Loewenstein (1996) describes this difference as the "empathy gap" suggesting we are not good at predicting how we will feel in altered states. A number of studies have shown this effect in relation to craving for cigarettes (Sayette et al., 2008), hunger and food choice (Read & Leeuwen, 1998) and sexual arousal (Loewenstein et al., 1997). Conner et al. (2008) had students, who were or were not intoxicated with alcohol, complete measures based on the TPB in relation to having sex without a condom. Being intoxicated increased men's but not women's intention to have unprotected sex. Interestingly intoxication also changed the relationship between thoughts and feelings about unprotected sex (i.e., a moderation effect). In women, intoxication significantly increased the importance of affective atti-tudes on intentions to have unprotected sex. In other words being intoxicated made the women place more emphasis on how they thought the behavior would make them feel in deciding whether to have unprotected sex.

The importance of altered states needs to be considered in develop-ing interventions to change behavior (see MacDonald et al., 2000, for an example in relation to promoting condom use in young people).

BURNING ISSUE BOX 5.2

ARE SINGLE ITEM MEASURES REALLY THAT BAD? (ALLEN ET AL. 2022)

When might it be ok to use single item measures?

Not so long ago, use of single item measures in questionnaires were outlawed. Well, not quite, but they were looked at negatively: "You can't capture the construct in a single item"; "Your measure is not valid"; "You should use a multi-item measure." However, are there instances when it's okay to use single items? In a recent editorial, Allen et al. (2022) suggest that single items can be suitable in some instances, when the construct is unidimensional, narrow in scope and clearly defined. So, while they may not be suitable to assess personality, for instance, they may be suitable for other constructs.

Are some single item measures better than others?

There can obviously be good and bad single item measures, and some of this can be considered with tests of reliability (test-retest reliability: in constructs not expected to vary over time, are respondents responding similarly to the item at different timepoints?) and validity (e.g., convergent validity: does the single item measure correlate sufficiently with a multi-item equivalent?; predictive validity: does the single item measure correlate sufficiently with an outcome that the construct is anticipated to relate to?; face validity: is the item relevant, unambiguous and easy to respond to?). Of course, internal consistency (how much related items correlate with one another) cannot be tested in a single item measure.

Are single item measures sometimes preferable to multi-item measures?

Yes. Reliable and valid single item measures can be particularly helpful when designing large surveys (or in any scenario where you want to limit cost/resource requirements and/or demand on participants, such as vulnerable people who may have difficulty participating in long study sessions). By reducing demand in studies involving data collection across multiple timepoints, dropout may be minimized too. So, perhaps, it's not all bad news for single item measures after all.

BURNING ISSUE BOX 5.3

IS COLLECTING QUESTIONNAIRE DATA ONLINE WORTH IT?

During the COVID-19 pandemic, it became increasingly popular for data collection via companies who provide access to individuals who are prepared to take part in paid online studies. Labs were closed and face-to-face data collection methods were not possible for most given social distancing restrictions and lockdowns. Platforms like Prolific and Amazon's Mechanical Turk (MTurk) filled the void. They enabled researchers to quickly gather data. On the surface, such platforms are amazingly efficient as you can run studies in a fraction of the time it would take if you recruited participants in traditional ways, meeting participants individually as they completed their questionnaires. Moreover, there are options to ensure you have samples that are representative on certain parameters such as age (though it is worth keeping in mind that those individuals who sign-up to complete online surveys may differ in important ways than those who do not). As long as the quality and robustness of the data Is up to scratch thon this approach can work well. Is this the case though?

One issue is the use of bots. Bots can complete surveys much faster than humans can, they may give out of range answers or answer open-ended questions in ways that don't make sense. Bots threaten the integrity of research data and can lead to researchers wasting money paying "fake participants." Many platforms offer some protection against bots and, as a researcher, steps can be taken to minimize the risk of "bot attacks," such as using time stamps (to identify impossibly quick responses), requiring answers to some open-ended questions (to identify bizarre looking responses or identical responses across participants), requiring answers to questions where only one response can possibly be correct, using skip logic so that you can see whether questions that shouldn't be answered based on previous question responses have not been responded to, using attention-check items, using the same question (e.g., how many siblings do you have?) at different points to check the same answer is acquired, preventing or identifying responses from the same IP address or using captcha to protect your survey against bots.

Another potential issue is that more true participants fail to engage with the material properly and respond particularly quickly and erratically. Some of the steps noted above can be taken (e.g., adding in attention-check items or looking at how long participants took to complete the survey). Additional strategies such as ensuring the survey is not overly lengthy and does not require participants to read whole chunks of text that they might be tempted to skip over could also help. This issue could affect the type of study that you wish to run online with studies that use vignettes, for example, potentially more risky than studies that just require the completion of simple questionnaires. Moreover, there are issues around how to identify such participants, how to treat them in your analyses and the potential impact on your findings of including or excluding such participants. Plans around these participants and how they are to be treated should be preregistered ideally. Given the additional "noise" it is also perhaps worth anticipating smaller experimental effects compared to equivalent studies that are completed offline and powering your study, a-priori, on this basis. Studies conducted by one of the authors, Andrew, have shown generally smaller effect sizes for online (Prestwich, in press) versus in-person (Prestwich et al., 2021) surveys.

As data collection can happen very rapidly, potentially in a few minutes, this creates additional issues around timing of data collection. Would findings markedly differ when based on data collected at 10am (where many people who are employed could be working) compared to data collected outside the relatively common 9am–5pm working window? Would data collected at 11pm (capturing the "night owls") differ to data collected at 7am (capturing the "early birds")?

Another potential ramification of quick data collection from online methods is that sample sizes of online studies can become very large. The drive for large sample sizes aids confidence in estimates of effects and replicability; however, one potential issue is that very small, trivial effects are treated as significant and important.

One final point is that not all platforms are equal. Peer et al. (2022) present evidence that platforms such as Prolific outperform other platforms such as MTurk in terms of data quality. They showed in their first study that Prolific users were more likely to pass attention check questions (68.7% vs. 22.1% for the worst performing platform), answered specific questions correctly (81% vs. 42% for the worst performing platform) and were honest more often regarding not solving an unsolvable problem (84% vs. 55% for the worst platform). To enhance confidence in this platform, Peers et al. showed Prolific was also one of the top performing platforms in their second study.

OBSERVATIONAL METHODS

Sometimes we can't ask people questions; babies, for instance, can't complete questionnaires or surveys but we can observe them. In these cases, observational methods, whereby behavior is observed within its natural environment, could be a useful option. We refer to observational methods here in the literal sense (where people are watched) rather than the broader sense often used in epidemiology which covers measuring and collating information about people (through health records, surveys, etc.). There are different types of these observational methods such as cohort studies that involve recruiting people with similar characteristics and comparing those who are exposed to a particular risk factor against those who are not over time. The Framingham Heart Study is one example that has followed people from a town in Massachusetts, USA, over time and across multiple generations to help identify risk factors for cardiovascular disease. Other common types of this broad group of observational methods are case control studies (that compare people with vs. without a specific condition) and cross-sectional (where information on people is collated at a single point in time).

Anyway, we digress. For the (literal) observational method that we cover here, people are viewed and all variables are typically free to vary with little interference. This lack of interference helps maximize **ecological validity**, the extent to which the findings can be generalized to other real world settings. Just as with survey methods, behavioral scientists can use observational methods to identify co-occurring events which can provide an insight into the factors underlying behavior. For example, they can attempt to identify features of green space that influence levels of physical activity.

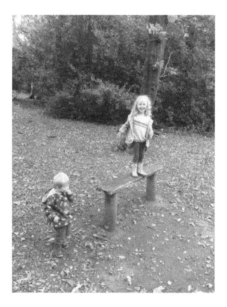

FIGURE 5.1 Young Milla and Sonny enjoying local green space.

There are different types of naturalistic observation: undisclosed and disclosed. **Undisclosed observation** prevents the right to informed consent but has the advantage that people should behave naturally. Under **disclosed observation**, observed individuals are informed beforehand, running the risk that one's thoughts and actions are affected.

In addition, observational methods can be combined with other approaches. For example, experimental methods (see next section) can be used with observational methods in the form of **natural experiments** to examine the impact of fewer elevators being available on certain days on stair use (see, for example, Olander & Eves, 2011) or to assess the influence of other environmental influences on health behavior (e.g., music played in a supermarket; discounting healthy foods, etc.). They can usefully be applied to consider the impact of policy such as the implementation of more cycle lanes comparing areas where the policy has been implemented versus where it hasn't.

CRITICAL SKILLS TOOLKIT 5.3

ADVANTAGES AND DISADVANTAGES OF OBSERVATIONAL METHODS

Advantages

1. High ecological validity
2. If the experimenter isn't detected then many biases can be overcome such as:
   a) demand effects: participants behaving in a way that they feel the experimenter wants them to act
   b) experimenter bias: an experimenter acting in a way that may encourage the participant to act in line with the hypothesis
   c) bias associated with the participant being worried about being observed.
3. Can provide an accurate account of spontaneous behavior.
4. If conducted purely through undisclosed methods, observational methods can be conducted quickly and at low cost.
5. It can be used with young children where other methods might be unreliable.

Disadvantages

1. Can be prone to observer-bias in which the observer sees what they want to see to support their chosen hypothesis.
2. Different observers may see different things. A good strategy when using observational methods is to use at least two observers and then compare their rates of agreement (to assess the inter-rater reliability).
3. On the flipside of enhanced ecological validity is a possible reduction in experimental control which may reduce **internal validity** (where one can confidently deduce that one variable causes a specific outcome).
4. Disclosed observation may cause an individual to act unnaturally thus off-setting many of the potential benefits of observational methods.

EXPERIMENTAL METHODS

While survey/questionnaire and observational methods help identify co-occurring factors, experimental methods help to identify the causes of behavior as well as the effects of various manipulations to the environment, individuals or related factors such as social groups (see Chapter 7, for example, for applications to different types of health behaviors).

There are three common types of experimental design: **between-subjects, within-subjects** and **mixed-design**. The advantages and disadvantages of these different types of experimental design are reported in the next chapter (see Critical Skills Toolkit 6.1). Examples of the three types of design are provided next in relation to assessing the effect of a complex intervention against a basic intervention on exercise:

a) Between-subjects (independent groups) designs: *different* participants are allocated to different experimental groups (e.g., one group of participants receive the complex intervention and one group of participants receive the basic intervention before completing a measure of how much they exercise, say, one month later).
b) Within-subjects (repeated measures) designs: where the *same* participants take part on multiple occasions (e.g., all participants receive the basic intervention and then complete a measure of how much they exercise one month later before being exposed to the complex intervention. Another month later they complete the measure of how much they exercise for a second time).

c) Mixed-design: this uses both between-subjects and within subjects elements. For example, half of the participants receive the basic intervention and half of the participants receive the complex intervention. Exercise behavior is measured twice (once before being exposed to either of the interventions and for a second time one month later). As one group of participants receive the basic intervention while a different group of participants receives the complex intervention, there is a between-subjects element. As participants complete the **dependent variable** measure (of exercise) more than once (twice in total, before and after intervention exposure), there is a within-subjects element. Putting these together results in a mixed-design.

CRITICAL SKILLS TOOLKIT 5.4

ADVANTAGES AND DISADVANTAGES OF EXPERIMENTAL METHODS

Advantages

1. Allows behavioral scientists to identify causal relationships (high internal validity).
2. Laboratory based experiments present a high degree of control that helps minimize the impact of **extraneous variables** (background variables that can influence the outcome of the study).
3. Tightly controlled experiments should be replicable. Many effects in health behavior change can be relatively small thus replicating significant effects can be more difficult compared to studies that yield large effects. To increase the likelihood of replication, the exact same procedures should be used across studies, similar participants should be sampled and the researchers should ensure there is a large sample size (larger sample sizes, everything else being equal, should increase the precision of the estimated experimental effect sizes). In Burning Issue Box 5.4, we present fuller consideration of issues around replicability.
4. Experimental methods can be used inside and outside of the laboratory. Conducting experiments outside the laboratory should increase ecological validity (the extent to which the results reflect real life) although it can reduce internal validity (the degree to which we can conclude the experimental effect was caused by the independent variable).

Disadvantages

1. Due to the sampling of specific participants and testing within specific, controlled environments (e.g., laboratories), ecological validity/**external validity** (the extent to which results can be generalized) can be limited. Field experiments can partially reduce this.
2. Conducting certain types of experiments can introduce participants to scenarios or stressors that they may not typically encounter (or want to encounter!).
3. Informed consent and minimizing deception can be important to protect the participants. However, letting participants know what they will do and the purpose of the experiment can introduce demand effects – whereby participants behave in the way that they feel the experimenter wants them to act.
4. If the experimenter knows which experimental condition the participant is in when they interact with them before or during the study, this can lead to experimenter effects. These effects can be minimized through **blinding** the experimenter to condition (so that the experimenter does not know which study condition the participant is in). When blinding is done successfully, the experimenter is unable to consciously or unconsciously affect the behavior of the participant in line with the experimental hypothesis.
5. If used alongside other methods (survey/questionnaire or observation), the accompanying methods need to demonstrate high levels of reliability and validity (see Critical Skills Toolkit 5.2).

When using experimental methods, behavioral scientists would deliberately try to produce a change in one variable (the independent variable) and record the effect this change has on other variables (the dependent variables). To ensure that conclusions relating to these causal effects are valid, the researchers should be sure that they manipulate only the **independent variable** of interest, thus ruling out the effects of **extraneous variables**. This is just one risk of bias in experimental studies (see Critical Skills Toolkit 5.5 for other risks). When the risk of bias is reduced, the accuracy of the results should increase.

CRITICAL SKILLS TOOLKIT 5.5

IDENTIFYING RISK OF BIAS IN EXPERIMENTAL TRIALS

1. Non-random allocation to conditions or other bias arising from the randomization process
   Random allocation of participants to experimental conditions should increase the likelihood that the participants in each group are similar to one another (which helps to ensure that any comparisons between the two groups, after manipulating the independent variable, are fair). Studies in which participants choose which experimental condition they wish to be in can introduce **self-selection bias** because the type of person who chooses group A may be different to the type of person who chooses groups B. Even in randomized trials, there can be issues with randomization leading to differences in the study groups at baseline (before participants have been exposed to different interventions or manipulations thus before any differences are expected to emerge).

2. Incomplete outcome data should be adequately addressed.
   Often, particularly in studies that follow-up participants at a later date, participants can drop out of your study. The percentage of participants that drop out is known as your **attrition rate** and can introduce bias into your study. Attrition rates should ideally be low and be similar across experimental conditions. Higher attrition rates within an experimental group versus a control group could suggest that the manipulation employed in the experimental group is not acceptable or harmful in some way. Moreover, the type of person who drops out should be similar to the type of person who remains in the study to permit wider generalizations of your study findings.

   One way to address incomplete outcome data is to employ **intention-to-treat analysis** (ITT) (see Chapter 6 for more details). In ITT, participants who drop out of the study are treated as if they did not drop out by carrying across their scores from baseline to follow up (i.e., treating them as if they did not change from baseline to follow up) or using other forms of ITT (such as multiple imputation in which missing scores are replaced with plausible, estimated scores).

3. Blinding research staff and participants.

   Blinding those individuals who screen participants entering the study is important. If a researcher can see the **allocation sequence** which determines the order which participants entering the study are allocated to experimental or control groups, the allocation sequence is not concealed. Lack of **allocation concealment** can bias the likelihood that the researcher accepts or rejects the individual onto the trial. For example, if the researcher, upon meeting a potential participant feels they may not be influenced by the experimental manipulation/intervention, they may be more likely to reject the participant if they know the next person accepted onto the trial will be allocated to the experimental condition (or increase the likelihood of accepting the person onto the trial if they are to be allocated to the control condition). Similarly, blinding the researcher delivering the intervention or interacting with the participant can minimize the risk of experimenter effects; blinding to condition the statistician analyzing the data can reduce bias in the selection of statistical tests; blinding observers can minimize observational bias; blinding participants to condition can reduce demand effects. However, it may not always be possible to blind researchers and/or participants to condition.

4. Selective outcome reporting.

   Researchers may be more inclined to report outcomes on which there were significant differences between the experimental and control groups. The primary and all secondary outcomes taken in the study and the results for each of these should be reported (i.e., reporting of results should not be selective). Pre-published trial protocols in which all of the measures to be taken in the study and how these will be analyzed are specified prior to the study being conducted can be particularly helpful. This practice is becomingly increasingly more common in studies of health behavior change.

5. Could you be manipulating other variables beyond your identified independent variable?

   When variables are similar to one another (e.g., the respect we have for our local doctor (GP) may be related to how much we like them), conclusions are stronger (i.e., more valid) if you are able to demonstrate that you have only manipulated the independent variable (e.g., respect) and not related variables (e.g., liking). These can be done by a series of manipulation checks whereby the researcher tests for changes in the independent variable and lack of changes in related variables shortly after the attempt to manipulate the specific independent variable.

6. Dependent variables should be measured reliably and validly (see Critical Skills Toolkit 5.2: Designing a reliable and valid rating scale questionnaire).

7. Bias from deviation from intended intervention.

   If an intervention is not delivered as intended, either because the participant did not receive what they should have received, or they deviated from what they were supposed to do, this has implications for the analyses and conclusions that can be drawn. For example, if the goal is to consider the effect of *assignment* of participants to condition, then this should be analyzed using intention-to-treat analysis in which all participants randomized to condition are included and analyzed based on the treatment to which they were assigned (which may be different from the treatment they actually received). If the goal is to consider the effect of *adhering* to the intervention then participants can be analyzed based on the treatment that they received or restrict the analyses to those who adhered to the protocol. Such analyses are problematic, however, because people who adhere to what they should do are likely to differ in important ways from those who do not adhere, and this can then confound the interpretation of the effects of adherence to the intervention.

PARALLEL GROUPS, CROSSOVER AND STEPPED WEDGE DESIGNS

There are different types of experimental trial designs and here we focus on three: parallel groups, crossover and stepped wedge.

In a parallel groups design, participants are assigned to a single condition (e.g., intervention vs. control) and they will remain allocated to that same condition throughout the study duration. In a crossover trial, participants are randomized to groups (intervention/control) but then at a later point during the study, those allocated to the control will receive the intervention and vice-versa. The stepped wedge design is a special case of crossover design; all participants begin without the intervention but then (typically) different clusters (or individuals) receive the intervention at randomized points in time (see Figure 5.2).

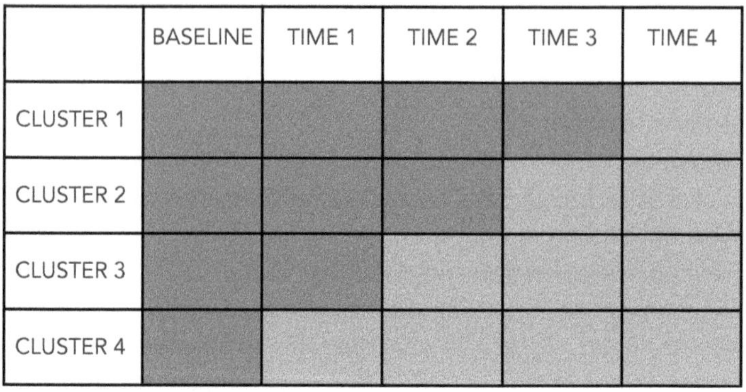

	BASELINE	TIME 1	TIME 2	TIME 3	TIME 4
CLUSTER 1					
CLUSTER 2					
CLUSTER 3					
CLUSTER 4					

FIGURE 5.2 Stepped Wedge Cluster Randomized Trial.
Note: Darker block = control exposure/pre-intervention; Lighter block = intervention exposure/post-intervention

The crossover points in a stepped wedge design flow in one direction, from the control to the intervention. There are different types of stepped wedge design depending on factors such as whether recruitment is continuous with participants recruited over a period of time even after the trial has started (vs. not) and whether exposure to the intervention is brief or delivered continually after participants enter the intervention condition. In some stepped wedge designs, participants take part throughout the study and eventually receive the intervention. In others, some participants may only take part briefly in either the intervention or control (e.g., when they visit the doctor).

Stepped wedge designs are often used when policy decisions have already been made to implement an intervention and this also ensures that the intervention can be more rigorously evaluated compared to a simple pre-post test (how things were before vs. after the intervention). As such, it can enable simultaneous implementation and evaluation. This type of design is also useful when it is difficult to implement an intervention to an entire group or population all at once, enabling a more staggered start across groups or sites.

In Critical Skills Toolkit 5.6, we compare parallel, crossover and stepped wedge designs but focus specifically on the type of stepped wedge design in which all participants eventually receive the intervention.

CRITICAL SKILLS TOOLKIT 5.6

ADVANTAGES AND DISADVANTAGES OF DIFFERENT TYPES OF EXPERIMENTAL TRIAL DESIGNS

	Parallel	Crossover	Stepped Wedge
Ease of administration	Relatively easy	Easier than stepped wedge	Hardest but can be useful if the intervention is time-consuming/resource heavy making it difficult to deliver to lots of groups at a time
Ethics/acceptability	Weakest as relatively high number of participants do not receive the intervention	Better than parallel as all receive the intervention	Better than parallel as all receive the intervention albeit, for some participants, this could be very much delayed
Duration	Typically shorter than stepped wedge	Typically shorter than stepped wedge	Typically requires longer than the other type of design to ensure participants can receive the intervention at different times
Recruitment/drop out	Can be harder to recruit than other designs	Good for recruitment as all receive the intervention; dropout potentially lower than other designs	While all participants receiving the intervention at some stage aids recruitment and can help minimize dropout, this is offset by a typically longer study duration

	Parallel	Crossover	Stepped Wedge
Confounding	Participants in the intervention and control may differ in important ways leading to confounds	As all participants go into each condition, they act as their own control (which also has benefits for statistical power), eliminating confounding from uneven participant characteristics across groups	Similar to crossover but there is a risk of confounding with factors that change over time (e.g., age)
Analyses/ reporting/ sample size planning	Typically least complex	Moderately complex	Typically most complex
Carryover effects (effects of being in one condition transfer to another when participants change groups)	None	Possible issue	Possible issue

RANDOMIZED CONTROLLED TRIALS, PILOT STUDIES AND FEASIBILITY STUDIES

In randomized controlled trials (RCTs), participants are randomly allocated to an experimental group receiving an intervention and a control group that does not receive this intervention. These groups are later compared on key outcomes (e.g., motivation to adherence to medication; medication adherence rates) to determine whether the intervention has been successful.

While the key aim of an RCT is to determine whether an intervention works or is successful, this is not the case for pilot or feasibility studies. As such, you should resist the temptation to statistically test hypotheses when using these types of study. Instead, the main goal for pilot or feasibility studies is to support the development of a main study (such as an RCT) and are smaller in scale (using fewer participants, etc.).

Feasibility studies really answer whether the main (larger) study can be done. They can be used to identify how likely participants are to take part (i.e., how difficult it would be to recruit and how long the process of recruitment might take) and dropout, whether an intervention can be delivered in the way it is intended (i.e., with fidelity) and to what extent participants adhere to an intervention and/or complete the outcome measures (e.g., are there too many outcome measures or items?). In addition, feasibility studies can inform whether randomization to condition is feasible, which particular outcomes are important to people and how acceptable a particular intervention is. They can use quantitative methods (e.g., rating scales), qualitative methods (e.g., interviews) or a combination of the two (**mixed methods**). **Pilot studies** have been argued to be a particular form of feasibility study in which the pilot study mirrors the main study or trial, using the same design albeit on a smaller scale (Eldridge et al., 2016).

As the main goal of feasibility and pilot studies is to inform whether conducting the main study is worthwhile, they should incorporate pre-specified criteria or rules regarding whether or not to progress and actually conduct the main study (and, if they are to progress, whether any amendments are needed). There is some debate regarding whether they can be used to inform the sample size of the main trial. On the one hand, they could be used to inform how variable the scores are on planned outcome measures. However, basing the effect size estimate on few participants will mean that it is likely to be too imprecise to inform the sample size of the main study. As an alternative, the sample size for the main trial could be determined based on estimates of clinically meaningful differences and could involve consultation with key people (e.g., patients, policymakers) to find out what type of difference would be important for them.

To what extent might findings from pilot or feasibility studies be similar to findings from the main trial? Well, it is worth keeping in mind that as pilot and feasibility studies have so few participants, estimates of effect sizes are likely to be imprecise. As such, there is a fair chance that the magnitude of effects in the preliminary pilot/feasibility study and final study differ. However, there are other factors (or biases) that increase the risk that findings from these types of study differ in substantial ways. These biases have been neatly summarized by Beets et al. (2020) and include things like "intervention intensity bias" (pilot/feasibility studies test an intervention that is delivered more (or less) often than in the main study), "intervention delivery agent bias" (does the person delivering the intervention in the pilot/feasibility study have the same level of expertise as the person doing this in the main study?), "target audience bias" (are the characteristics of the participants in both types of study the same?) and "setting bias" (are the settings used for both types of study the same?).

RISK OF BIAS

The Cochrane Collaboration has put forward a tool to assess the risk of bias in randomized controlled trials (RCTs). The Cochrane Collaboration Risk of Bias tool can be used to judge whether adequate steps have been taken to minimize various risks of bias such as those outlined in the Critical Skills Toolkit 5.5. This tool has been recently revised and updated (to create a second version, known as RoB 2, a little *Star Wars*-esque!) and now focuses on bias of a particular result rather than bias of a particular study and includes a means to judge the overall risk of bias for a particular result (low risk of bias, some concerns, high risk of bias). If you are tempted to use this tool, however, be warned, it is quite complex and there is evidence that inter-rater agreements can be low with the tool even for those experienced in systematic reviews (Minozzi et al., 2020). Extensive training is likely necessary to improve how reliably and accurately the tool is used to assess bias.

REPORTING TRIALS

Take a journal article reporting the results of a randomized controlled trial (RCT). Give it a cursory read. Probably everything, at first glance, looks in order. Take a closer look, especially if it is an article that was published several years ago and/or is located in a journal that does not require authors to adhere to the CONSORT (CONsolidated Standards Of Reporting Trials; Schulz et al., 2010) guidelines. Key details that would allow you to fairly and accurately assess the methodological quality of the trial could be missing. For example, were research staff dealing with participants aware of which condition (intervention or control group) the participant was allocated to when they dealt with them (i.e., were the research staff blinded to condition)? The CONSORT group, by providing their guidelines, strive for transparency in the reporting of RCTs. As a result, readers should be able to more accurately judge the reliability of the trial taking into account methodological limitations that could lead to bias.

More and more journals (particularly those related to health) require researchers conducting RCTs to adhere to these guidelines when writing up the results of their study in a journal article. By requiring behavioral scientists to clearly report information linked to the risk of bias/study quality, it is likely that behavioral scientists will more often employ the types of procedures that minimize bias (such as concealing the allocation sequence and blinding researchers to experimental conditions). A similar reporting guideline for nonrandomized designs is also available (TREND: Transparent Reporting of Evaluations with Nonrandomized Designs) and there is also an extension to the CONSORT guidelines for randomized pilot and feasibility trials. Moreover, there is a reporting guideline for trial **protocols** called SPIRIT that can be very helpful in addressing issues around replicability (see Burning Issue Box 5.4).

BURNING ISSUE BOX 5.4

ISSUES AROUND REPLICABILITY

What is replicability?

If findings in one study are consistent with the findings of a second study that adopted the same key methods, then the findings can be argued to have shown replicability. How replicability is measured, however, is not an exact science and can involve comparison of p-values (preferably in equivalent sized studies), effect sizes (when sample sizes differ), meta-analyses (when several attempts have been made to replicate a study) or some form of subjective assessment. Stanley et al. (2018) distinguish replicability from reproducibility; an aspect of replicability relating to whether the same results can be achieved if the same dataset and method of data analyses are used, as well as from generalizability which is whether consistent effects are found in different contexts (e.g., in samples drawn from different countries). Nosek et al. (2022) also differentiate replicability from robustness. Robustness, like reproducibility, involve re-analyses of the same dataset but involve different analytic methods rather the same analytic methods.

How widespread is the problem of failing to replicate?

In a landmark paper, the Open Science Collaboration (2015) attempted to replicate 100 psychology studies which used either correlational or experimental designs. In the original studies, nearly all (97%) found significant results but this fell to 36% in the replication studies. The effect sizes that they found were roughly half the size of the original studies and only 47% of the effect sizes in the replication attempts fell within the 95% confidence intervals for the effect sizes of the original studies. The Many Labs Replication Project (Klein et al., 2014) adopted a different approach, conducting the same study multiple times, and revealed 10 out of 13 studies largely replicated. This project has since been expanded in the form of Many Labs 2 (Klein et al., 2018) involving more studies, more labs and more diverse samples. In this latter attempt, about half of the studies achieved significant effects in the same direction and three quarters of the replication studies achieved smaller effect sizes than the original studies.

Certain types of effects may be harder to replicate than others. For instance, the Open Science Collaboration reported that only 22% of interaction effects were replicated compared to 47% testing main effects.

What has led to issues around replicability?

There are a great number of issues that can impact on whether a particular study can replicate ranging from scientific fraud to random or systematic error which can cause even studies that have been conducted using robust methods to fail to replicate. Original studies may be false positives; replications may be false negatives (or vice-versa). However, several other factors that are more controllable also play a role:

- *Proportionally few replication attempts.* Scientists have been incentivized to discover novel findings with new studies that attempt to replicate old studies seen as being of less value. This picture is gradually shifting in the light of the replicability crisis, however, with high-powered replications seen as important for enhancing certainty around original findings and thus the advancement of science.
- *Questionable research practices (QRPs) and researcher degrees of freedom (RDF).* Manapat et al. (in press) identify a range of factors that contribute to the replicability crisis. They distinguish between two types of practices – what they describe as acceptable (researcher degrees of freedom, RDF) and unacceptable (questionable research practices, QRPs) – that arise due to the choices that researchers can make when conducting their research.
- According to them, RDF include sample size planning and measuring additional variables that can be used as covariates or independent or dependent variables.

QRPs include analyzing the data and then deciding whether or not to continue collecting data/using optional stopping during data collection, dropping participants, measures or conditions from analyses (p-hacking) and using inappropriate measures or analyses to obtain significant findings.

They also describe conditional RDF/QRP which can be either RDF or QRP in different situations. These include selecting dependent variables, conducting exploratory studies without hypotheses (which can become HARKing (Hypothesizing After the Results are Known) if these post-hoc hypotheses (that come after analyzing) are presented as a-priori hypotheses (that come before the research was conducted), dealing with violations of assumptions in statistical tests. Their final category related to reporting issues (noting how the data was processed prior to the main analyses; whether all methods and results are reported and falsifying research data).

- *Selective outcome reporting.* In any one study, several outcomes could be measured. If significant findings are more likely to be reported than non-significant findings, or if significant findings are more likely to be used as the basis for effect size estimates in power calculations, the consequence is that the estimated size of the effect of interest is likely to be inflated. The knock-on effect of this is that this inflated effect size will then be used in further research (including for replications) that uses too few participants and is consequently underpowered and unlikely to replicate.
- *Differences between the original and follow-up study.* Using the same study materials and consulting with the researchers from the original study can help minimize the differences between the original and follow-up study though may not eliminate them; differences in the sample, setting and potentially in procedures remain. For studies that deliver interventions using verbal rather than written procedures, this issue may be greater with differences in the interactions between participants and researchers as well as the sequence, timing and duration of behavior change techniques harder to control.
- *Design.* Between-subjects designs lead to different people being allocated to different conditions, and this can potentially contribute to some significant (and null) effects depending on who is allocated to which conditions. Within-subjects designs are helpful here as the

same participants are used in each condition acting, in effect, as their own control.

- *Underpowered studies/publication of marginal findings.* It has been argued that the vast majority of psychology studies are underpowered (about 7 out of 8 according to Stanley et al., 2018). In their paper, the Open Science Collaboration (2015) reported that while 63% of studies replicated (achieved $p < .05$ in the replication attempt) when the original finding had a p-value below .001; only 18% replicated when the p-value was greater than .04.

- *Publication bias/file drawer problem.* The overwhelming amount of studies that are published report at least some positive effects. Studies with purely null effects are difficult to publish and researchers may be less inclined to try to publish them. Null effects are important as they can provide evidence regarding what does not work. In health behavior change terms, this is important because investing in interventions or techniques that are not effective is wasteful in terms of resources.

- *Human error and inter-researcher variability.* Individuals and research teams are not infallible, they can make mistakes. For instance, in a study that required 85 independent research teams to try to replicate the results of a study by reconducting analyses based on either transparent information (which even included the statistical code used by the original authors) or less clear information (the methods section of the report, rough description of the results and no code for analyses), 4.3% and 10.7% did not replicate the same p-value and sign, respectively (Breznau et al., 2021). This error rate increased to nearly 25% and over 50%, respectively, if numbers were compared to the second decimal place. Breznau et al. also highlight variation across research groups that can lead to differences in findings such as how missing data is treated or how certain variables are coded, prior experience with particular statistical tests/packages as well as use of different statistical packages. The example here relates to just a couple of steps of the research process (statistical analyses conduct and reporting) with errors and variability possible throughout the research chain.

How can issues around replicability be addressed?

- *Adopting more stringent significance level thresholds.* By requiring tests to achieve lower significance levels (e.g., $p < .01$) the risk of false positives (detecting a significant effect in error) is reduced.

- *Using a-priori powered/more powerful original studies.* Planning the required sample size for a study in advance of actually conducting the study (i.e., a-priori) and then sticking to this target sample size is important to ensure that studies are not underpowered (such studies provide ambiguous evidence) and prevents researchers from continuing to collect data until at least some of their effects become significant. Such processes can inflate effect size estimates, meaning that researchers attempting to replicate studies are anticipating finding larger effects than the size of the true effect, consequently underpower the study (as studies trying to find larger effects require fewer participants) with a high risk of not replicating the results of a previous study.
- *Preregistration and better reporting.* Templates such as the PRP-Quant Template (Bosnjak et al., 2022) provide guidance on what information to preregister covering things like how to deal with participants who drop out during the study, missing data and planned exclusions (e.g., because responses were too fast, outliers, etc.) in the analyses. Reporting checklists can ensure that all key information is reported in articles.
- *Open Science can facilitate sharing of materials and datasets to* facilitate replication attempts and the verification of analyses by others, respectively.
- *Automate research processes* and be aware of how characteristics of the experimenter and aspects of the testing environment can impact on how similar replication attempts are to the original study (Ellefson & Oppenheimer, in press). Variations in the characteristics of the experimenter (e.g., how friendly they are, how clearly they speak, how attentive they are to following the experimental procedures) and the testing environment (e.g., time of the day or temperature can lead to participants being more or less tired and stressed which impacts how attentive they are). Blinding researchers can reduce the risk of treating participants in different conditions in different ways (beyond the manipulation) to influence their responses or how decisions around analyses are made.
- *Multiple replication attempts.* One replication attempt is insufficient to conclusively determine whether an effect is meaningful or negligible; multi-site replication attempts can provide much more confidence.
- *Incentivizing and facilitating publication of papers reporting exclusively null findings* is important given the importance of null

findings. This is likely challenging; researchers have limited time, so they are inclined to focus their efforts on publishing work that has produced significant effects that are likely to be better received and easier to publish. General incentivization of researchers (e.g., from virtual badges to promotion/recruitment decisions) can encourage them to engage in open science practices.

- *The Transparency and Openness Promotion (TOP) Guidelines* provide a set of standards that academic journals can sign up to show the steps they have taken to implement open science practices such as posting data, analysis code and materials to a trusted repository, requiring study preregistration and enabling registered reports for replication studies and having reporting guidelines. Journals requiring such standards enable and promote the awareness and uptake of open science practices towards a 'new norm'.
- *There have been calls for better training in methods and statistics* for researchers and/or involving methodologists/independent overseers (Munafo et al., 2017).

Will the suggested approaches fix the problem?

The promising news is that when studies showing novel findings adopt optimal methods, including pre-registration and large samples (around 1,500+), they can be replicated much more often. For example, Protzko et al. (2020) reported that over 86% of these types of studies were replicated (achieving $p < .05$) and their effect sizes were around 97% of the original effect sizes. For anybody who likes cookies, one of these studies found that people who are offered free cookies and take three of the same kind are viewed as greedier than somebody who takes three different types of cookie!

Less promising is that, despite preregistration, sometimes studies deviate from the preregistration to the published study suggesting that some issues remain. For instance, in a review of 136 registered trials with publications between the years 2011–2015, only 16 of the publications were both registered before the study began and reported outcomes and methods that were consistent with the preregistration (Taylor & Gorman, 2022). It is possible that these issues are now less pronounced. Moreover, these issues are not limited to psychology. For instance, the COMPare (CEBM Outcome Monitoring Project) has shined a light on these issues in relation to clinical trials.

Are there any drawbacks to open science and other issues noted above?

Some researchers may be reluctant to share materials and datafiles that they have developed and resourced (in terms of time, energy and funds). Furthermore, by making data open-access and available to all, there is an increased risk that others use the datafile for "redundant or inappropriate question formulation or data analysis activities" (Hekler & King, 2020).

A movement to lower p-value thresholds from .05 can lead to less power and increased Type II errors (failing to find an effect in a sample when it should exist). This is problematic as, it has been argued, null effects are less likely to be subjected to replication attempts than significant effects so false negatives remain. As Carlin et al. (in press) argue, trying to resolve the replication crisis may contribute to a Type 2 error crisis.

To better address the issue of poor reporting regarding the content of interventions, an extension of one of the CONSORT items (item 5) was made in the form of the Template for Intervention Description and Replication (TIDieR; Hoffmann et al., 2012). This 12-item checklist attempts to ensure that authors consistently report more detailed information regarding the content of interventions to help ensure that the intervention can be implemented by others (e.g., clinicians) and researchers can replicate or build on the reported interventions. The checklist includes items relating to what content was delivered (including any physical or informational materials used with electronic links to the full set of

BURNING ISSUE BOX 5.5

WHAT ARE PLACEBO AND NOCEBO EFFECTS AND CAN THEY AFFECT HEALTH EQUITY?

Placebo effects relate to individuals in a "control" group who respond positively to an inert drug, sham device or medical intervention; nocebo effects are the equivalent but represent negative symptoms or effects. Whether placebo or nocebo effects emerge have been argued to be driven in some way by the patients' expectations and whether these are beneficial (for placebo) or harmful (for nocebo).

In their review of the literature, Webster et al. (2016) overview three broad factors that can lead to nocebo effects: negative expectations (arising from how the treatment has been communicated or other factors related to the individual such as their level of pessimism), misattribution (where symptoms that existed before are misattributed to the new treatment) and learning (e.g., through observing how others who have been treated in the same way respond). Following their review of 89 studies, they concluded that the strongest predictors of nocebo effects were patients perceiving they had taken a higher dose, explicit suggestions that the treatment leads to symptoms or arousal, seeing how others respond to the same treatment and having higher expectations of symptoms.

Given nocebo effects can be influenced by factors related to negative expectations, and negative expectations can be influenced by how the treatment is communicated to patients (including the communication style, attitudes and subtle cues from the healthcare provider), past experiences or observing others go through the same treatment, there is a risk of inequity if these factors vary across different groups of patients (Yetman et al., 2021).

materials), as well as who provided it, how, where, when, how much and why (including reference to any underlying theory). In addition, the TIDieR checklist includes items relating to tailoring (i.e., whether the materials were personalized in any way), any modifications made, and intervention adherence/fidelity (the extent to which the intervention was delivered as planned).

CONSENSUS METHODS

There are different types of consensus methods such as nominal group technique, Delphi, RAND/UCLA appropriateness method and consensus development panels or conferences each of which involves experts attempting to form agreement, or consensus, regarding a particular topic.

The nominal group technique is a structured, face-to-face, small group discussion that first requires individuals to work independently in addressing the problem and write down their ideas before these ideas are recorded in a "round robin" format with each person sharing an idea in turn for later group discussion/grouping of ideas and clarifications, before ranking/voting of the top ideas and final group discussion of the results.

The Delphi method is typically run remotely over several weeks with multiple rounds of voting. In the first stage, participants respond to a series of Likert-type questions adding, where necessary, written comments should they feel like they wish to justify their response or to note that the item is not relevant or unclear. In a second round, participants respond to the same questions but this time with information about how they responded individually last time, how the group responded on average and relevant text comments that were provided by the group in the first round. There can be multiple rounds until consensus (ideally based on a pre-specified criteria) is reached. By using questionnaires, the approach can maintain anonymity.

The RAND/UCLA appropriateness method combines elements of both the nominal group technique and Delphi and aims to combine the latest scientific evidence and expert opinion. To ascertain the latest scientific evidence, the approach begins with a literature review of the evidence. The results of the review are then sent to the panel members along with a series of statements that are rated on 1–9 scales, in terms of appropriateness, individually at home without input from others. In the second round, participants receive their original responses and those of the group, and then these are discussed as a group face-to-face, focusing on disagreements, before re-rating. Additional rounds may take place to consider necessity. On the scales, average ratings of at least 7 are needed to be judged appropriate or necessary. It has been described more as a technique to identify when experts agree rather than for the experts to reach a consensus.

Consensus development panels typically involve experts meeting in person, discussing the issues at hand and reaching agreement. They have been used to develop influential guidelines such as CONSORT guidelines for report-ing (as covered earlier in this chapter).

Which of these approaches is taken can depend on a range of factors including the goal of the project and resources available. For example, if the generation and exploration of ideas is important than the nominal group technique is useful as idea generation is an important aspect. If the goal is to develop guidelines than the Delphi method or consensus development panels may be more useful. The Delphi method can be flexible as it does not require face-to-face meetings but can take place over a longer period of time; consensus development panels and the nominal group technique can be quicker but potentially more expensive if conducted in person.
The advantages and disadvantages of consensus methods are overviewed in Critical Skills Toolkit 5.7.

CRITICAL SKILLS TOOLKIT 5.7

ADVANTAGES AND DISADVANTAGES OF CONSENSUS METHODS

Advantages

1. Can be a useful means to form agreement in areas where empirical evidence is lacking.
2. Can be used to generate a lot of ideas or comments including potentially minority views that can be considered to some degree.
3. Can be a relatively quick method to draw upon the views and opinions of a range of experts to form influential guidance.
4. Given advances in technology, hosting consensus panels online rather than in-person can reduce costs substantially.

Disadvantages

1. Consensus methods are often seen as being a "fall back" or "low quality" option where other, more "credible" or "rigorous" methods are not suitable.
2. In the absence of clear guidelines about how different types of consensus methods should be conducted, there has been wide variability in how researchers have used these methods *and* how the outcomes or processes have been reported.
3. It is not always clear which consensus method is the best to use and when.
4. It can be difficult to know how many people and/or rounds are needed to form a consensus. This can be particularly difficult if the panel comprises of different groups of people (e.g., patients, researchers, policymakers, healthcare professionals, etc.). If the panels are too large or heterogeneous then communication can be difficult; if they are too small they become less representative and potentially less creative.
5. Consensus development panels or conferences can be dominated by a few vocal members (we've all been in scenarios like that) though this is less true of other methods (e.g., nominal group technique). Relatedly, the outcomes can be driven by who is and who is not involved.
6. By selecting who is and who is not involved, there is a risk that these methods lead to inequity.

7. Approaches that show participants how their responses compare to the average response of others can encourage artificial agreement, lessen diversity in views and remove outlying perspectives. Methods that include divergent views have been encouraged (e.g., Blazey et al., 2022).
8. Reliability/validity of the outcomes from such methods are not always assessed.

N-OF-1 STUDIES

The majority of methods used in psychology focus on comparing groups of individuals against other groups of individuals. Specifically, they're focused on differences or changes *between* individuals (e.g., which individuals smoke and which do not?). An important aspect to consider are changes *within* individuals (e.g., when does an individual smoke a cigarette and when do they not?). More generally, what leads an individual to do specific health behaviors at some points but not others? How long after a change in a determinant does change in health behavior occur? Given psychological models relevant to health behaviors concern individuals there is clear potential for N-of-1 studies.

N-of-1 studies (also known as "single case studies") involve repeated measurements of an individual or a cluster of individuals (e.g., a family) to test the effects of interventions (in N-of-1 *experimental* trials) or to consider the interrelationships between variables that do not involve a manipulation or intervention (in N-of-1 *observational* studies). They often make use of **ecological momentary assessment** which can assess people's thoughts, feelings and behaviors in real time in their own natural environment outside of the laboratory. In experimental studies, participants can be given different behavior change techniques (BCTs) in a fixed or random order to work out which BCTs work best for them. In observational studies, N-of-1 studies can help unpick which variables precede others (e.g., does anxiety lead to more chocolate consumption and/or does scoffing more chocolate increase anxiety?), as well as identify the time lags and/or strength of relationships over time between determinants and behaviors or other outcomes.

Analyzing data from N-of-1 studies can bring some challenges. For example, there may be time-related patterns within the dataset and periodic or cyclical processes such as time of day, day of the week, menstrual cycles or weather season: people may be in a more positive or negative mood depending on the time of day (one of the authors, Andrew, for example, tends to feel better in the afternoon or evening compared to the morning!)

or whether it's a weekday or weekend. Unless the researcher accounts for such patterns, incorrect conclusions can be drawn. Another issue is that how somebody responds earlier can influence how they respond later. For example, how depressed somebody is on one day can be associated with how depressed they were the day before. In such instances, the datapoints are not independent of one another and this violates an important assumption of some statistical tests. Fortunately, time–series analyses techniques exist to deal with these types of issues. McDonald et al. (2020) provide a useful overview of how to analyze data from N-of-1 studies that work around these types of issues. There are other useful resources related to N-of-1 studies that can support the design, conduct and reporting of such studies (see https://www.nof1sced.org/) which includes links to approaches to evaluate the risk of bias in these types of studies such as the RoBiNT scale (Tate et al., 2013). The CONSORT guidelines have been extended to support the reporting of N-of-1 trials (CENT) and there is a single case reporting guideline for behavioral interventions (SCRIBE).

CRITICAL SKILLS TOOLKIT 5.8

ADVANTAGES AND DISADVANTAGES OF N-OF-1 STUDIES

Advantages

1. *A different type of change.* Allows consideration of changes *within* individuals; this is important because theories concern individuals.
2. *Flexibility.* They can be used to consider: a) how determinants (e.g., motivation), behaviors (e.g., whether somebody exercises or not) and other types of health outcomes (e.g., symptoms) change over the time; b) relationships between variables (e.g., do intentions predict behavior?) including how they vary over time and c) the effect of interventions on psychological variables and behavioral outcomes in individuals.
3. *Focus on individuals.* Experimental studies focused on groups may indicate that a particular intervention or behavior change strategy works, on average, for the group. However, this can mask the fact that some individuals may not benefit or are adversely affected. N-of-1 methods circumvent this issue by looking at the effects of interventions on individuals rather than groups.

4. *Tailoring.* By identifying which predictors or determinants of behavior are important for one person (e.g., negative feeling states), and which predictors or determinants are important for another person (e.g., feelings of self-efficacy), they can help to inform interventions tailored to an individual's needs.

5. *Precision.* Rather than relying on people to recall what they did in the past or how they feel on average, N-of-1 studies utilize methods (e.g., Ecological Momentary Assessment) to make these types of assessment in real-time, which can enhance the accuracy of measurement.

6. *Ecological validity.* Another advantage of using methods which assess individuals' thoughts, feelings and behaviors in real time, in their own environment (such as ecological momentary assessments) is that it helps to maximize ecological validity.

7. *Timely.* Given technological developments that enable collation of huge amounts of data from an individual over time, N-of-1 studies are well-positioned to make use of such developments.

8. *Useful when studying rare cases.* In instances where there are few eligible participants (e.g., who have a rare diseas), N-of-1 are a more appropriate option than alternatives that require many participants such as RCTs.

9. *Time and cost.* Given participants provide lots of data and data from multiple N-of-1 trials can, in some instances where they are sufficiently similar, be pooled, they can reduce time and cost.

Disadvantages

1. *Carryover effects.* By measuring an individual multiple times, and possibly subjecting them to multiple interventions to compare their effectiveness, these can have knock-on effects either directly or in some form of interaction with previous measures or manipulations. Put simply, what was found may be as a direct result of everything that came before (not just immediately before). This is particularly relevant here given that the goal of behavior change interventions and techniques is to obtain long-lasting changes in behavior and the determinants that cause behavior change.

2. *Unlikely to be suitable for many types of behavior change techniques.* Given the risk of carryover effects, BCTs that are likely to have a sustained effect over time or help an individual to learn

something (such as instructions or information on consequences) are unlikely to be testable using N-of-1 trials. BCTs that are time specific (such as using prompts and cues) or can be time-restricted in other ways (e.g., using goal setting over a set period of time) may be suitable, however (Kwasnicka et al., 2019).

3. *Compliance and missing data.* As the approach tends to be more intensive for individuals, relative to alternative methods of data collection, there are concerns that some studies can have issues with low compliance. This introduces complexities around how to deal with missing data, an under-researched area in the N-of-1 literature.

4. *Generalizability.* As these methods are focused on few individuals, it can be argued that the findings are less generalizable to groups of people than alternative methods. It should be noted, however, that methods can be applied to generalize findings from individuals to groups. For example, findings from multiple similar N-of-1 studies can be aggregated to consider differences between groups (as well as within individuals). Such approaches may be cheaper than running traditional RCTs.

5. *Power calculations can be complex.* For other types of studies, researchers calculate how many participants are needed in a particular study based on the underlying effect size, desired power and significance level. For N-of-1 trials, power is determined by the number of repeated assessments. Although there are tools out there to help calculate power for N-of-1 studies, they often require the researcher to use educated guesses for certain aspects of the calculation (although this is often true also for other types of designs such as RCTs).

6. *Evidence base.* For certain types of N-of-1 studies (e.g., intervention studies that test multiple interventions within the same participants), there are relatively few published studies (Kwasnicka et al., 2019).

MEGASTUDIES

At the other end of the spectrum to N-of-1 studies are megastudies. Megastudies are a new type of approach that addresses the problem of trying to compare and combine results from several studies that may test different behavior change techniques or the same behavior change techniques using different measures, forms (e.g., type of delivery) and timeframes. Rather than test different techniques in different studies or the same techniques multiple times, a megastudy throws everything into the mix by evaluating different manipulations or interventions at the same time using the same outcome measures. Megastudies have been conducted to identify, for example, that strategies such as providing microrewards for returning to the gym after missed sessions appears helpful for exercise promotion while many other strategies do not (Milkman et al., 2021).

CRITICAL SKILLS TOOLKIT 5.9

ADVANTAGES AND DISADVANTAGES OF MEGASTUDIES

Advantages

1. *Comparability of interventions.* As outcomes and other study features are matched, relative to collating evidence across studies, it is easier to make comparisons of different interventions or behavior change techniques.
2. *Power and accuracy of estimate of effect size.* Given the large number of participants involved, there will be large amounts of statistical power and the estimated effect size of a particular intervention or behavior change technique (under the specific conditions of the study) will be more precise.
3. *Reducing the file drawer.* Given significant results are more likely to be published, by simultaneously testing a large number of interventions, details regarding those that "do not work" are published alongside those that do.
4. *Aids efficiency.* They can be used to, relatively quickly, identify strong candidates for potentially effective techniques (at least compared to conducting multiple studies each testing one intervention at a time). The results from these megastudies can be further evaluated in follow-up trials rather than interventions that may be likely to be less effective.

Disadvantages

1. *Expensive.* Recruiting thousands of participants into a trial is costly not just financially but also in terms of time and effort.
2. *Generalizability.* Compared to collating data from smaller studies that each test the same behavior change technique in slightly

different contexts and/or using different outcomes in different samples over different timeframes, the generalizability of the findings from a megastudy is weaker.

3. *Choice of comparator.* While a megastudy can be used to compare different behavioral interventions against one another, to test whether an intervention works, there is still a need to select a control or comparison group. If this comparison group also contains effective behavior change content, otherwise effective behavior change interventions may appear to be ineffective.

4. Effect sizes of top-performing interventions will likely be overestimated, and effect sizes for the worst-performing interventions will likely be underestimated (Milkman et al., 2021).

SYSTEMATIC REVIEWS AND META-ANALYSES

Systematic reviews identify a set of studies tackling a specific issue (e.g., ways to prevent young adults from exceeding the speed limit while driving) and then attempt to synthesize evidence from these studies. A systematic review follows various stages.

First, researchers think about the topic they wish to review as well as the type of studies (e.g., RCTs, qualitative studies, etc.) and populations that they wish to investigate. This then leads to a research question defined in terms of the Population, Intervention, Comparator, Outcome and Study design (PICOS). In accordance with these, the reviewer will produce a set of search terms that they will enter into database search engines (such as PsycINFO, Embase or Medline) to identify a set of studies that are potentially of interest. These search terms are used to look for articles within database search engines that use those specific terms (typically in their title or abstract). An example of this is "Do competition-based interventions (I), compared to interventions not comprising this technique (C), increase physical activity (O) in adults (P) based on randomized trials (S)?" Search terms would be included relating to the intervention (competition), outcome (physical activity) and study design (randomized controlled trials). In this example, as the comparator is not a specific intervention (it is an intervention that just doesn't comprise competition), adding terms to reflect a comparator would likely restrict the number of studies identified in your review in a way that it misses eligible studies; not a good idea! You may add terms relating to the population (adults) but given studies may not specify terms related to "adults" in their title or abstract, you may be best advised not to use terms linked to adults for the same reason (i.e., you'll miss eligible studies). Once you have developed a provisional set of search terms, the PRESS checklist can be used to help ensure that the quality and comprehensiveness of the search is as high as possible.

Next, screening the potential papers identified by the search terms against inclusion/exclusion criteria allows the systematic reviewer to decide which studies should be included in their review and which studies should be excluded (e.g., because they do not address the topic of interest, do not include the relevant population of people or do not employ the desired methods). Once the reviewer has identified the studies that meet the desired criteria, information (data) from each study can be taken.

In a systematic review, the same types of information should be consistently taken (extracted) from each paper. To help reviewers to do this, a data extraction sheet (listing various items relating to the conduct of the study, the population tested, how the manipulation was delivered, the methodological quality of the study, the study findings, etc.) is typically used. The data extracted as part of this process will then be brought together (synthesized) to draw overall conclusions on the basis of the studies included in the review. When this synthesis is statistical, the review becomes a **meta-analysis**. Meta-analyses are statistical versions of systematic reviews in which the results (effect sizes) across various studies are combined and contrasted (see Chapter 6 for further details).

REPORTING AND RISK OF BIAS

Similar to the CONSORT guidelines which encourage the standard reporting of key methodological details from RCTs, the PRISMA (Preferred Reporting Items for Systematic Reviews and Meta-Analyses) statement encourages the standard reporting of key methodological details for systematic reviews and meta-analyses such as how the studies were selected, how the results from the studies were synthesized and the risk of bias of the studies. The PRISMA guidelines were updated in 2020 to accommodate advances in technology (e.g., using machine learning to help identify eligible studies) and methods (e.g., how to synthesize evidence when meta-analyses are not possible such as Synthesis Without Meta-Analysis (with the pretty neat acronym, SWiM); and new methods to assess risk of bias such as the Cochrane Risk of Bias Tool v2 and ROBINS-I to evaluate bias in non-randomized trials).

In addition to such advances and methods to evaluate the studies included *within* systematic reviews (i.e., the primary studies), there are also methods now to assess the methodological quality of the systematic review itself

(AMSTAR-2) and the risk of bias within the review (ROBIS). AMSTAR-2 contains items relating to things like whether the search strategy was comprehensive, whether one or more reviewers independently screened papers to identify whether studies are eligible or not and likewise, when extracting data from included studies, was this done by one person or in duplicate and, if so, was agreement sufficient (at least 80%)? ROBIS has items that cover whether there is likely to be bias in the study eligibility criteria (e.g., were the eligibility criteria ambiguous in any way?), study identification (e.g., were an appropriate range of databases used? Were the search terms likely to identify as many eligible studies as possible?), data collection/study appraisal (e.g., were attempts made to minimize inaccuracies in risk of bias assessment?) and synthesis (e.g., Was there little variation between the studies synthesized and, if not, was this addressed in the analyses?).

INTERVENTION SYNTHESIS

Once a systematic review or meta-analysis has been completed, how should its results be used? This is an important question to address to ensure that the evidence gathered from the review/meta-analysis is appropriately used to develop or implement evidence-based health behavior change interventions. Typically, in this field, a systematic review or meta-analysis is based on poorly reported descriptions of health behavior change interventions (problem 1) and different studies have closely related but rarely identical interventions which may differ in various ways such as intensity of intervention (how often and how frequently an individual is exposed to a particular intervention component), setting (e.g., hospital, school, community) or mode of delivery (e.g., leaflet, mobile app) (problem 2). As a result, people (clinicians, researchers, etc.) who would like to develop and deliver a specific health behavior change intervention on the basis of the findings of the review/meta-analyses have a difficult task in deciding what to implement. **Intervention synthesis**, described by Glasziou, Chalmers, Green, and Michie (2014), is a process to help translate the results from systematic reviews into practical treatments. Glasziou et al. (2014) highlight three basic approaches to intervention synthesis:

1. Single Trial-Based Choice
    An intervention is developed based on only one study included in the review. The intervention selected has the best trade-off between factors such as likely effectiveness, acceptability, feasibility and cost. The selection criteria regarding which intervention to choose should be made explicit and it should also be established who will rank the trial

interventions and how consensus will be achieved. When considering the effect sizes from single trials, one should also take into account the sample size from the trial and, where possible, try to avoid basing decisions on a single trial with a small sample size (larger sample sizes will provide a more precise estimate of the effect size). Relative to the other approaches (Common Components Hybrid & Model-Guided Synthesis), the Single Trial-Based Choice approach requires the least effort.

2. Common Components Hybrid
   Rather than selecting a complete intervention as used in a previous study, this approach leads to a "new" intervention based on various components (e.g., specific behavior change techniques (see Chapter 3), mode, intensity, etc.), picked and mixed from various studies included in the systematic review. One way to do this is to specify the requisite information using relevant taxonomies (e.g., BCTv1; Michie et al. 2013) and then use statistical approaches (e.g., meta-regression) to identify the effective ingredients that could be combined in the "new" intervention. For this approach to work, there needs to be a sufficient number of studies with the relevant information regarding components clearly reported.

3. Model Guided Synthesis
   This approach is a variant of the Common Components Hybrid approach but draws on theory to determine which components should be combined and how. Like the Common Components Hybrid approach, it requires a sufficient number of studies to be included in the review that clearly reports the components of the intervention. In addition, across the studies included in the review, there should be tests of all of the relevant elements of the theory/model so that the studies in the review can be used to test the theory. If supported, the theory can then be used to guide the selection of the intervention components.

QUALITATIVE METHODS

Qualitative methods allow behavioral scientists to go beyond numbers. Behavioral scientists can collect qualitative data using open-ended questions through methods such as interviews or focus groups. Whereby more quantitative methods attempt to minimize the impact of the researcher, qualitative methods tend to embrace more the role of the researcher. The focus of qualitative work can be broader and more process oriented, exploring the experiences of participants in a non-judgmental fashion and from this generate theories, whereas quantitative methods are narrower in scope, focused on testing hypotheses and controlling extraneous variables in an attempt to provide concrete answers.

Although qualitative methods have been traditionally viewed as something that is most relevant at the start of the research process, in the context of health behavior change, qualitative methods can be helpful throughout the process. As well as helping to understand the problem or difficulties to be addressed, they can help to understand the context within which an intervention will be delivered including potential barriers, identify potential solutions or intervention components from a range of stakeholders, as well as identify issues with implementing behavior change interventions. For example, they can help to figure out whether health behavior interventions were unsuccessful because they were not implemented correctly and help to understand why such difficulties emerged. Thus, qualitative methods can be of use throughout the research lifecycle from study or intervention development to evaluation and implementation.

Qualitative methods can take different forms including written responses to open questions in surveys and case studies. However, for the purpose of this chapter, we focus on two common methods: interviews and focus groups.

INTERVIEWS

Interviews are a classic form of qualitative method that involves researchers asking questions of their participants. These can range from being very unstructured (much like a conversation between the interviewer and interviewee) to very structured (where the interviewer follows a strict schedule of questions only). Semi-structured interviews, where a set of questions is used only as a guide for discussion and can be deviated from, are often utilized.

CRITICAL SKILLS TOOLKIT 5.10

ADVANTAGES AND DISADVANTAGES OF INTERVIEWS

Advantages

1. It can be a quick and relatively cheap way to obtain in-depth data.
2. Can be useful for obtaining detailed information regarding a little known topic; sometimes few people are affected by the issue/illness, so obtaining detailed information from a small number of interviewees can be vital.
3. Can be a way of identifying unexpected but useful information regarding a topic; highlighting ideas and issues not previously considered by the research team.

4. The process (e.g., being directly asked questions on a topic and perhaps challenged to explain or justify their views) may help participants to strengthen or change their views on topics or issues that they were uncertain about.

5. Compared to focus groups, they can be more flexible to organize as multiple diaries do not need to be managed.

Disadvantages

1. Some participants may be reluctant to disclose information in interviews, particularly when done face-to-face where anonymity is not maintained.

2. How successful these are might be dependent on the skills and characteristics of the interviewer (e.g., whether or not they're perceived to be warm and friendly).

3. Data may vary depending on the context within which the interviews took place. What an individual says in a GP practice may differ to what they say at home, for example.

4. Transcribing and analyzing interviews can be time-consuming and complex.

5. Confidentiality can sometimes be difficult to maintain. This issue can arise, for example, if the people interviewed are prominent, well-recognized figures or what they said is intrinsically linked to something else (e.g., job role) that is unique to one person in the sample.

FOCUS GROUPS

Focus groups are an alternative to interviews that involve discussion between a group of people around a topic selected by the research team. They are run by a moderator who leads the discussion and keeps it on track (focused on achieving the research goals) and often an observer who monitors non-verbal aspects of the group. Ideally, members of the focus groups should feel comfortable and interested enough to contribute to discussion as well as feel equal to one another to avoid power imbalances. This can be aided by ensuring that the group is somewhat homogeneous on certain important characteristics; which characteristics are important depends on the topic and goals of the research. Conversely, the group should be somewhat heterogeneous to encourage different viewpoints.

Focus group moderators should try to facilitate rather than dictate, introducing a particular topic and letting the participants freely discuss it rather than asking each participant sets of questions. The dynamics and interactions at play are between the moderator and participants as well as between the participants themselves with the latter being of particular interest (Acocella, 2012). The moderator needs to ensure that interactions between the participants themselves (rather than the moderator and each individual participant) is most prominent. It is generally recommended, in order to help with confidentiality, that individuals in focus groups do not know each other beforehand and that between 8–10 people is ideal (though generally 4–12 people take part in typical focus groups; Secor, 2010).

CRITICAL SKILLS TOOLKIT 5.11

ADVANTAGES AND DISADVANTAGES OF FOCUS GROUPS

Advantages

1. It can be a quick and a relatively cheap way to obtain in-depth data.
2. Compared to individual interviews, the information generated can be more in-depth because points raised by members of the focus group may prompt/cue additional points within participants that may not have emerged in individual interviews.
3. As they involve multiple people, they can give insight into how certain topics are debated between people.
4. Can be useful for obtaining detailed information regarding a little known topic; sometimes few people are affected by the issue/illness, so obtaining detailed information from this small pool of people can be vital.
5. Can be a useful way of identifying unexpected but useful information regarding a topic; bringing ideas and issues not previously considered by the research team.
6. In a similar vein, the process (e.g., being challenged by others to explain or justify their views) may help participants to strengthen or change their views on topics or issues that they were uncertain about.

Disadvantages

1. They can be difficult to run and coordinate given the involvement of several people. Sometimes, because participants needed for focus groups need to represent particular roles/jobs (e.g., bosses

of companies; line managers, etc.), the participant pool might be restricted making the project unfeasible or difficult to recruit into.
2. Given the social elements to the method, participants may be reluctant to share particular views and opinions, especially if they perceive these to be divergent from the rest of the group. This can lead to overly conformed viewpoints.
3. Particular dynamics within the group (certain people dictating conversation; certain participants being unable to get their views or points out quickly enough before the discussion moves on) can influence the data generated.
4. They may be anxiety-inducing for some participants.
5. They may not be suitable for topics that can be particularly sensitive.
6. Transcribing and analyzing focus group discussions can be time-consuming and complex.
7. Confidentiality can be difficult to ensure given the involvement of multiple interacting participants.

REPORTING

As with quantitative-based methods, reporting guidelines exist for studies that use qualitative methods. COREQ (Tong, Sainsbury & Craig, 2007) is a checklist comprising 32 items that covers characteristics of the research team and their relationship with participants, theoretical framework (e.g., grounded theory, content analysis), participant selection, setting, data collection (e.g., interview guide, duration), data analysis (e.g., software used, number of data coders) and reporting (e.g., were quotes used to illustrate themes?, were themes clearly presented?). A more recent guideline, SRQR, was also developed for reporting of qualitative research (O'Brien et al., 2014). Most recently, the American Psychological Association (APA) developed guidelines for qualitative primary studies, qualitative meta-analysis and mixed methods research (Levitt et al., 2018).

CRITICAL SKILLS TOOLKIT 5.12

ADVANTAGES AND DISADVANTAGES OF QUALITATIVE METHODS IN GENERAL

Advantages

1. Qualitative-based studies tend to be based on fewer people than quantitative studies so could be more straightforward in terms of recruiting participants and running studies.

2. Despite being based on fewer people, qualitative methods can lead to "rich" (in-depth) data-sets that can be used to uncover more about people and their experiences.
3. On the basis of uncovering such experiences, qualitative methods can be used to generate hypotheses (that could be tested through other methods such as experimental approaches).
4. They may offer unique insights and theories and thus can be complementary to quantitative methods.

Disadvantages

1. A drawback of being based on fewer participants is that it can be more difficult to make generalizations about how your data applies to other people.
2. Can be difficult to analyze and can rely on differing levels of subjectivity; different analyzers may draw different interpretations from the data (this can also be true of quantitative methods).
3. Questions can be leading and this can threaten validity.
4. People who participate in qualitative-based studies (such as interviews or focus groups), and are particularly vocal in such studies, may not be very representative of other groups of people. This reflects potential risks of sampling bias.
5. How people respond in qualitative studies can be influenced by the social context. While this can be seen as advantageous, social desirability (responding in a way that they feel they should) can be a problem causing people to be reluctant to give their true, personal opinion.

GUIDANCE FOR INTERVENTION DEVELOPMENT AND EVALUATION

In this section, we will cover some guidance and recommendations for developing and evaluating health behavior change interventions. The UK Medical Research Council (MRC) updated their guidance for developing and evaluating complex interventions in 2021. Behavior change interventions are typically complex, comprising different behavior change techniques, delivered in different contexts (e.g., different settings, different modes, to and from different people) and potentially tackling multiple behaviors so these guidelines can be useful in the area of health behavior change.

The MRC guidance was updated to incorporate four different questions, four different phases of research and six different components to be incorporated in each phase.

Questions: The MRC guidance differentiates between four different types of questions relating to efficacy (does an intervention work in ideal/experimental/tightly controlled settings?), effectiveness (does an intervention work in the real-world?), theory (what works in an intervention, when and why?) and systems (how does the intervention and the context in which it is delivered/received impact one another?).

Phases: It also notes four phases of research: development or identification of the intervention (identifying an existing intervention and considering how it will be evaluated, developing a new intervention, refining an existing one for a new context); feasibility testing (is the intervention and how it will be tested feasible and acceptable?); evaluation of the intervention; and implementation of the intervention (how can the impact of an intervention be enhanced and how can uptake of the intervention be encouraged in practice?). The four phases do not need to be completed sequentially and it is possible to start at any phase depending on what is already known and where the key problem lies.

Components: Each of the four phases has the following six components relating to 1) considering context (e.g., different physical, social and cultural contexts can influence whether an intervention is likely to work or not); 2) program theory (outlining how and when an intervention is likely to have an effect); 3) stakeholder involvement (involving patient and healthcare professionals, policymakers, etc.); 4) working out what is unknown or uncertain; 5) intervention refinement; and 6) economic factors (e.g., do the benefits outweigh the costs?). It is expected that all six components will be considered before moving to the next step or going back to a previous step (as frustrating as that might be, it may be necessary for achieving an effective and impactful intervention for health behavior change!).

ADAPTING INTERVENTIONS TO NEW CONTEXTS

Is it easier to take an intervention that has evidence to support its use in one context (e.g., to promote physical activity in low-income women from the United States who have recently given birth) and apply it, with relevant adaptations, to a new context (e.g., to promote physical activity in low-income women from a different country who have recently given birth) or develop a new intervention from scratch? Part of the answer may lie in how similar or different the two contexts are and how easy it is to adapt the intervention to the new context: Would the intervention fit with local norms? Will people delivering/receiving the intervention in the new context find the intervention acceptable? Is the intervention similar to what has been used in the new context in the past given similar interventions may be easier to implement?

The ADAPT guidance (Moore et al., 2021) was recently developed to provide a framework for how candidate interventions can be first identified, later adapted to fit a new context (e.g., to work with a different population or setting), evaluated, implemented and later reported. These adaptations can be made before the intervention is delivered or later, while the intervention is being delivered, to adapt to any changes in the context. Throughout, the involvement of stakeholders (including those with expert knowledge of the intervention and its evidence base (perhaps researchers) and those who understand the new context (perhaps patients, members of the public, policymakers, etc.) is critical and can often make use of coproduction methods (see later in this chapter).

ADAPT guidance points to following four key steps which are also overviewed in Figure 5.3:

> Step 1: *Rationale for intervention and intervention-context fit.* What is the problem that is being addressed and why is intervention needed? Does the team already have an intervention in mind and is this the best choice? If not, are there reviews comparing the effects of different interventions across relevant contexts available? How robust is the evidence that the intervention works in different contexts, or indeed works at all? Is a new review needed? Can process evaluations of interventions give insights into how the intervention worked and, if so, are these mechanisms likely to be relevant in the new context? How similar or different are the original and new contexts and can any differences likely affect how the intervention is implemented or how effective it is? For example, if the intervention is unlikely to be acceptable to those delivering or receiving the intervention, the implementation and ultimately the effectiveness of the intervention is likely to be adversely affected. Is there sufficient resource to deliver the intervention in the new context? Does it fit with the norms and delivery systems within the new context? Qualitative research (see earlier in this chapter) can be helpful in identifying similarities and differences across contexts and thus the possible adaptations required.
>
> Step 2: *Plan and make adaptations.* What are the factors that might impede or facilitate the translation of the existing intervention to the new context? Such factors could affect how effective the intervention is,

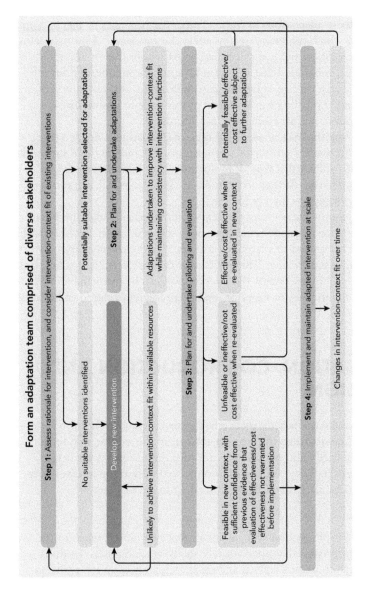

FIGURE 5.3 The ADAPT approach for adapting interventions to a new context.

Moore G., Campbell M., Copeland L., Craig P., Movsisyan A., Hoddinott P. et al. (2021). Adapting interventions to new contexts—the ADAPT guidance. BMJ, 374:n1679. doi:10.1136/bmj.n1679

how widely it's adopted, as well as how successfully it is implemented or maintained. A team is required to come up with a list of possible adaptations to ensure that any potential barriers are overcome and any potential facilitators are made use of. Do the intervention materials need to be adapted and what is the rationale for these changes? Are any of these adaptations likely to change the processes or mechanisms through which the interventions affect the outcome? Who will deliver the intervention and can this be achieved within their existing roles? It is also recommended that the team monitor throughout for any potential adverse consequences arising from the adapted intervention. Economic modelling can be useful at this stage to ensure that the intervention, and its evaluation, are affordable.

Step 3: *Piloting and evaluation.* What type of evaluation is needed (e.g., pilot, effectiveness, cost-effectiveness, process) and are there sufficient funds to conduct this type of evaluation? Can piloting be used to identify whether further adaptations are likely needed? Are further changes needed as the context changes?

Step 4: *Implement and maintain the adapted intervention at scale.* The intervention to be adapted should have been selected, in part, as it is scalable and can be applied to a large population. Are the partnerships between the various stakeholders sustainable over the long term and what plans are in place to ensure that the intervention can be maintained? What systems are in place to monitor long-term implementation and effects?

CO-CREATION, CO-PRODUCTION AND CO-DESIGN

Arguably these are not strictly methods. However, we were keen to cover **co-creation**, **co-production** and **co-design** in this edition due to their increasing popularity and potential to improve the relevance, quality and impact of research. They can be commonly used to develop interventions and may be particularly helpful when needing to develop new interventions.

Co-creation, co-production and co-design represent an approach to the whole research process that does not rely solely on researchers. In this approach, patients are not viewed as passive recipients of an intervention. Instead, patients along with other stakeholders/members of the "co-creation team" (e.g., researchers, patients, service providers, policymakers) play a key role in identifying and prioritizing the problem, contribute to design and deliver research to develop products or systems to address the problem and improve the healthcare experience. In addition, the team interprets, shares and implements the findings. The bottom line is that these approaches help to ensure the questions that matter to key people (e.g., patients, clinicians) are identified and addressed with workable solutions: more use, less waste.

Co-creation, co-production and co-design are often used interchangeably though they are distinguishable. Vargas et al. (2022) describe co-creation as an overarching term that incorporates both co-design and co-production. Co-design comes earlier in the process than co-production.

There is no fixed "one-size fits all" approach to co-design or co-production, so what follows in this section should be seen as a set of general, rather than prescriptive, principles and steps. Co-design begins with identifying relevant stakeholders as well as seeking opportunities where working collaboratively can be valuable, identifying relevant problems and solutions. For this to work effectively, there is a need to analyze and understand the various stakeholders' experiences and ideas and how the different groups work together. Next, the problems are prioritized and next steps and actions are outlined cumulating in a design, generation or selection of materials (e.g., selecting outcome measures that best represent the problem from the perspective of the users; ensuring the language used in the materials are appropriate for the target users), evaluation plan and allocation of resources in order to test the initiative/solution to the problem. Effectively, co-design covers the study planning phase rather than testing and would exclude recruitment, data collection and analysis and dissemination activities (Slattery et al., 2020). There are many methods that can be used for co-design including, but not limited to, interviews, surveys, focus groups, nominal group technique and Delphi methods (as covered earlier in this chapter).

Co-production involves the steps of testing the initiative, taking on-board feedback for implementation of the initiative in wider practice and suggestions for improvements. The final steps ensure the initiative is fully evaluated along with consideration of what can be learned from the various stakeholders in the previous steps and how the initiative can be sustained in the future.

In co-creation, the balance of power shifts from researchers to the team as a whole and, in this way, is different from a research project that just uses PPI (Patient & Public Involvement rather than Payment Protection Insurance). It requires the building of trust and mutual respect for the skills, knowledge and perspectives of each team member. It is thought that increasing the participation of key groups such as users (interventionists and patients or recipients) and policymakers can improve innovation, implementation and overall success of an intervention.

CRITICAL SKILLS TOOLKIT 5.13

ADVANTAGES AND DISADVANTAGES OF CO-CREATION, CO-DESIGN AND CO-PRODUCTION

Advantages

1. By involving a wider group of stakeholders throughout the process, the approach has the potential to improve the relevance (ensuring the intervention fits the context within which it will be applied), acceptability, quality and impact of the research.
2. Involving those who will ultimately use, deliver or receive the intervention/service/product should aid participant recruitment including for hard-to-reach groups.
3. By working together, there is the potential to build trust, empathy and understanding between researchers and other groups (e.g., service providers, service users, policymakers, etc.).
4. The approaches can be flexible to ensure it meets the needs of the various stakeholders and helps develop an initiative that is fit for context.
5. The approach has direct benefits for the users (e.g., patients) directly involved in the research process in terms of enhancing their understanding of the research process, being able to better manage their condition and reporting positive emotional responses to taking part.

Disadvantages

1. There is no fixed rule-book regarding how co-creation should be done, and no guidance on how many people should be involved (Slattery et al., 2020).
2. Relatively few studies have examined whether co-design/ co-production leads to better outcomes or tried to identify when it'd be useful and when it is not. Evaluations tend to use qualitative methods based on perceptions of benefit of the users and researchers (Slattery et al., 2020). Better quality evaluations – ideally pre-registered prior to the study – are needed.
3. Co-creation takes longer and requires more resources (including money) than other forms of research.
4. It may work well in some contexts but not others.

5. The process can be difficult and challenging in that divergent views can arise and need to be aligned. Sometimes researchers may need to forego academic rigor to meet the needs of the users.
6. Relatedly, if done badly, it can be a process that evokes conflict between the various groups of people involved and leads to frustration with voices not being heard. It is important to ensure that users involvement is not "tokenistic."
7. Co-production has rarely been used in low and middle-income countries; more than 98% of the literature has been focused on high-income countries (Ageypong et al., 2021).

ACCEPTABILITY

One of the potential advantages of co-creation methods for health behavior change is that it leads to interventions that are acceptable to the users (this could include those who are being targeted for health behavior change such as patients, as well as the those delivering the intervention such as healthcare professionals). But how do we know whether or not an intervention is acceptable?

When trying to answer whether an intervention is acceptable or not, we should first try to define what is meant by acceptability. Fortunately, Sekhon and colleagues help us here with the following formal definition: "A multi-faceted construct that reflects the extent to which people delivering or receiving a healthcare intervention consider it to be appropriate, based on anticipated or experienced cognitive and emotional responses to the intervention" (Sekhon et al., 2017). Their Theoretical Framework of Acceptability comprises of the following seven constructs:

- Affective attitude: the feelings somebody has regarding the intervention

- Burden: how much effort or burden somebody feels it takes to use the intervention

- Ethicality: whether or not the intervention is consistent with somebody's values

- Intervention coherence: whether an individual can understand the intervention and how to use it

- Opportunity costs: what are the costs to the individual of using the intervention?

- Perceived effectiveness: will the intervention be effective?

- Self-efficacy: does the individual feel that they have the ability to use the intervention?

These seven constructs are assessed in a measure of acceptability that comprises largely of single items for each construct (for ethicality and affective attitudes, researchers are offered a choice of using one of two items) plus an item assessing overall acceptability (Sekhon, Cartwright, & Francis, 2022).

Over time, studies can be conducted to identify which constructs in the Theoretical Framework of Acceptability are most strongly related with overall acceptability and help to identify at which thresholds an intervention becomes acceptable or unacceptable. The measure can be used to assess acceptability prospectively (before the intervention is used), concurrently (while using the intervention) and retrospectively (after the intervention has been used). This measure is offered as an alternative to other means of trying to infer acceptability such as dropout rates. While people may drop out of a study that tests an intervention because they find the intervention not acceptable, they may dropout for a host of other reasons (lack of time, illness, etc.). As such, assessing acceptability more directly through this questionnaire offers a convenient and potentially more useful alternative to ways in which acceptability has been considered in the past.

IMPLEMENTATION SCIENCE

So, you have developed an intervention that seems to work. It changes health behavior in the target sample, maybe a set of patients, university students or workplace employees, and this has been evidenced in studies such as randomized controlled trials. The next step is widespread implementation/worldwide dominance (well, not quite but you get the idea). How is this gap between identifying an effective intervention and implementing it on a bigger scale bridged? Is the intervention ready for implementation? How can the intervention be feasibly delivered, in an acceptable manner, consistently and as effectively on a sustained basis on the bigger stage to improve healthcare services? Can this be done within routine practice and can it be evaluated in routine practice? Can it be integrated into policy?

Implementation science deals with these type of issues described at multiple levels, taking into account the behaviors of various people at various levels of the healthcare system. Utilizing a range of methods highlighted in this chapter such as randomized controlled trials, questionnaires, qualitative methods, process evaluations and stakeholder engagement, as well as **pragmatic trials** (as defined by the **PRECIS-2** tool), it seeks to identify which behaviors to change in which people as well as potential barriers (and/or facilitators) to implementation. This is done for both those receiving or contributing in some way to the delivery of the intervention. When identifying behaviors to change, the potential impact of changing the behavior, as well as the ease of changing the behavior, and its underlying determinants, should be taken into account. Implementation scientists also develop and test strategies to overcome these barriers (or make use of the facilitators) in the real world.

To provide an illustration, healthcare professionals may be less likely to recommend or refer certain patients (e.g., from lower socio-economic groups; older patients, etc.) to particular programs. Possible solutions include automated referrals or prompts to the healthcare professional. Factors such as whether an individual can afford to travel to the treatment sessions or lack of childcare provision could be two barriers preventing access to treatment programs. Strategies to resolve these could include providing sessions online enabling wider access that does not require travel and may, in some circumstances, help address childcare issues.

Implementation interventions can be informed by behavior change theories (to identify intervention content and how an intervention might change behavior, i.e., mechanisms) as well as broader frameworks for intervention development such as the Behavior Change Wheel (see Chapter 2) and Intervention Mapping (see Chapter 4). These frameworks can be used to identify whose behaviors and what behaviors, plus their determinants, to change and how.

Normalization Process Theory (NPT; May & Finch, 2009) considers how individuals and groups work together to reach a point where an intervention becomes "normal"; part of everyday routine. It can also be used as a framework to ensure that interventions that are being developed are suitable for widespread implementation and that evaluations are appropriate for determining the effectiveness of the intervention. According to this theory, there are four core components which can influence how easily an intervention becomes part of routine. These components are the same for developing, evaluating and implementing interventions and they interact with each other and the wider working environment. These four components are overviewed in Table 5.2 and highlight the various issues to

TABLE 5.2 Overview of Normalization Process Theory (May & Finch, 2009).

Component	For Development & Implementation	For Evaluation
Coherence	Is the intervention easy to describe?	Is the trial easy to describe?
	Does it fit with organization activities?	Does the trial fit with activities of the organization?
	Will it produce clear benefits?	Do participants in the trial directly benefit?
	Is the purpose clear for all people?	
Cognitive Participation	Do users think it's a good idea?	Will users think the trial is a good idea? Will they invest time and effort into the trial?
	Do they want to engage/ commit to it?	There are many methods that can be used for code-sign
Collective Action	Will it help/impede users' work?	How will the trial affect the work of users? Will it help or impede? Is training needed?
	Does it fit with existing practice?	
	Is training needed?	
	Does it affect how work, resources, responsibilities are split across groups?	Will the trial affect how work, resources/responsibilities are split across groups?
Reflexive Monitoring	Will it be viewed positively in the future?	Will the trial be viewed positively after it has been running for a while?
	Can users offer feedback?	
	Can feedback be used to modify/ improve the intervention?	Can users offer feedback on trial procedures and can these be refined accordingly?

Adapted from Murray et al. (2010).

consider in an NPT analysis when designing, evaluating and implementing an intervention that is to be delivered in real-world settings.

THE MARRIAGE OF BEHAVIORAL SCIENCE/HEALTH PSYCHOLOGY & IMPLEMENTATION SCIENCE

To maximize the impact of health psychology/behavioral science research, it is important that steps are taken to translate effective health behavior change interventions into routine practice. There is a concern, however, that at the moment there is a real gap. To help address this, Presseau and colleagues have developed a set of recommendations regarding how health psychology can aid implementation science and vice-versa and these are summarized in Table 5.3.

TABLE 5.3 Recommendations regarding how health psychology and implementation science can inform one another (Presseau et al., 2022)

How implementation science can inform health psychology	How health psychology can inform implementation science
1. Incorporate into systematic reviews discussion of how ready for implementation different interventions are taking into account whether the underpinning evidence has been generated in ideal (efficacy) or real world (effectiveness) settings.	1. At multiple levels, identify whose behavior (e.g., health providers, managers, government leads), and which behaviors, should change to ensure interventions can be implemented into practice.
2. When developing an intervention (or as soon as possible thereafter), consider barriers and facilitators regarding how the intervention can be implemented in the real world by other people outside the research team. Take into account whether the necessary resources and infrastructure for implementation are in place and whether delivery fits within the routines of those who have been identified to deliver the intervention in the real world.	2. Utilize relevant theories/techniques regarding stopping behaviors when deciding which low-value care to stop implementing. Consider the environmental features that can trigger behaviors automatically.

(*Continued*)

TABLE 5.3 (Continued)

How implementation science can inform health psychology	How health psychology can inform implementation science
3. Consider how the behaviors of people involved at multiple levels of health behavior change can be altered including those delivering the interventions. Which theories are the best to use and can theories from implementation science and health behavior change be combined?	3. Utilize relevant theories/techniques/methods when considering how positive changes in care can be maintained.
4. Build implementation science capacity within health psychology (e.g., via implementation science training for health psychologists; funding health psychology positions within healthcare settings; involving implementation scientists in health psychology societies and journals; providing grant opportunities for collaborations).	4. Utilize relevant theories/methods to consider how implementation interventions change outcomes (mechanisms) and how they can be delivered and received as intended (fidelity).
	5. Build health psychology capacity in implementation science (using the same sort of approaches detailed in point 4. in the opposite column).

SUMMARY

In this chapter we introduced a range of different methods and evaluated their strengths and weaknesses. There is no perfect method, each approach has some form of weakness. Methodological quality, when poor, hinders the development of the science of health behavior change. Researchers need to minimize the risks posed by different sources of bias when conducting their research and need to follow relevant guidelines such as CONSORT and PRISMA when reporting the results. When developing and evaluating interventions, frameworks such as those provided by the MRC can help. Ultimately, acceptable, credibly effective interventions need to be developed and implemented to benefit the health of the population. Utilizing the methods and approaches covered in this chapter should help to achieve this ultimate aim.

FURTHER READING

Hoffmann, T., Glasziou, P., Boutron, I., Milne, R., Perera, R., Moher, D., Altman, D., Barbour, V., Macdonald, H., Johnston, M., Lamb, S., Dixon-Woods, M., McCulloch, P., Wyatt, J., Chan, A., & Michie, S. (2014). Better reporting of interventions: template for intervention description and replication (TIDieR) checklist and guide. *BMJ*, 348, g1687. Explains the key elements that should be consistently and clearly reported for studies testing behavioral interventions.

Weinstein, N. (2007). Misleading tests of health behaviour theories. *Annals of Behavioral Medicine*, *33*, 1–10. This paper clearly highlights the issue of using correlational designs to test health behavior theories.

Wolfenden, L. et al. (2021). Designing and undertaking randomised implementation trials: guide for researchers. *BMJ*, *372*, m3721. Provides useful guidance on how implementation interventions should be developed, evaluated and reported.

The EQUATOR Network strives to improve the transparency of reporting in health/medical-related fields: http://www.equator-network.org/.

For issues relating to the incorporation of randomized controlled trials to inform government policy see: http://onthinktanks.org/2012/03/08/making-policy-better-the-randomisation-revolution-how-far-can-experiments-lead-to-better-policy/.

The NIH provides a great overview of different study designs and associated resources to aid study planning: https://researchmethodsresources.nih.gov/.

For those readers who are particularly interested in co-production, the *BMJ* has published a collection of articles specific to this topic: https://www.bmj.com/content/372/bmj.n434/related.

GLOSSARY

Allocation concealment: a list of which experimental condition participants will be assigned to (following a review of whether the participant is eligible or ineligible for the study) is known as the **allocation sequence**. Allocation concealment refers to whether this sequence is hidden from the researchers deciding whether a particular participant should enter the study or not.

Attrition: whether a participant drops out of the study or not. The proportion of participants who dropout (withdraw) during a study reflects the **attrition rate**.

Between-subjects design: a type of design where different groups of participants do different things depending on the experimental condition/group to which they have been assigned.

Blinding: whether the participant/member of the research team is aware of the condition to which the participant has been assigned.

Co-Creation: an overarching term incorporating co-design and co-production.

Co-Design: a collaborative approach to identifying needs or problems, potential solutions and a design to test them involving a team that comprises not only researchers but users (e.g., patients, healthcare professionals) and other groups (e.g., policymakers).

Co-Production: a collaborative approach to testing the initiative, taking on-board feedback for implementation of the initiative in wider practice and suggestions for improvements.

Content validity: the extent to which the measure covers all aspects of the construct that it aims to assess.

Convergent validity: the extent that a measure correlates with other related measures that have been previously validated.

Criterion-related validity: the extent to which the measure can differentiate between different groups of people who should differ on the measure.

Dependent variable (DV): the outcome measure and reflects what is observed following changes in the independent variable.

Dimensionality: whether the scale measures one underlying construct (unidimensional) or several related (but distinct) constructs (multidimensional).

Disclosed observation: observed individuals are informed beforehand.

Discriminant (divergent) validity: extent that responses on the

to-be-validated scale are unrelated to responses on other scales that should be unrelated to the to-be-validated scale.

Ecological momentary assessment: a method that can assess people's thoughts, feelings and behaviors in real time in their own natural environment outside of the laboratory using, for example, diaries or mobile phones.

Ecological validity: extent to which the study reflects real-life.

External validity: extent to which results can be generalized to different settings, populations, times, etc.

Extraneous variable: a third type of variable (after the IV and DV); these variables can potentially influence the DV. Unless controlled, these variables can confound the experiment such that it becomes more difficult to establish whether changes in the IV alone cause changes in the DV.

Face validity: whether the scale, on the surface, appears to appropriately assess what it is supposed to assess.

Feasibility Study: a particular type of "small-scale" study that helps establish whether it is possible and worthwhile to conduct a larger, main trial.

Independent variable (IV): the variable that is manipulated (changed) by the experimenter in a study. Changes in the dependent variable are observed consequently to establish whether the IV causes changes in the DV.

Intention-to-treat (ITT): Different researchers can mean different things when using this term. First: ITT could mean that data from participants are analyzed on the basis of which treatment group the participants were allocated to (rather than the treatment that the participants received, which could differ, particularly in large, complex experiments). Second: ITT could reflect an approach taken so that participants who dropout are still included in the analysis. ITT could mean either or both of these things.

Internal reliability: the extent to which a measure yields similar responses to related items.

Internal validity: extent to which one can confidently deduce that one variable causes a specific outcome.

Intervention synthesis: a process to help translate the results from systematic reviews into practical treatments.

Meta-analysis: A statistical procedure used to combine, compare and contrast the findings of studies on a related topic.

Mixed-design: a type of experimental design that contains at least two independent variables (IV) one of which is a between-subjects IV and the other of which is a within-subjects IV.

Mixed methods: an approach that involves collecting, analyzing and interpreting data drawn from both quantitative and qualitative methods in the same study.

Natural experiment: a type of observational, quasi-experimental method in which the researcher does not control which participants are allocated to which condition. Instead, it compares groups who have been naturally exposed to some manipulation/intervention (e.g., to a particular policy) against a group that has not.

Pilot study: a type of feasibility study that is consistent with the main study but on a smaller scale (a miniature version of a main study or trial).

Pragmatic trials: trials which mirror, as far as possible, how the tested intervention would be delivered in usual practice.

PRECIS-2: Measures the extent to which a trial is pragmatic (usual care) vs. explanatory (intervention tested in ideal conditions) taking into account factors such as eligibility criteria (are the participants eligible for the trial typical of those who would receive the treatment in practice?), setting (is the setting equivalent to that in which the intervention will be delivered in the real world) and primary outcome (how relevant is this to participants?).

Predictive validity: whether the response on a measure predicts future events that one would expect it should predict.

Protocol: a record that specifies what a research team will do before they actually do it.

Reliability: the extent to which a measure yields consistent responses

Self-selection bias: a bias that arises when participants can choose which group to join (or a study compares two groups that differ on an existing variable). This bias is problematic as participants who choose to join one group/condition may differ on many (unmeasured) variables to participants who choose to join another group/condition.

Systematic review: a rigorous and replicable approach to identify, and synthesize evidence from, studies tackling a specific issue.

Test-retest reliability: extent to which responses are similar across time-points.

Undisclosed observation: a form of observational method in which participants are unaware that they are being observed.

Validity: extent to which a measure assesses what it is supposed to measure.

Within-subjects: a type of design in which the same participants complete different conditions/manipulations.

REFERENCES

Acocella, I. (2012). The focus groups in social research: advantages and disadvantages. *Quality & Quantity, 46*, 1125–1136.

Ageypong, I.A., Godt, S., Sombie, I., Binka, C., Okine, V., & Ingabire, M. (2021). Strengthening capacities and resource allocation for co-production of health research in low and middle income countries. *BMJ, 372*, n166.

Allen, M.S., Iliescu, D., & Greiff, S. (2022). Single item measures in psychological science: A call to action. *European Journal of Psychological Assessment, 38*, 1–5.

Beets, M.W. et al. (2020). Identification and evaluation of risk of generalizability biases in pilot versus efficacy/effectiveness trials: a systematic review and meta-analysis. *International Journal of Behavioral Nutrition and Physical Activity, 17*, 19.

Blazey, P., Crossley, K.M., Ardern, C.L., van Middelkoop, M., Scott, A., & Khan, K.M. (2022). It is time for consensus on "consensus statements". *British Journal of Sports Medicine, 56*.

Bosnjak, M., Fiebach, C.J., Mellor, D., Mueller, S., O'Connor, D.B., Oswald, F.L., & Sokol-Chang, R. I. (2022). A template for preregistration of quantitative research in psychology: Report of the joint psychological societies preregistration task force. *American Psychologist, 77*, 602–615.

Breznau, N., Rinke, E., Wuttke, A., Nguyen, H.H.V., Adem, M., Adriaans, J., … Żółtak, T. (2021, May 18). How Many Replicators Does It Take to Achieve Reliability? Investigating Researcher Variability in a Crowdsourced Replication. https://doi.org/10.31235/osf.io/j7qta

Carlin, M.T., Costello, M.S., Flansburg, M.A., & Darden, A. (in press). Reconsideration of the type 1 error rate for psychological science in the era of replication. *Psychological Methods*.

Drapeau, M. (2002). Subjectivity in research: Why not? But... *The Qualitative Report*, 7, 1–15.

Eldridge, S.M., Lancaster, G.A., Campbell, M.J., Thabane, L., Hopewell, S., Coleman, C.L., & Bond, C.M. (2016). Defining feasibility and pilot studies in preparation for randomised controlled trials: Development of a conceptual framework. *PLoS One*, *11*, e0150205.

Ellefson, M.R. & Oppenheimer, D.M. (in press). Is replication possible without fidelity? *Psychological Methods*.

Glasziou, P.P., Chalmers, I., Green, S., & Michie, S. (2014). Intervention synthesis: A missing link between a systematic review and practical treatment(s). *PLoS Medicine*, *11*, e1001690.

Grant, A.M., & Hofmann, D.A. (2011). It's not all about me: Motivating hand hygiene among health care professionals by focusing on patients. *Psychological Science*, *22*, 1494–1499.

Hekler, E., & King, A. C. (2020). Toward an open mechanistic science of behavior change. *Health Psychology*, *39*, 841–845.

Hoffmann, T., Glasziou, P., Boutron, I., Milne, R., Perera, R., Moher, D., ... & Michie, S. (2014). Better reporting of interventions: template for intervention description and replication (TIDieR) checklist and guide. *BMJ*, 348, g1687.

Klein, R.A. et al. (2014). Investigating variation in replicability. A "Many Labs" replication project. Social Psychology, 45, 142–152.

Klein, R.A. et al. (2018). Many labs 2: Investigating variation in replicability across samples and settings. *Advances in Methods and Practices in Psychological Science*, 1, 443–490.

Kwasnicka, D., Inauen, J., Nieuwenboom, W., Nurmi, J., Schneider, A., Short, C. E., ... & Naughton, F. (2019). Challenges and solutions for N-of-1 design studies in health psychology. Health Psychology Review, 13, 163–178.

Levitt, H.M., Bamberg, M., Creswell, J.W., Frost, D.M., Josselson, R., & Suárez-Orozco, C. (2018). Journal article reporting standards for qualitative primary, qualitative meta-analytic, and mixed methods research in psychology: The APA publications and communications board task force report. *American Psychologist*, *73*, 26–46.

Loewenstein, G. (1996). Out of control: Visceral influences on behavior. *Organizational Behavior and Human Decision Processes*, *65*, 272–292.

Loewenstein, G., Nagin, D., & Paternoster, R. (1997). The effect of sexual arousal on expectations of sexual forcefulness. *Journal of Research in Crime and Delinquency*, *34*, 443–473.

MacDonald, T.K., MacDonald, G., Zanna, M.P., & Fong, G.T. (2000). Alcohol, arousal, and intentions to use condoms in young men: Applying the alcohol myopia theory to risky sexual behavior. *Health Psychology*, *19*, 290–298.

Manapat, P.D., Anderson, S.F., & Edwards, M.C. (in press). A revised and expanded taxonomy for understanding heterogeneity in research and reporting practices. *Psychological Methods*.

May, C., & Finch, T. (2009). Implementing, embedding, and integrating practices: An outline of Normalization Process Theory. *Sociology*, *43*, 535–554.

McDonald, S., Vieira, R., & Johnston, D.W. (2020). Analysing N-of-1 observational data in health psychology and behavioural medicine: a 10-step SPSS tutorial for beginners. *Health Psychology and Behavioral Medicine, 8*, 32–54.

Milkman, K.L. et al. (2021). Megastudies improve the impact of applied behavioural science, *Nature, 600*, 478–483.

Minozzi, S., Cinquini, M., Gianola, S., Gonzalez-Lorenzo, M., & Banzi, R. (2020). The revised Cochrane risk of bias tool for randomized trials (RoB 2) showed low interrater reliability and challenges in its application. *Journal of Clinical Epidemiology, 126*, 37–44.

Moore, G., Campbell, M., Copeland, L., Craig, P., Movsisyan, A., Hoddinott, P., ... & Evans, R. (2021). Adapting interventions to new contexts, the ADAPT guidance. *BMJ, 374*, 1679.

Munafo, M.R., Nosek, B.A., Bishop, D.V.M., Button, K.S., Chambers, C.D., Percie du Sert, N., ... & Ioannidis, J. P. A. (2017). A manifesto for reproducible science. *Nature Human Behaviour, 1*, 0021.

Murray, E., Treweek, S., Pope, C., MacFarlane, A., Ballini, L., Dowrick, C., ... & May, C. (2010). Normalisation process theory: a framework for developing, evaluating and implementing complex interventions. *BMC Medicine, 8*, 63.

Nosek, B., Hardwicke, T.E., Moshontz, H. et al. (2022). Replicability, robustness and reproducibility in psychological science. *Annual Review of Psychology, 73*, 719–748.

O'Brien, B.C., Harris, I.B., Beckman, T., Reed, D.A., & Cook, D.A. (2014). Standards for reporting qualitative research: A synthesis of recommendations. *Academic Medicine, 89*, 1245–1251.

Olander, E.K., & Eves, F.F. (2011). Elevator availability and its impact on stair use in a workplace. *Journal of Environmental Psychology, 31*, 200–206.

Open Science Collaboration (2015). Estimating the reproducibility of psychological science. *Science, 349*(6251):aac4716.

Peer, E., Rothschild, D., Gordon, A., Evernden, Z., & Damer, E. (2022). Data quality of platforms and panels for online behavioral research. *Behavior Research Methods, 54*, 1643–1662.

Presseau, J. et al. (2022). Enhancing the translation of health behaviour change research into practice: a selective conceptual review of the synergy between implementation science and health psychology. *Health Psychology Review, 16*, 22–49.

Prestwich, A., Lalljee, M., & Laham, S.M. (2021). The Morality-Agency-Communion (MAC) model of respect and liking. *European Journal of Social Psychology, 51*, 1019–1034.

Prestwich, A. (in press). A test of the Morality-Agency-Communion (MAC) model of respect and liking across positive and negative traits. *British Journal of Psychology*.

Protzko, J., Krosnick, J., Nelson, L.D., Nosek, B.A., Axt, J., Berent, M., ... Schooler, J. (2020, September 10). High Replicability of Newly-Discovered Social-behavioral Findings Is Achievable. https://doi.org/10.31234/osf.io/n2a9x

Read, D., & Leeuwen, B. (1998). Predicting hunger: The effects of appetite and delay on choice. *Organizational Behavior and Human Decision Making, 76*, 189–205.

Sayette, M.A., Loewenstein, G., Griffin, K.M., & Black, J.J. (2008). Exploring the cold-to-hot empathy gap in smokers. *Psychological Science, 19*, 926–932.

Schulz, K.F., Altman, D.G., Moher, D., for the CONSORT Group. (2010). CONSORT 2010 Statement: updated guidelines for reporting parallel group randomised trials. *Annals of Internal Medicine, 152*, 726–732.

Secor, A.J. (2010). Social survey, interviews, and focus groups. In B. Gomez and J.P. Jones III (Eds.) (pp. 194–205), *Research Methods in Geography*. Wiley-Blackwell.

Sekhon, M., Cartwright, M., & Francis, J. J. (2017). Acceptability of healthcare interventions: an overview of reviews and development of a theoretical framework. *BMC Health Services Research, 17*, 88.

Sekhon, M., Cartwright, M., & Francis, J. J. (2022). Development of a theory-informed questionnaire to assess the acceptability of healthcare interventions. *BMC Health Services Research, 22*, 279.

Sigall, H., & Mills, J. (1998). Measures of independent variables and mediators are useful in social psychology experiments: But are they necessary? *Personality and Social Psychology Review, 2*, 218–226.

Slattery, P., Saeri, A. K., & Bragge, P. (2020). Research co-design in health: a rapid overview of reviews. *Health Research Policy and Systems, 18*, 17.

Stanley, T.D., Carter, E.C., & Doucouliagos, H. (2018). What meta-analyses reveal about the replicability of psychological research. *Psychological Bulletin, 144*, 1325–1346.

Tate, R.L., Perdices, M., Rosenkoetter, U., Wakim, D., Godbee, K., Togher, L., & McDonald, S. (2013). Revision of a method quality rating scale for single-case experimental designs and *n*-of-1 trials: The 15-item Risk of Bias in N-of-1 Trials (RoBiNT) Scale. *Neuropsychological Rehabilitation, 23*, 619–638.

Taylor, N.J., & Gorman, D.M. (2022). Registration and primary outcome reporting in behavioral health trials. *BMC Medical Research Methodology, 22*, 41.

Tong, A., Sainsbury, P., & Craig, J. (2007). Consolidated criteria for reporting qualitative research (COREQ): a 32-item checklist for interviews and focus groups. *International Journal for Quality in Health Care, 19*, 349–357.

Vargas, C., Whelan, J., Brimblecombe, J., & Allender, S. (2022). Co-creation, co-design, co-production for public health – a perspective on definitions and distinctions. *Public Health Research & Practice, 32*, e3222211.

Webster, R.K., Weinman, J., & Rubin, G.J. (2016). A systematic review of factors that contribute to nocebo effects. *Health Psychology, 35*, 1334–1355.

Yetman, H.E., Cox, N., Adler, S.R., Hall, K.T., & Stone, V.E. (2021). What do placebo and nocebo effects have to do with health equity? The hidden toll of nocebo effects on racial and ethnic minority patients in clinical care. *Frontiers in Psychology, 12*, 788230.

6

CHAPTER 6
ANALYZING HEALTH BEHAVIOR CHANGE DATA

OVERVIEW

Following on from Chapter 5, this chapter covers statistical tests often used on data from studies concerning health behavior change and illustrates a number of key statistical issues. Regarding statistical tests, we provide a flow-diagram to help identify which statistical test to use and when (Figure 6.1). The chapter also covers reasonably advanced, but important, tests such as **mediation** and **moderation**. These tests really lie at the heart of health behavior change research because mediation helps to identify *why* certain interventions affect outcomes (or why variables are related with one another) and moderation identifies *when* interventions affect outcomes and when they do not (or when variables are related with one another and when they are not related). Regarding statistical issues, we consider different types of design, sample sizes and non-linear relationships, all of which will help you expand your critical skills toolkit!

THE RESEARCH AND ANALYTICAL PROCESS

Just as in other areas of science, when considering health behavior change, we formulate predictions (hypotheses) on the basis of previous research. We may predict that what somebody *intends* to do will be associated with what they *actually* do (see Ajzen, 1991) or that individuals exposed to a particular intervention will change their behavior more than those who were not. Such predictions, where we predict an association between variables or a difference between groups, represent **alternative hypotheses**. Where we predict there will be no association or no differences, these are known as **null hypotheses**.

DOI: 10.4324/9781003302414-7

After formulating a prediction, we next design a study to test the prediction. The study may require the researcher to only *measure* variables (e.g., what somebody intends to do (intentions) and what they actually do (behavior)), in which case we adopt a **correlational design**, or we need to *manipulate* variables (e.g., whether somebody is allocated to a behavior change intervention condition or to a control condition that is not exposed to behavior change content), in which case we adopt an **experimental design**. In an experimental design, we may formulate independent groups (such as exposing participants *either* to a behavior change intervention or not before measuring their behavior at a later point in the future). In this instance, we have used a between-subjects design (see Chapter 5; also known as an independent groups design or an unrelated design). Alternatively, we may have a single group of participants but measure their behavior when they are exposed to multiple conditions (e.g., during a period in which they are not exposed to behavior change content and, at a later period of time, after they have been exposed to behavior change content). This is known as a within-subjects design (see Chapter 5; also known as a repeated measures design or, for good measure, a related design). We may also have a more complex design that incorporates both between-subjects and within-subjects elements known as a mixed design (see Chapter 5). For example, we may manipulate participants into two independent groups, one that is exposed to behavior change content and another group which is not (this is the between-subjects/independent groups/unrelated aspect of our design). In addition, all of the participants are required to complete a measure assessing their behavior twice – once at the beginning of the study (before any behavior change content is delivered) and once at the end (after some of the participants have been exposed to the behavior change content; this is the within-subjects/repeated measures/related aspect of our design). Each of these designs has its own advantages and disadvantages (see Critical Skills Toolkit 6.1).

CRITICAL SKILLS TOOLKIT 6.1

ADVANTAGES AND DISADVANTAGES OF WITHIN-SUBJECTS, BETWEEN-SUBJECTS AND MIXED DESIGNS

Within-subjects designs tend to be more powerful than between-subjects designs. Having more **power** means they are more likely to detect significant effects with the equivalent number of participants than between-subjects designs. This is because within-subjects designs involve the same participants minimizing individual differences across conditions (whereas between-subjects designs involve different participants) and each individual provides multiple data under different conditions.

Within-subjects designs are at risk of learning, carry-over and order effects. **Learning effects** (e.g., what participants learn on the first task can be used to assist them in the second task), **carry-over effects** (where performance on one task has an impact that is still persistent on a later task), **fatigue effects** (where performance diminishes in later tasks due to tiredness), or **order effects** (the order in which the tasks are completed is important: e.g., task A influences task B, but task B doesn't influence task A) are potential problems for within-subjects designs. For example, assessing participants' behavior, in a single group design, after they have been exposed to behavior change content and then again at a later date could bias the results (people may still have changed their behavior as a result of their earlier exposure to the behavior change content, i.e., there is a carry-over effect). If you are worried about learning, carry-over or order effects, you can do a number of things to mini-mize these risks of bias: a) adopt a between-subjects design; b) increase the amount of time between completion of the tasks; c) include a distracter task between the critical tasks that can help people to unlearn, forget, disrupt the influence of one critical task on another; d) counterbalance the order of the tasks (so half of your participants complete task A before task B, and the other half of your participants first complete task B then task A). Counterbalancing the order of the tasks introduces a between-subjects element thus creating a mixed design. *Mixed designs that counterbalance therefore allow the experimenter to assess the impact of order effects.* As the same participants provide data under multiple conditions rather than under a single condition (as in a between-subjects design), *mixed designs are more powerful than between-subjects designs* (assuming there are no strong over-riding biases such as learning effects, order effects, etc.).

Between-subjects designs deal with various types of bias such as learning effects as participants complete only one task in a single condition (other participants in a different experimental group will either complete a different task or the same task but under a different condition). The drawback is that relative to within-subjects designs, where participants complete measures under multiple conditions, these designs require more participants (due to having less power to detect significant effects). With between-subjects designs, there is a risk that the independent groups are not equivalent on some unmeasured, but important, characteristic that impacts on your study in some unknown way.

After collecting data consistent with our design, we then need to analyze the data. The design that you've adopted will determine the statistical test that you should use (see Figure 6.1). For instance, if you measure attitudes towards eating healthily (what people think and feel about eating healthily) and healthy eating behavior because you are interested in whether these variables are related, you would adopt a correlational design. If you fail to meet relevant (parametric) assumptions, then you should conduct a Spearman's Rho test. If you have a correlational design, you meet parametric assumptions, you have three or more variables (attitudes towards eating healthily, intentions to eat healthily, healthy eating behavior) and you think one variable (intentions to eat healthily) helps explain why two other variables (attitudes towards eating healthily and healthy eating behavior) are related, you would conduct a mediation analysis (see "Mediation and Moderation" section).

Based on our analysis, we will either find evidence to support our prediction (supporting our alternative hypothesis) or not (supporting our null hypothesis), a process called null hypothesis significance testing (NHST). In this process, the statistical test that we conduct (e.g., a t-test, ANOVA, chi-square, see Figure 6.1) will produce a test statistic. Next, this test statistic is compared against a known distribution of values of this statistic. From this, we can determine the likelihood of getting a test-statistic of the size that we have, or greater, if there were no effect in the population. If this probability is less than .05, then we conclude that the effect that we have found is "statistically significant" thus accepting our alternative hypothesis and rejecting our null hypothesis. If the probability is greater than .05, then we describe the result as non-significant and accept our null hypothesis and reject our alternative hypothesis.

Studies may be designed to look at health behavior change in ideal, typically tightly controlled laboratory settings to consider **efficacy**, or in real-world settings to consider **effectiveness**. As efficacy trials take place in ideal conditions (with potentially more experienced intervention deliverers, higher levels of fidelity in delivery, greater adherence to the intervention, more homogeneous samples and settings, etc.), interventions in efficacy trials can appear to change behavior more compared to when they are tested in effectiveness, real-world trials.

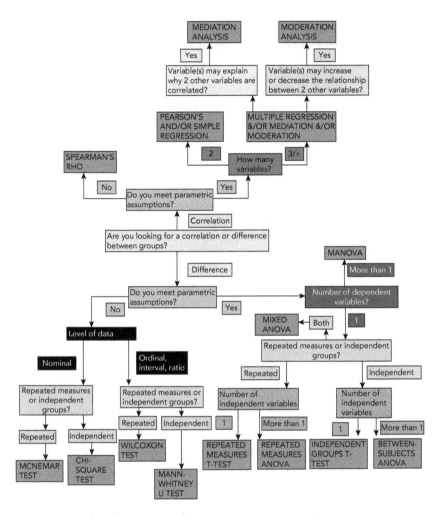

FIGURE 6.1 Flow diagram to select appropriate statistical test.

PROBLEMS WITH NULL HYPOTHESIS SIGNIFICANCE TESTING (NHST)

A major problem with NHST is that it is influenced by the number of people included in the analysis (i.e., the sample size). For example, when the difference in scores between two groups of participants is the same across two studies, everything else (e.g., the variability of the scores) being equal, the study with more people included in the analysis will be more likely to achieve a significant result (i.e., $p < .05$), meaning that you will accept the alternative hypothesis and reject the null hypothesis. The opposite is also true; when you have a particularly small sample size, it is difficult to achieve a significant result, meaning that you are more likely to reject the alternative hypothesis and accept the null hypothesis. So, in a nutshell, a very large sample size (e.g., 500,000 participants) is problematic because even a tiny, or trivial, difference between groups will be concluded as being significant; a small sample size (e.g., 10 participants) is problematic because a large, or important, difference between groups is likely to be concluded as being non-significant: sample size bias conclusions drawn from NHST.

A second problem is the obsession within the scientific community (including those interested in health behavior change) with the critical p-value of .05. If a statistical test generates a p-value of less than .05 (such as .04), then we conclude the effect is significant (accepting the alternative hypothesis and rejecting the null hypothesis); if the p-value is greater than .05 (such as .06), then we conclude the effect is non-significant (rejecting the alternative hypothesis and accepting the null hypothesis). There are two things to note here: 1) The fine lines: p-values of .04 and .06 are very similar but are associated with very different conclusions; 2) The p-value of .05 is somewhat arbitrary, for example, one may argue that the cut-off point for judging whether the effect is significant or not should be $p = .10$ or $p = .01$, or some other p-value!

So, what are the alternatives to NHST? One option is to use Bayes Factors, and an alternative is to calculate and report an effect size.

BAYES FACTORS

Bayes Factors, a form of Bayesian statistics, compare two alternative models (e.g., model A (null): that the intervention has no effect compared to a control group vs. model B (alternative): the intervention has a benefit over the control group) and enable conclusions of whether there's more support for model A (no effect) or B (benefit) and how much stronger the evidence is for one model compared to the other.

Unlike the NHST approach described earlier in which a p-value greater than .05 means we cannot reject the null hypothesis (which equates to we cannot support it), an advantage of Bayes Factors is that it can enable tests of support for the null or alternative hypothesis relative to one another; it will tell you how many times more (or less) likely the data would have been produced under one model than another (e.g., the support in the data is five times larger for the null hypothesis than the alternative hypothesis). Moreover, sensitivity analyses can be conducted to compare the "null hypothesis/model" against a variety of different alternative hypotheses/ models (that can specify different sized effects with different distributions) and vice-versa. As both the null (e.g., no difference; scores within a small range either side of zero) and alternative hypotheses (e.g., not 0, greater than 0, greater than a minimum specified sized effect) can be specified in different ways, Bayes Factors can be used flexibly.

EFFECT SIZES

An alternative option is to calculate **effect sizes**. Effect sizes are a useful way of reflecting the standardized treatment effect. There are many different types of effect sizes – each calculated in different ways. Two of the most common effect sizes are Cohen's d (representing the standardized difference between two means) and Pearson's r (representing the correlation between the independent and dependent variables). For both of these measures, a larger number represents a larger effect. Moreover, both Cohen's d and Pearson's r can be negative (representing a negative effect, e.g., control group outperforms the intervention group) or positive (representing a positive effect, e.g., intervention group outperforms the control group). Cohen's d can be of any size (with $d = 0.2$ reflecting a small effect size; $d = 0.5$ reflecting a medium effect; and $d = 0.8$ or greater reflecting a large effect); while Pearson's r varies between -1 and +1 (with, regardless of sign, $r = .1$ reflecting a small effect; $r = .3$ a medium effect; $r = .5$ a large effect).

Effect sizes are independent of sample size: they can stay the same regardless of whether the sample size becomes larger or smaller. They are useful in making direct comparisons across studies while it is difficult to make such comparisons using p-values (because studies tend to have different sample sizes and sample sizes influence p-values). Given they are useful for making comparisons across studies, effect sizes represent the building blocks of meta-analyses.

META-ANALYSIS

Meta-analysis is a useful means to combine the findings of studies on a related topic (producing an overall average effect size). Meta-analyses have been conducted widely within health behavior change (see, for example,

Table 3.1, in Chapter 3). Meta-analyses are based on effect sizes. Given studies will produce different effect sizes (reflecting **statistical heterogeneity**), meta-analyses can also compare and contrast findings across studies tackling the same topic, identifying factors that explain why some studies produce larger effects than others. Statistical heterogeneity may occur because studies use different participants, interventions or outcomes (**clinical heterogeneity**) or because they have used different designs or carry different levels or types of risk of bias (**methodological heterogeneity**). The sources of statistical heterogeneity can be investigated through **sub-group analyses** or **meta-regression**.

Sub-group analyses are typically used where studies fall into categories (such as studies with young participants and studies with old participants). They compare the effect sizes of studies falling into each category to examine whether the effect sizes of studies falling into one category (e.g., studies recruiting participants under the age of 18) differ to the effect sizes of studies falling into another category (e.g., studies recruiting only participants over the age of 60). Meta-regressions can be used when studies measure a variable on a scale (such as mean age of participants in a study) and also when variables comprise groups (e.g., comparing studies that blinded experimenters to condition versus studies that did not blind experimenters to condition). In meta-regressions, these scale or categorical (group) variables are used to predict study effect sizes.

When investigating statistical heterogeneity, it is important to specify in advance what sub-group analyses and/or meta-regressions were planned prior to conducting the meta-analysis. Given a very large number of sub-group or meta-regressions could be conducted, there is a high-risk of making **type 1-errors** (incorrectly concluding that a particular moderator or sub-group is influential/significant when it is not). Thus, specifying in advance the analyses to be conducted encourages the researcher only to test moderators that are theoretically or methodologically important which minimizes the number of tests to be conducted and, in turn, minimizes the risk of type 1 errors.

CRITICAL SKILLS TOOLKIT 6.2

POWER CALCULATIONS – WHAT IS THE RIGHT SAMPLE SIZE?

To avoid problems of under-sampling (recruiting too few participants and inflating the likelihood of making a **Type 2 error** (incorrectly accepting the null hypothesis) and over-sampling (recruiting too many participants and inflating the likelihood of making a **Type 1 error** (incorrectly accepting the alternative hypothesis), it is useful to conduct an a-priori sample size calculation to determine how many participants you should recruit into your study. Recruiting too many participants is potentially a waste of time, effort and money, so a-priori sample sizes really are useful (see Farrokhyar et al., 2013)!

Conducting a-priori sample size calculations involves the following concepts:

1. Type 2 or β error: reflects the probability of accepting the null hypothesis when it is false. $\beta = .20$ is commonly used in sample size calculations (see point 2. power).
2. Power: ability to detect a significant effect within the sample of participants used in a study when a significant effect truly exists (i.e., within the entire population). Power $= 1 - \beta$. For sample size calculations, this is typically set at .80 (reflecting 80% power).
3. Type 1 or α error: the probability of rejecting the null hypothesis when it is true/accepting the experimental hypothesis when it is false. For sample size calculations, this is typically set at .05 for health behavior change studies as with many other areas of science. For issues that are of critical importance (e.g., testing the effects of specific drugs on health-related outcomes) a more stringent value may be set (such as .001) to minimize the likelihood that a study incorrectly supports the drug when the drug is in fact not useful. When multiple tests are conducted relating to the same hypothesis, the α could be divided by the number of tests (e.g., where there are five tests of the same hypothesis, the α could be set at .01, i.e., .05/5).
4. 1-tailed vs. 2-tailed: using one-tailed testing (where the direction of the effect is specified: e.g., treatment A will be better than treatment B) produces greater power than two-tailed testing (where the direction of the effect is not specified: e.g., treatment A will be worse or better than treatment B). Thus, one-tailed tests require fewer participants than two-tailed tests.
5. Effect size: the standardized difference between groups. For sample size calculations, the effect size can estimated based on (a) effect sizes generated in similar studies or (b) conducting a pilot study or (c) deciding what would be the minimum meaningful effect size for the planned study.

6. The number of participants allocated to the experimental and control groups: the more these differ, the less power the study has (i.e., for the same total sample size, power is greatest when the number of participants in each group is the same)

7. Type of design: within-subjects (repeated measures or related) designs are more powerful than between-subjects (independent groups or unrelated) designs.

So, when conducting a sample size calculation, the researcher will need to decide (1) power (linked to type 2 or β error), (2) type 1 or α error, (3) whether they will use a one-tailed or two-tailed test, (4) estimate the likely (or desired) effect size, (5) the proportion of people allocated to each group and (6) study design. As long as these decisions are all justified then the *planned* sample size calculation is justified. The next step is to ensure that the *planned* sample size matches the *actual* sample size and, if not, the sample size is open to criticism!

MEDIATION AND MODERATION

Both mediation and moderation involve (at least) three variables: a predictor variable, a mediator or moderator, and an outcome variable.

MEDIATION

What is it?

Mediation assesses *how* two variables (the predictor and outcome) are related. Specifically it tests whether these two variables are related through a third variable (the mediator) that is related to both the predictor and outcome. Running mediation analysis allows us to understand the processes through which the predictor may influence the outcome. For example, in a large randomized trial, Bricker et al. (2010) tested whether an intervention encouraged smoking cessation in adolescents relative to a control group and tried to identify why the intervention was effective in promoting smoking abstinence. They found that self-efficacy to resist smoking in social and stressful situations mediated the effect of the intervention on smoking abstinence. In particular, being in the intervention increased participants' self-efficacy in resisting smoking in social and stressful situations and, in turn, increased the likelihood of abstaining from smoking. So, the increase in self-efficacy helps explain why the intervention increased smoking abstinence. In sum, think of mediated relationships as involving (at least)

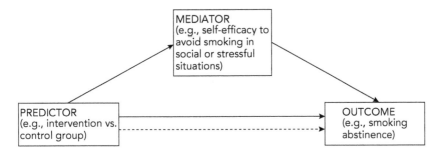

FIGURE 6.2 Mediation based on study by Bricker et al. (2010).

three variables that flow from the predictor to the outcome via the mediator (see Figure 6.2).

As well as identifying factors that help explain how, for example, a smoking cessation intervention promotes abstinence, mediation analysis (by identifying non–significant mediators) can also be used to rule out potential explanations regarding how the smoking cessation intervention works.

How to test for mediation

Analyses can be conducted in statistical programs (e.g., SPSS) to test for mediation. To identify whether you have a significant mediated relationship there are various different approaches that you can take. A particularly common approach, and the one outlined in detail here, is the method suggested by Baron and Kenny (1986). To establish mediation, according to Baron and Kenny (1986), the following conditions should be met:

1. The predictor (e.g., the intervention vs. control group) should significantly predict the outcome (e.g., smoking abstinence).

   - To test this condition, the predictor (e.g., the intervention vs. control group) should be entered as the predictor variable and the outcome (e.g., smoking abstinence) should be entered as the outcome variable in a simple linear regression.

2. The predictor (e.g., the intervention vs. control group) should significantly predict the mediator (e.g., self-efficacy).

   - To test this condition, the predictor (e.g., the intervention vs. control group) should be entered as the predictor variable and the mediator (e.g., self-efficacy) should be entered as the outcome variable in a simple linear regression.

3. The mediator (e.g., self-efficacy) should significantly predict the outcome (e.g., smoking abstinence) while controlling for the predictor (e.g., the intervention vs. control group).

- To test this condition, the predictor (e.g., the intervention vs. control group) and the mediator (e.g., self-efficacy) should both be entered as predictor variables and the outcome (e.g., smoking abstinence) should be entered as the outcome variable in a multiple regression.

4. The predictor (e.g., the intervention vs. control group) should *no longer* significantly predict the outcome (e.g., smoking abstinence) when controlling for the mediator (e.g., self-efficacy).

- To test this condition, the same multiple regression used to test condition 3 can be used.

If all four conditions are met, then this is consistent with the conclusion that the mediator (e.g., self-efficacy) *fully mediates* the relationship between the predictor (e.g., the intervention vs. control group) and the outcome (e.g., smoking abstinence).

If the first three conditions are met, but not condition 4, then this is consistent with the conclusion that the mediator (e.g., self-efficacy) *partially mediates* the relationship between the predictor (e.g., the intervention vs. control group) and the outcome (e.g., smoking abstinence).

If either condition 1, 2 or 3 is not met, then one should conclude that the mediator (e.g., self-efficacy) *does not mediate* the relationship between the predictor (e.g., the intervention vs. control group) and the outcome (e.g., smoking abstinence). An alternative approach to mediation simply examines the significance of the indirect effect (the relationship between the independent variable (e.g., treatment/control variable) and mediator (e.g., motivation) multiplied by the relationship between the mediator and the outcome (e.g., fruit and vegetable intake). Andrew Hayes' PROCESS macro can be used to test mediation in this way.

BURNING ISSUE BOX 6.1

WHEN SHOULD WE MEASURE MEDIATORS?
Sigall and Mills (1998) suggest that measures of mediating (or explanatory) variables have become increasingly common to check the assumptions that the experimental treatment successfully manipulated

those variables that it intended to change. However, they also argue that such measures are not always necessary in experiments. In particular they argue that if no plausible alternative explanations exist, data from such measures are not needed and that plausible alternative explanations are not eliminated by data from such measures. Let's look at the study by Grant and Hofmann (2011).

Grant and Hofmann (2011) looked at how simple changes to signs made health professionals more or less likely to engage in hand hygiene behaviors (i.e., using sanitizing gels). They showed that signs that emphasized personal consequences ("Hand hygiene prevents you from catching diseases") were not as effective as signs that emphasized patient-consequences ("Hand hygiene prevents patients from catching diseases"). The title of their paper focused on motivating change ("It's not all about me: Motivating hand hygiene among health care professionals by focusing on patients") yet just measured changes in behavior. Classic measures of motivation like intentions (I intend to wash my hands) were not measured and so they could only speculate on whether their interventions produced changes in behavior through changing motivation. If they had also measured motivations they could have more directly tested this mediation effect (i.e., did the patient-consequences message produce more change in intentions for hand washing than the personal-consequences message?).

So would measuring intention as a potentially mediating variable have been a valuable addition to Grant and Hofmann's study? According to Sigall and Mills (1998) the answer to this question would turn on whether change in intentions (or motivation) is the only plausible mechanism behind the changes in behavior they observed. If it is the only plausible mechanism then no value would be added by measuring intentions. A further problem is that we know that measuring intentions can itself change behavior (see the Question-Behavior Effect discussed in Chapter 7). So measuring intentions to hand wash might obscure rather than reveal any effects of presenting different messages on hand washing. How might we resolve this problem?

One way out of this problem is to use a Solomon four group design where we assess each of the combinations. For example, we have a "no intervention" group, a group where the message is present, a group where the mediator is measured, and a group where the message is presented and the mediator is measured.

MODERATION

What is it?

In moderation, the analysis tests whether the relationship between two variables (the predictor and outcome), or the effect of one variable (the independent variable) on another variable (the dependent variable), is changed by a third variable (the moderator). It directly answers questions relating to *when* are two variables (predictor and outcome) related or when are two variables (predictor and outcome) related more or less strongly. For instance, Prestwich et al. (2016) ran moderation analyses to identify for whom a feedback-based intervention compared to other interventions was most effective in promoting physical activity. They identified that the effect of the feedback intervention (versus the other study conditions) on levels of physical activity was moderated by intentions to do physical activity at baseline. In particular, the feedback intervention compared to the other interventions was most useful in promoting physical activity for those individuals who were less likely to intend to do physical activity at baseline. Thus, baseline intentions moderated (influenced) the effect of the feedback intervention on physical activity levels: the feedback intervention had a stronger effect on physical activity *when* baseline intentions were weak; the feedback intervention had a weaker effect on physical activity when baseline intentions were strong.

In another example, de Vet, Oenema, Sheeran and Brug (2009) tested whether an intervention encouraging people to plan the days, time, where and how long they would do physical activity (called implementation intentions, see Chapters 3 and 7) increased physical activity more for individuals intending to increase their physical activity compared to individuals not intending to increase their physical activity. In this example, whether participants were asked to form implementation intentions or not was the predictor/independent variable, the number of days they were active was the outcome/dependent variable, and how much the participants intended to increase their physical activity was the moderator.

De Vet et al. (2009) found that forming implementation intentions significantly increased physical activity more for those who intended to increase their physical activity compared to those who did not intend to increase their physical activity. In other words, how much an individual intended to increase their physical activity influenced whether the implementation intention intervention increased physical activity or not.

How to test for moderation

Analyses can be conducted in statistical programs (e.g., SPSS) to test for moderation. To identify whether you have a significant moderator, you can run moderation analyses through regression. In your regression analyses, you need to enter the following variables as your predictors: predictor (e.g., the intervention versus control group variable), moderator (e.g., baseline intentions) and the interaction between predictor and moderator (e.g., intervention/control group variable multiplied by baseline intention scores). You then enter your outcome variable (e.g., level of physical activity) as your outcome in the regression analysis. After running this analysis, you need to study the output. If the interaction term (e.g., intervention/control group variable multiplied by baseline intention scores) is significant then you have a moderated relationship (it doesn't matter whether your predictor or moderator variables are significant, what is required for a significant moderation is for the interaction term to be significant).

That isn't the end of the story, however. At this stage, you do not know the exact nature of the moderated relationship. For instance, having weaker baseline intentions to do physical activity may increase the effect of the intervention on physical activity or having weaker baseline intentions may decrease the effect of the intervention on physical activity. It may be that the intervention *always* significantly increases physical activity (and strengthening (or weakening) intentions only makes the effect of the intervention on physical activity even more significant) or it may be that the intervention *only* significantly increases physical activity levels when intentions are strong (or weak). To examine the exact nature of the relationship you need to conduct simple slopes analysis; conducting this analysis will answer all of the questions relating to the nature of the moderation in your dataset. Simple slopes analysis can be conducted through various programs (see Further Reading section for details regarding an online calculator and Andrew Hayes's PROCESS approach; Hayes, 2021).

CRITICAL SKILLS TOOLKIT 6.3

VARIABLES MAY BE RELATED BUT NOT LINEARLY

Simple correlations/regressions work on the assumption that two variables may be linearly related (i.e., for each unit increase in one variable, there is a corresponding increase in a second variable (see Figure 6.3a) or a corresponding decrease in a second variable (see Figure 6.3b)).

Variable X and Y may be unrelated (e.g., $r = 0$) based on Pearson's correlation but may be related non-linearly. For example, in a study looking at the relationship between task conflict (sample item: "How often do the members of your team disagree about how things should be done?") and team creativity (sample item: "Indicate the extent to which the team output was original and practical"), Farh, Lee and Farh (2010) revealed that the two measures demonstrated a non-significant linear relationship but that there was a significant quadratic relationship. This indicated that as task conflict increased, team creativity also increased up to a turning point whereby further increases in task conflict were associated with reduced team creativity (see Figure 6.3c).

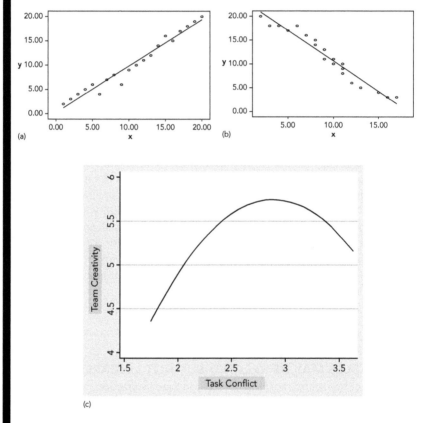

FIGURE 6.3 (a): Positive, linear relationship. (b): Negative, linear relationship. (c): Curvilinear relationship between task conflict and team creativity (Farh et al., 2010).

Farh, J-L., Lee C., & Farh, C.I.C. (2010). Task conflict and team creativity: A question of how much and when. *Journal of Applied Psychology, 95*, 1173–1180.

COMMON STATISTICAL ANALYSES IN HEALTH BEHAVIOR CHANGE INTERVENTION STUDIES

In this section, we highlight statistical analyses and statistical issues that are regularly encountered when conducting studies relating to health behavior change. In particular, we focus on analyses and issues that relate to randomized controlled trials of health behavior interventions.

RANDOMIZATION CHECKS

It is hoped that by randomizing participants to conditions, the type of person in condition A is similar to the type of person in condition B. However, this is not guaranteed. A set of analyses are regularly conducted to identify whether the participants in condition A differ to the participants in condition B on any measured variable. A chi-square test, for instance, could examine whether the proportion of men and women differ across intervention and control groups. A MANOVA analysis can be used to check whether participants in two or more conditions differ on a group of different measures that are measured along a scale such as age, intentions, self-efficacy, past behavior, etc. Where baseline differences are detected, these variables are often statistically controlled in the main study analyses that compare the study conditions (e.g., intervention versus the control) on the main study outcome variables.

However, this practice of testing for baseline differences and later statistically controlling variables for which there are baseline differences has been criticized on a number of grounds including that some baseline differences could be achieved by chance; for instance, if you use $p < .05$ as a benchmark of significance, and compare two groups on 20 baseline measures, you'd expect one difference, on average. Moreover, controlling for baseline differences can increase the risk that unimportant covariates (i.e., those that are not associated with the outcome) are considered (when there are baseline differences on these measures), and important covariates (i.e., those that are related to the outcome) are not considered (when there are no significant baseline differences on these measures) in the main analyses (see de Boer et al., 2015, for further discussion). For these reasons, testing for baseline differences and controlling for any observed differences is becoming less commonly used when reporting randomized controlled trials.

SAMPLE SIZE, RECRUITMENT AND ATTRITION ANALYSES

Planning the required sample size a-priori (in advance of the study) is a useful means to help address the replicability crisis (see Chapter 5) and helps to ensure that resources are not wasted by overrecruiting or underrecruiting. Sample sizes are planned taking into account the underlying effect size/difference between groups, statistical power (probability of detecting a significant effect in your sample when one exists in the population) and p-value (the level at which an effect is judged to be significant) (see Critical Skills Toolkit 6.2). For correlational designs, Schönbrodt and Perugini (2013) demonstrate that with small sample sizes, correlations between variables can fluctuate widely but, in typical circumstances, the correlations become much more stable with around 250 or more participants (see Figure 6.4). As such, correlational studies with sample sizes of at least 250 participants are likely to become more replicable compared to studies with, say, fewer than 50 participants. Guidance for sample sizes in experimental studies can be found in the recommended reading at the end of this chapter. Lakens (2022) also provides guidance and a resource covering issues and means to justify sample size calculations, including basing sample sizes on the smallest effect size of interest, expected effect sizes and other reasons.

Being able to calculate recruitment and attrition rates are useful in feasibility type studies to give an indication of the time and cost required to run a larger study that is better equipped to more clearly determine the impact of an intervention on health-related outcomes (i.e., a fully-powered trial).

The number of people approached, the number meeting eligibility criteria and the number of people agreeing to participate within a particular timeframe can be recorded to infer recruitment rates. Similarly, considering

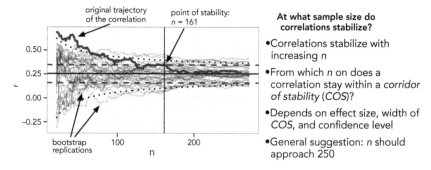

FIGURE 6.4 How stability of correlation estimates increases as sample size increases.

Schönbrodt, F. D., & Perugini, M. (2013). At what sample size do correlations stabilize? *Journal of Research in Personality, 47*(5), 609–612. https://doi.org/10.1016/j.jrp.2013.05.009

the attrition rate (the proportion of participants who withdraw once accepted onto a trial) and whether this varies across condition is useful. The rate of recruitment should be equivalent across groups. If not, especially if the dropout rates are higher in the intervention/treatment condition than in the control condition, then it is possible that there are issues relating to the acceptability of the intervention; in other words, for whatever reason, participants are at increased risk of not liking or engaging with the intervention. Such results would suggest that your intervention may not be viable to deliver in the "real world" without some form of modification to address the issues. The rate of attrition and whether it varies across conditions can be determined through chi-square analyses (or equivalent).

The type of participants who complete the study should be similar to those who do not complete the study. If there are detectable differences such that, for example, the people who complete a physical activity study are more likely to have strong intentions to do physical activity, then the generalizability of the findings are compromised and may not relate to specific groups of people (such as those with weaker intentions to do physical activity). MANOVA can be conducted to test whether those who completed the study differ in any measured variables (measured on a scale) compared to those who did not complete the study. Chi-square can be used to compare dropouts against completers on categorical variables (such as sex of the participants, educational qualifications, etc.).

An alternative approach to planning sample size in advance of the study is to use a group-sequential design in which data can be analyzed at interim stages (rather than just at the end of the study). This approach is seen as more efficient than analyzing data only when the final sample size is reached because studies that do not appear to be working, and those that have larger effects than initially expected (and provide support for alternative hypotheses) can be stopped earlier with fewer participants recruited and tested. An obvious risk of analyzing the data in this way is that the Type 1 error risk increases. To address this issue, researchers need to plan, in advance, when and how often they will look at the dataset and adjust their p-values accordingly. One simple (Bonferroni-type) option is to divide the alpha value (the value at which the effect is deemed to be significant) by the number of planned tests. Other, less conservative approaches are recommended, however (Lakens et al., 2021).

MAIN ANALYSES

The main analyses will test the main hypotheses. In health behavior change research, common scenarios include examining whether specific variables correlate with or predict health-related behaviors (which require correlational analyses, see the top segment of Figure 6.1) or whether interventions change the behavior of individuals (which require tests of difference as indicated in the bottom segment of Figure 6.1). If individuals are clustered into groups – for instance in cluster randomized trials in which groups such as whole schools, classes within schools, hospital wards, etc., are randomized into conditions – then more sophisticated analyses are required (e.g., multi-level modeling). Multi-level modeling is one way of taking account of such clustering of data. For example, Conner and Higgins (2010) used multi-level modeling to analyze data from a cluster randomized controlled trial of an intervention to reduce smoking initiation. The multi-level modeling allowed the analysis to assess the impact of the intervention on rates of smoking initiation and control for the fact that adolescents were clustered within different schools in different conditions. Another example is that of O'Connor et al. (2008) who were interested in the relationship between stress and between meal snacking. They took measures of stress and snacking behavior on a number of consecutive days within the same individuals. They then used multi-level modeling to assess the relationship between stress and eating after controlling for the fact that each individual provided multiple days of data. In effect this analysis answered the question of whether individuals tended to eat more snacks on days when they were more stressed compared to days on which they were less stressed. Hoffman and Walters (2022) provide a useful review of the use of multi-level modelling in psychology research.

HANDLING MISSING DATA

When running a study related to health behavior change, you will more than likely encounter several instances of missing data. This could be as a result of participants intentionally, or unintentionally, not completing a particular measure or because a participant withdraws from a study part way through (as can happen when the study involves more than one time-point). Missing data can be handled in two main ways: 1) live with it and analyze your data using only the responses provided; 2) conduct **intention-to-treat (ITT) analyses**, in which the missing data is replaced with estimated values. The advantages and disadvantages of ITT analyses are considered in Critical Skills Toolkit 6.4. A couple of common approaches to intention-to-treat analysis are: a) last observation carried forward in which data from a previous timepoint is carried across to the timepoint in which data are missing; b) multiple imputation that is designed to replace missing values with plausible estimates.

CRITICAL SKILLS TOOLKIT 6.4

INTENTION-TO-TREAT (ITT) ANALYSES

Intention-to-treat analyses, in which all participants who have been randomized to condition are analyzed regardless of whether they deviated from the protocol or withdrew from the study, have a number of advantages and disadvantages. Being aware of these is useful when thinking about the strengths and weaknesses of the analytical approach taken within a particular study:

Advantages

1. By analyzing data from all participants, ITT can reduce the risk of generating overly optimistic results that may be produced when only conducting analyses on those who completed the study (reducing the risk of making a Type 1 error; concluding that an intervention is effective when it is not).
2. Linked to the above, people may withdraw from a study because of something adverse about the treatment. The impact of this would be detected through ITT but not through non-ITT analyses in which only study completers are considered.
3. By including all participants in the analyses, statistical power could be somewhat maintained (but see Disadvantage 2 below).
4. May provide a better estimation of how effective the intervention is in the real world/clinical type settings (and have greater general-izability of results) where participants/patients may not always receive the correct intervention, receive only part of the interven-tion or, in some other way, deviate from what was intended.

Disadvantages

1. ITT can "muddy the waters" by putting together data from participants who followed the protocol and completed the study; participants who followed the protocol and withdrew; participants who did not follow the protocol (possibly receiving the materials intended for those assigned to a different study condition) and completed the study; and possibly even participants who did not follow the protocol and did not complete the study. As a result, particularly by including data from individuals or groups who did

not receive the intervention, it is difficult to accurately estimate the effect of the intended intervention on the outcome.

2. Linked to the above, there could be an increased risk of making a Type 2 error. In this context, this would mean that there is an increased risk of concluding that a particular health behavior change intervention was ineffective when it actually is effective.

IDENTIFYING AND HANDLING OUTLIERS

Statistical **outliers** are data-points that lie particularly far from other data points. Sometimes they can occur through data-entry error and can thus be corrected by the data analyst or person entering the data in the dataset. However, in practice, it is more likely that the data point(s) represent genuine responses (accurately or inaccurately) provided by, or related to, the participant.

In correlational/regression-based analyses, approaches such as Mahalanobis's distance and Cook's distance can be used to identify the impact of specific cases on the dataset. In experimental analyses, an outlier can be identified by standardizing the scores on the dependent variable (e.g., through z-scores).

Once identified, outliers can be eliminated (or Winsorized to the nearest non-outlier score) when any scores to be judged to be too high (e.g., often researchers classify standardized scores greater than 3.5 or less than -3.5 as outliers). The impact of eliminating or Winsorizing outliers can be examined by comparing the results from these approaches against the results produced when the outliers are not removed or Winsorized. For transparency, any similarities or differences in the conclusions drawn from these two basic approaches (remove/treat vs. keep in) should be reported in academic papers.

PROCESS EVALUATION

Not only can researchers establish whether an intervention changes health behavior, there are ways to establish how or why an intervention changes health behavior. Process evaluations can play a role here. As well as identifying the mechanisms (e.g., how motivated an individual feels about performing a health behavior) that change or do not change as a result of an intervention, and using this data to potentially explain why an intervention "worked" (by successfully changing health behavior) or didn't work, process evaluations also consider how the intervention was implemented. This is important because if you want to make any claims about how an intervention worked, you need to know how the intervention was delivered or implemented. Process evaluations also consider the context in which the intervention was delivered. In process evaluations, context is defined as anything outside of the intervention itself so it could include a variety of things such as features of the setting that the intervention was delivered in and the characteristics of the people delivering or receiving the intervention. By assessing and understanding the context in which the intervention was delivered, researchers can identify the contexts within which the intervention works or does not work. Process evaluations can use quantitative methods, qualitative methods or a combination of the two (mixed methods).

Figure 6.5 overviews the United Kingdom's Medical Research Council (MRC) "recommended" approach to conducting process evaluations (Moore et al., 2015). We say "recommended" like this because it is acknowledged, even within the guidance, that there are many different ways to conduct process evaluations, so there is some degree of flexibility in how they are conducted – one size does not fit all! However, as alluded to earlier, there are three central components to include:

- Implementation. This concerns what is delivered and how. Aside from measuring whether the actual content of the intervention was delivered or not, this element can consider the *implementation process* including the training and support that is provided for those delivering the intervention plus communication and management strategies to help garner support for, or aid the delivery, of the intervention. There are other key elements of implementation including *reach* (how many members of the target population received each part of the intervention), *dose* (how much of the intervention did they receive), *fidelity* (was the intervention delivered as it was supposed to) and considering any *adaptations* that were needed to ensure that the intervention could be delivered in a specific context;

- Mechanisms of action. Changes in these mechanisms of action can be measured using quantitative measures and/or qualitative methods to help establish *how* the intervention worked and to provide a means of checking whether an intervention can be replicated with similar effects in the future. Mechanisms of action common in health behavior change can include the kind of constructs considered in the various theories and models overviewed elsewhere in this book (Chapter 2 in particular) such as motivation, normative beliefs and self-efficacy (see also Chapter 7);

- Contextual factors. These are any factors, external to the intervention, that could influence the size of the intervention effects, such as setting (where the intervention took place), the characteristics of the person(s) delivering the intervention, the characteristics of the people receiving the intervention, etc. An intervention that is implemented in the same way across two different contexts may be effective in one but not another.

It is worth keeping in mind that approaches to process evaluations vary from one study to the next; there is not one standard approach. The actual act of doing a process evaluation can be tricky and throw up some difficult questions and issues that require careful planning and thought. For example:

- Does an observer who spots an error while monitoring implementation (maybe an element of an intervention isn't being delivered well or is not being delivered at all) just observe or also act to address the problem? Whether the observer is to take a passive or more active role should be decided in advance and will also depend on whether the intervention is at an early stage of development (e.g., feasibility testing) or whether effectiveness is being evaluated. During feasibility testing, MRC guidance (2015) states that taking an active approach is more appropriate compared to when effectiveness is being evaluated (given an active approach here would threaten the external validity of the evaluation).

- What happens if different members of the team have different views on how the intervention should work? In such instances, can the team back up their views with evidence? Can all of the views be integrated together in a logic model (a visual representation of what is being delivered, its effects and how these effects are achieved)?

- Will including process measures be off-putting to participants in your study and/or those delivering the intervention? Will it lead to more people dropping out of the study? Will it lead to components of the intervention not being delivered? Feasibility/pilot testing can be helpful to address these types of questions.

- Given the variety of methods available for process evaluations, what methods should be used? A useful step towards the start of planning a process evaluation is to look for similar studies that can be used as a guide for what methods to use.

- Can existing theories or models, such as those overviewed in Chapter 2, be used as a framework for assessing and testing mechanisms of action? Using such theories or models can be appealing as they often make clear what mechanisms of action to measure and how these relate to one another; they may also have an existing evidence base. However, do they provide a full account of how your intervention will work in your context? Does this account make sense to those delivering and/or receiving the intervention, or does the model need to be adapted in some way to account for possible differences in views? Exactly what the intervention is and how it is anticipated to have its effects on outcomes (including for us, as authors of a health behavior change textbook, measures of health behavior!) should be agreed before the process evaluation plan is finalized.

As well as these types of issues, Moore et al. (2015) also provide other guidance regarding how to conduct a process evaluation. Importantly, they argue that a process evaluation should be conducted prior to analyses that identify whether the intervention was effective or not to minimize the risk of biased interpretation. They also note that process evaluations should report quantitative information on reach, dose and fidelity; this can enable tests to identify whether features of the context (e.g., the socioeconomic status of the targeted population) affects, for example, how much of an intervention an individual receives (dose), how aligned the intervention delivery was with the planned delivery (fidelity) and if it affected whether they received the intervention at all (reach). If, for example, those from low socioeconomic groups receive less of the intervention, there is a risk that the intervention increases inequalities and steps should be taken to address this limitation.

Process evaluations can be conducted for different types of studies. Process evaluation of feasibility/pilot studies are useful in helping to understand how feasibly the intervention can be implemented and tested, its acceptability and identifying how the design and evaluation can be strengthened. At the full trial stage, a process evaluation is useful to strengthen confidence in the effectiveness of the intervention (by taking account of the quality and quantity of what was delivered within the intervention) and its generalizability (by taking account of context).

RE-AIM

RE-AIM (standing for Reach Effectiveness Adoption Implementation Maintenance) is a framework that can be used to consider the extent to which an intervention has the potential to lead to public health benefits (Glasgow et al., 1999). Interventions may appear to be effective in changing behavior but if they are not widely adopted, for example, then they are unlikely to achieve widespread public health benefits. Interventions with high reach (high proportion of the target population are exposed to the intervention), effectiveness (the intervention is successful), adoption (high proportion of eligible settings, target staff or organizations take up and use the intervention), implementation (the intervention is implemented as intended) and maintenance (the intervention becomes integrated within the routine practice of the organization and the effects of the intervention are maintained over time) represent the interventions most likely to generate public health impact.

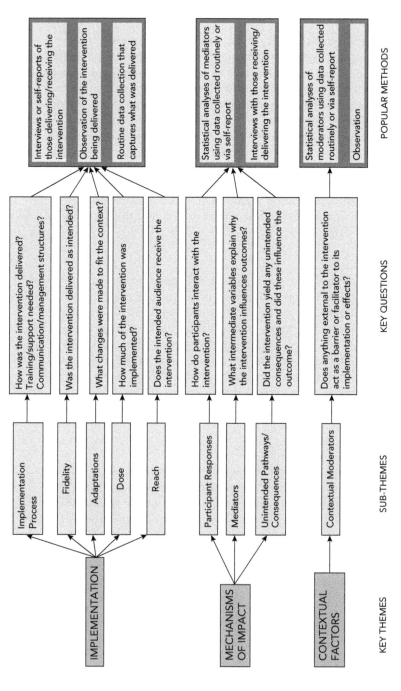

FIGURE 6.5 Overview of the key elements of process evaluation of complex evaluations. (based on Moore et al., 2015).

QUALITATIVE ANALYSES

Just as quantitative (numerical) data can be analyzed in different ways, qualitative (more descriptive) data can also be analyzed in various ways. For example, thematic analysis involves the researcher presenting, or categorizing, the qualitative material into themes often based around the general research questions. Alternatively, grounded theory involves the researcher coding elements of the text before grouping similar codes together into categories in an attempt to generate a theory which is consistent with the content of the text. Analyzing qualitative data can be deemed subjective (though some may approach analysis in a more neutral, objective way), and this subjectivity can be seen as a potential limitation with different people potentially drawing different inferences from the same dataset. However, subjectivity has also been argued to have some advantages; for example, it allows the researcher to draw on their own experiences to better understand the participant and serves to ensure that the participant is not kept at a distance (Drapeau, 2002).

SUMMARY

Analyzing the results of studies related to health behavior change is important to understand the potential for health benefits, to explain why relationships between variables such as exposure to health behavior interventions and health behaviors emerge (via mediation) and when such relationships are stronger or weaker (via moderation). Behavioral scientists have a variety of statistical approaches that they can use to analyze data, and it is essential that an appropriate statistical approach is selected. While the most common approaches were overviewed in Figure 6.1, other statistical approaches are required in some instances such as in cluster trials/group randomized trials when approaches such as multilevel modelling are more suitable. A number of hurdles need to be cleared in the statistical analysis procedures such as how best to handle missing data and outliers and we have highlighted key issues in relation to these. As well as considering the effectiveness of health behavior interventions, process evaluations provide additional information relating to how well the intervention is implemented, potential mechanisms, and context that can influence, positively or negatively, the effectiveness of the intervention. RE-AIM is a potentially useful framework to consider effectiveness and process-related factors in order to estimate the potential public health benefits that may accrue from a particular health behavior intervention.

FURTHER READING

Hayes, A. F. (2021). *Introduction to mediation, moderation, and conditional process analysis. 3rd Edition.* Guilford Press. Overviews and describes mediation, moderation and their integration plus introduces a macro called PROCESS that can be used within SPSS and SAS to conduct basic and more complex mediation and moderation analyses containing multiple mediators and moderators.

Kristopher Preacher has an excellent website that explains moderation analysis (including simple slopes analyses) in more detail and provides online calculators that you can use to run simple slopes analyses: http://www.quantpsy.org/interact/.

G★Power, a program that is useful to help calculate a-priori sample sizes and statistical power, can be downloaded for free: http://www.psycho.uni-duesseldorf.de/abteilungen/aap/gpower3/download-and-register.

A collection of articles considering ways in which sample sizes can be planned in advance of conducting studies can be found here: https://www.biomedcentral.com/collections/randomizedtrialsamplesize.

More about RE-AIM here www.re-aim.org/.

GLOSSARY

Alternative hypotheses: a prediction in which a significant difference across groups or significant relationship between variables is anticipated.

Carry-over effects: a bias linked with within-subject designs where performance on one task has an impact that is still persistent on a second task.

Correlational design: a design in which there is no manipulation of variables, i.e., the researcher is required only to *measure* variables.

Effectiveness: relates to whether an intervention works in real-world settings where a number of factors are free to vary.

Effect sizes: standardized treatment effect useful for comparing the impact of manipulations (or size of relationships) across studies.

Efficacy: relates to whether an intervention works in ideal (tightly controlled) settings.

Experimental design: a design in which the experimenter *manipulates* variables to identify whether changes in one variable (the independent variable, IV) cause changes in an outcome variable.

Fatigue effects: a bias associated with within-subjects designs where performance diminishes in later tasks due to tiredness.

Heterogeneity: reflect differences

Statistical heterogeneity: reflects differences in effect sizes across studies

Clinical heterogeneity: reflects differences in studies through use of different participants, interventions or outcomes

Methodological heterogeneity: reflects differences in studies due to using different designs or having different risks of bias

Intention-to-treat analyses: a statistical approach in which data from all participants are analyzed irrespective of whether they chose not to comply, deviated from the protocol or dropped out/withdrew from the study.

Learning effects: a bias linked with within-subject designs where participants' learning on the first task can be used to assist them in subsequent tasks.

Mediation: a statistical approach examining *why* two variables are related.

Meta-analysis: a statistical procedure used to combine, compare and contrast the findings of studies on a related topic.

Meta-regression: a statistical procedure in which measures are used to predict study effect sizes.

Moderation: a statistical approach that attempts to identify *when* two variables are related.

Null hypothesis: a prediction in which groups are anticipated not to differ or measures are anticipated to be unrelated.

Order effects: a bias linked with within-subjects design; the order in which the tasks are completed can influence the findings: e.g., task A influences task B but task B doesn't influence task A.

Outliers: data points that differ from the general trend of the data-set and consequently exert a potentially undue effect on the statistical findings.

Power: ability to detect a significant effect within the sample of participants used in a study when a significant effect truly exists (i.e., within the entire population).

Sub-group analysis: statistical procedure where the statistical test is conducted separately for different groups of participants or conditions to identify whether the findings differ across participants/ conditions.

Type 1 error: an instance in which an alternative hypothesis is accepted but should have been rejected.

Type 2 error: an instance in which an alternative hypothesis is rejected but should have been accepted.

REFERENCES

Ajzen, I. (1991). The theory of planned behavior. *Organizational Behavior and Human Decision Processes, 50*, 179–211.

Bricker, J.B., Liu, J., Comstock, B.A., Peterson, A.V., Kealey, K.A., & Marek, P.M. (2010). Social cognitive mediators of adolescent smoking cessation: Results from a large randomized intervention trial. *Psychology of Addictive Behaviors, 24*, 436–445.

Conner, M., & Higgins, A. (2010). Long-term effects of implementation intentions on prevention of smoking uptake among adolescents: A cluster randomized controlled trial. *Health Psychology, 29*, 529–538.

De Boer, M.R., Waterlander, W.E., Kuijper, L.D.J., Steenhuis, I.H.M., & Twisk, J.W.R. (2015). Testing for baseline differences in randomized controlled trials: an unhealthy research behavior that is hard to eradicate. *International Journal of Behavioral Nutrition and Physical Activity, 12*, 4.

De Vet, E., Oenema, A., Sheeran, P., & Brug, J. (2009). Should implementation intentions interventions be implemented in obesity prevention: the impact of if-then plans on daily physical activity in Dutch adults. *International Journal of Behavioral Nutrition and Physical Activity, 6*, 11.

Farh, J.-L., Lee, C., & Farh, C.I.C. (2010). Task conflict and team creativity: A question of how much and when. *Journal of Applied Psychology, 95*, 1173–1180.

Farrokhyar, F., Reddy, D., Poolman, R.W., & Bhandari, M. (2013). Why perform a priori sample size calculation? *Canadian Journal of Surgery, 56*, 207–2013.

Glasgow, R.E., Vogt, T.M., & Boles, S.M. (1999). Evaluating the public health impact of health promotion interventions: the RE-AIM framework. *American Journal of Public Health, 89*, 1322–1327.

Hayes, A. F. (2021). *Introduction to mediation, moderation, and conditional process analysis. 3rd Edition.* Guilford Press.

Hoffman, L., & Walters, R.W. (2022). Catching up on multilevel modelling. *Annual Review of Psychology, 73*, 659–689.

Lakens, D. (2022). Sample size justification. *Collabra: Psychology, 8*, 33267.

Lakens, D., Pahlke, F., & Wassmer, G. (2021). Group sequential designs: A tutorial. *PsyArXiv.* https://doi.org/10.31234/osf.io/x4azm

Moore, G.F., Audrey, S., Barker, M., Bond, L., Bonell, C., Hardeman, W., … Baird, J. (2015). Process evaluation of complex interventions: UK Medical Research Council (MRC) guidance. *BMJ, 350*: h1258.

O'Connor, D.B., Jones, F., Conner, M., McMillan, B., & Ferguson, E. (2008). Effects of daily hassles and eating style on eating behavior. *Health Psychology, 27*, S20–S31.

Prestwich, A., Conner, M., Hurling, R., Ayres, K., & Morris, B. (2016). An experimental test of control theory-based interventions for physical activity. *British Journal of Health Psychology, 21*, 812–826.

Preacher, K. J., Zhang, Z., & Zyphur, M.J. (2016). Multilevel structural equation models for assessing moderation within and across levels of analysis. *Psychological Methods, 21*, 189–205.

Schönbrodt, F.D., & Perugini, M. (2013). At what sample size do correlations stabilize? *Journal of Research in Personality, 47*, 609–612.

7

CHAPTER 7
BEHAVIOR CHANGE THROUGH TARGETING MECHANISMS OF ACTION
HEALTH PROMOTION, RISK AND DETECTION BEHAVIORS

OVERVIEW

The next three chapters of the book focus on different approaches to health behavior change applying what has been learned from the earlier chapters of the book. Chapter 7 considers approaches that focus on key determinants of health behavior (or mechanisms of action) identified in important theories. Chapter 8 considers environment- and policy-based approaches, while Chapter 9 considers technology-based approaches. There are clear overlaps between the material presented in the three chapters and this division is a fairly arbitrary one. In Chapter 7 a range of different health behaviors are considered, including **health promotion behaviors, health risk behaviors** and **health detection behaviors**. Burning Issue Box 7.1 provides an overview of these different types of health behavior and other ways health behaviors can be distinguished.

Models covered in Chapter 2 (e.g., the Theory of Planned Behavior, TPB) specify the determinants to try to change in order to promote health behavior change. These determinants are sometimes referred to as the *target for the intervention* or *mechanism of action*. The idea is that behavior change can be best achieved through changing a mechanism of action that determines that behavior (see Burning Issue Box 7.2). This is a mediational model of

DOI: 10.4324/9781003302414-8

behavior change (see Chapter 4) with the intervention or behavior change technique (BCT) producing change in behavior via change in the mediator (i.e., the mechanism of action or the target for the intervention such as intentions or self-efficacy). These mediators (e.g., intention and/or self-efficacy) are the targets that an intervention tries to change in order to change behavior.

Although the various models specify quite a long list of potential targets for intervention, only a limited number have received significant research attention and might be considered key determinants. The set of key determinants considered here comprise: risk perceptions, attitudes/outcome expectancies, norms, self-efficacy, intentions and implicit influences. Each appears in one or more key models/theories discussed in Chapter 2.

In subsequent sections of this chapter, for each key determinant, we highlight correlational evidence that indicates how important a determinant of behavior it is and intervention research targeting this construct and the observed effects on behavior. We also consider how these vary across different types of health behavior. This way of presenting the evidence is similar to the experimental medicine approach (Davidson et al., 2020; Sheeran et el., 2017) taken to understanding successful health behavior change in projects like the science of behavior change (https://scienceofbehaviorchange.org/) in the USA and the operating conditions framework (Rothman & Sheeran, 2021) (see Burning Issue Box 7.2 for an overview of these approaches). Chapter 7 considers these different stages in relation to six key targets for interventions to change health behaviors (risk perceptions, attitudes, norms, self-efficacy, intentions, implicit influences).

In the final section, we introduce the *Science of Health Behavior Change: In Action* feature which is used to evaluate studies testing a behavior change intervention to change health behavior. This feature illustrates how the scientific, critical approach that we introduced in the first six chapters can be applied in the context of different health behaviors.

BURNING ISSUE BOX 7.1

HOW BEST TO CLASSIFY HEALTH BEHAVIORS?
Health behaviors can be grouped in various different ways (Conner & Norman, 2019):

- *Health-promotion versus health risk* or impeding behaviors. The former are associated with decreased mortality and morbidity (i.e., death and illness), while the latter are associated with increased mortality and morbidity.
- *Preventive* (those which aim to prevent onset of ill-health and includes prevention and risk behaviors), *detective* (those which aim to detect potential problems), *curative* (those which aim to cure or treat a health problem).
- *Frequent versus infrequent*: more frequent health behaviors may be more habitual in nature.
- "*Easy immediate pay-offs* versus *effortful long-term pay-offs*"; "*private un-problematic* versus *public and problematic*"; "*important routines* versus *unimportant one-offs*" (McEachan et al., 2010).
- An interdisciplinary taxonomy of behavior (including health behaviors) included 250 behaviors classified into nine domains: engaging in learning and applying knowledge; communicating; moving/exercising; engaging in self-care behavior; engaging in domestic life activities; engaging in interpersonal interactions and relationships; engaging in behavior related to major life areas; engaging in behavior related to community, social and civic life; engaging in mood/state changing activities and behavior (Larsen et al., 2019).

The distinction used in this textbook is between promotion, risk and detection health behaviors and focuses on the target of the behavior:

- **Health promotion behaviors** help protect or maintain health when engaged in (e.g., physical activity, healthy eating).
- **Health risk behaviors** can damage or risk health when engaged in (e.g., smoking, alcohol consumption).

- **Health detection behaviors** help detect potential problems that when treated early can lead to better health outcomes (e.g., skin examination, screening attendance).

BURNING ISSUE BOX 7.2

THE EXPERIMENTAL MEDICINE APPROACH AND OPERATING CONDITIONS FRAMEWORK TO HEALTH BEHAVIOR CHANGE

The experimental medicine approach (Davidson et al., 2020; Sheeran et al., 2017) focuses attention on a mediational model of health behavior change (see Chapter 2). The first stage is the identification of the modifiable factor or factors that cause the behavior. This is sometimes called the target or mechanism of action and includes things like intentions and self-efficacy. The second stage assesses the impact of changing these modifiable factors on behavior change and is sometimes called the validation pathway (because it is about validating the effect of the target on the behavior). This may be experimental research that manipulates the modifiable factor and observes the effect on the behavior or correlational studies that observe how the modifiable factor and behavior covary. The third stage assesses the impact of different manipulations on the modifiable factor to identify the best way to change it. This is called the engagement pathway because it is about ensuring the manipulation leads to engagement with the target. The fourth and final stage tests whether an intervention produces change in the behavior through changing the modifiable factor (i.e., a mediation model). For example, research might identify intentions to get vaccinated against COVID-19 as the key modifiable factor influencing COVID-19 vaccination behavior (stage 1). Then research might focus on assessing the degree of vaccination intentions with subsequent vaccination behavior (stage 2). Additional research might then test different ways of changing intentions to get vaccinated (stage 3). This stage might identify that persuasive messages focusing on the safety of vaccination and efficacy of vaccination as the best means to change vaccination intentions. The last stage (stage 4) would involve assessing the effectiveness of these persuasive messages in changing vaccination behavior and the extent to which this effect on behavior change can be explained by changes in intentions.

Rothman and Sheeran (2021) extend the experimental medicine approach by considering moderators of the different paths and call this the operating condition framework. In particular, they discuss the idea of moderators of how strongly the modifiable factor influences behavior and the intervention influences the target. These are referred to as validity moderation and engagement moderation.

Validity moderation asks the question: Under what conditions do changes in the target elicit changes in the behavior? Rothman and Sheeran (2021) highlight aspects of the behavior, intervention, context and population as the key operating conditions. For example, there may be differences between risk and protection behaviors, between active and passive interventions, between high and low socio-economic status neighborhoods, or between different age groups in how well a target like intentions is associated with a health behavior. Population may be a particularly important operating condition that requires much more study. We know that intentions can be better predictors of behaviors like physical activity (e.g., Godin et al., 2010) in high compared to low education groups. But we know much less about whether intentions predict health behaviors to the same or a different extent in specific populations (e.g., those with mental health problems, those with physical disabilities).

Engagement moderation asks the question: Under what conditions does the intervention elicit changes in the target? Rothman and Sheeran (2021) again highlight aspects of the behavior, intervention, context and population as the key operating conditions. For example, in relation to context, public versus private recording of progress towards a goal leads to greater self-monitoring (Harkin et al., 2016). More research is needed on the impact of different operating conditions on how well different manipulations lead to different impacts on targets.

This experimental medicine/operating conditions framework may provide a useful way for thinking about research on health behavior change.

_____

RISK PERCEPTIONS AND HEALTH BEHAVIOR

Knowing that smoking, eating certain foods or being inactive leads to certain health conditions reflects general risk perceptions. These general risk perceptions, in themselves, are unlikely to lead to behavior change. Instead, an individual needs to feel at personal risk. These risk perceptions are an individual's perceived susceptibility or vulnerability to a threat (e.g., "How likely are you to catch COVID-19?"). They appear in important models of health behavior such as the Health Belief Model (HBM; there labelled perceived susceptibility, see Chapter 2) and Protection Motivation Theory (PMT; there labelled perceived vulnerability, see Chapter 2) as direct predictors of health behavior (in HBM) or as indirect predictors via intentions (in PMT). Avoiding risky but pleasurable behaviors (e.g., smoking, drinking alcohol) and engaging in healthy but inconvenient health promotion behaviors (e.g., physical activity, wearing a mask) are assumed to be partly driven by perceptions of the probability that a (positive or negative) health consequence will follow (Ferrer & Klein, 2015). This probability of a health consequence is the risk perception. A classic example would be the perceived risk of getting cancer from smoking (see Burning Issue Box 7.3 on adolescent smoking). Interestingly, there is evidence that such risk perceptions become stronger and increasingly important drivers of health behaviors as we age (Renner et al., 2007).

BURNING ISSUE BOX 7.3

ADOLESCENT SMOKING: DO E-CIGARETTES INCREASE OR DECREASE TAKING UP SMOKING?

The last few years have seen a dramatic rise in e-cigarettes use. E-cigarettes commonly comprise of a liquid containing nicotine and flavorings that are heated to produce a vapor that is inhaled (hence the term vaping). These were seen as a safer alternative to smoking (albeit not health risk free, especially in the long-term) because they contain the nicotine but not the many cancerous substances released when burning tobacco and a way to help people quit smoking. E-cigarettes have generally been judged to be a success in helping people quit smoking (the "off ramp" from smoking).

The effects of e-cigarette use on taking up smoking (the "on ramp" to smoking), particularly in adolescents, is something that has caused a great deal of debate. Adolescents who take up vaping seem to be much more likely to go on to smoke cigarettes than those who do not take up vaping. For example, Conner et al. (2018) showed that in a sample of nearly 3,000 UK adolescents those who tried e-cigarettes were five times as likely to start smoking cigarettes as those who did not try e-cigarettes. Two quite different explanations have been offered for this and many other similar findings. First, that this indicates a gateway into smoking with many who would never have taken up smoking doing so because they tried e-cigarettes. Second, that this simply indicates common liabilities, with those who try e-cigarettes being the same adolescents who would have first tried cigarettes if e-cigarettes had not been available. Distinguishing between these two potential explanations has proved difficult! One idea has been to control for various predictors of initiating smoking and then see if a relationship between trying e-cigarettes and then starting smoking remains. A number of studies have done this. For example, the Conner et al. (2018) study showed that controlling for various predictors like attitudes towards smoking and family and friends smoking only modestly reduced the impact of e-cigarette use on later smoking initiation (dropping from being five times more likely to four times more likely). However, the list of potential predictors of starting smoking is very long and it is unlikely that any one study can control for all such predictors. Nevertheless the studies that do control for more such predictors do report smaller effects for e-cigarettes on subsequent smoking initiation.

As e-cigarette use becomes more prevalent in adolescent groups it will be interesting to see the impact on cigarette use. If the common liabilities explanation is correct then more vaping might mean less cigarette use in young people, so reducing the risks from smoking, although we may then become more concerned about the health risks associated with long-term vaping. If the gateway explanation is correct then more vaping may lead to more cigarette use or at least a blunting of the downward trend in smoking rates that has been observed in many countries over the past 20 years.

Ferrer and Klein (2015) refer to the above type of risk perceptions as **deliberative risk perceptions** and distinguish them from **affective risk perceptions**. Deliberative risk perceptions are systematic, logical and rule-based and emphasize the idea that individuals rely on a number of reason-based strategies to derive an estimated likelihood that a negative or positive outcome will occur (e.g., "I don't know many people who have caught influenza so it is probably not very common and therefore I am unlikely to catch it"). In contrast, affective risk perceptions refer to the affect associated with risk. For example, affective reactions such as worry, anxiety or anticipated regret about a health behavior may be associated with thinking about engaging in that behavior (e.g., "I worry about catching influenza"). Ferrer and Klein (2015) also make the case for experiential risk perceptions that refer to rapid judgements made by integrating deliberative and affective information into an "intuition" or "gut feeling" (e.g., "My hunch is that I will not get influenza").

CORRELATIONAL STUDIES ON RISK PERCEPTIONS

Do risk perceptions correlate with different types of health behaviors and associated intentions? The short answer is yes, meaning they are usual targets for interventions designed to change health behaviors. However, these correlations may be stronger for affective risk perceptions than deliberative risk perceptions.

For deliberative risk perceptions, meta-analyses across multiple health behaviors using the PMT (Milne et al., 2000) indicate small-sized correlations with intentions and behavior (Table 7.1). Relatively few studies were included in this review, however. More focused reviews on specific health behaviors suggest slightly higher values but still in the small-medium magnitude effect size range (e.g., Brewer et al., 2016, on vaccination reported r_+ = .26, .24 and .16 for risk likelihood, susceptibility and severity, respectively, with vaccination behavior).

For affective risk perceptions, meta-analyses across various behaviors suggest medium-sized correlations with engaging in the behavior (Loewenstein et al., 2001). For health behaviors, anticipated regret has received particular attention. Regret is a negative affective reaction that most of us are familiar with in relation to negative outcomes following acting in a particular way (e.g., shouting at a friend). Anticipated regret refers to the idea of anticipating how we might feel if we performed a particular behavior such as smoking or binge drinking but before we actually act in that way. Anticipated guilt is a similar negative affective reaction, while anticipated pride and satisfaction are anticipated positive affective reactions. However, research in this area has tended to focus on anticipated regret to the exclusion of these other important anticipated affective reactions (see Conner et al., 2013a, for an exception in relation to blood donation).

Anticipated regret has been found to be a strong predictor of engaging in protection (e.g., fruit and vegetable intake: Caso et al., 2016), risk (e.g., avoiding smoking in adolescents: Conner et al., 2006) and detection (e.g., Sandberg & Conner, 2009) health behaviors. One meta-analysis (Sandberg & Conner, 2008) showed anticipated regret to have large-sized correlations with intentions to engage in health-behaviors (r_+ = 0.47), and medium-sized correlations with health behaviors (r_+ = 0.28). Interestingly these relationships remained significant when controlling for variables from the TPB suggesting that the TPB may benefit from being modified to incorporate anticipated regret. In the largest published meta-analysis of anticipated regret and health behaviors, Brewer et al. (2016) reported that across 81 studies containing over 45,000 participants, the correlation with intention was equivalent to a large-sized effect, while the correlation with behavior was equivalent to a medium-sized effect (Table 7.1). Interestingly

TABLE 7.1 Effect sizes for key determinants of health behaviors based on reviews of the literature.

	Correlational Studies				Experimental Studies					
	Intention		Behavior		Construct		Intention		Behavior	
Construct	N	r_+	N	r_+	N	d_+	N	d_+	N	d_+
Deliberative risk perception	2	0.16	<1	0.12	35	0.75	27	0.36	12	0.25
Affective risk perception	46	0.50	46	0.29	4	0.39	4	0.27	3	0.30
Attitude	65	0.49	59	0.27	35	0.47	59	0.48	67	0.38
Behavioral beliefs	21	0.39	18	0.22	3	0.39	-	-	-	-
Affective attitude	13	0.55	13	0.30	-	-	-	-	22	0.43
Cognitive Attitude	13	0.38	13	0.19	-	-	-	-	-	-
Norms	63	0.34	55	0.19	10	0.62	16	0.48	17	0.36
Normative beliefs	23	0.35	20	0.22	4	0.54				
Injunctive norms	18	0.39	12	0.22	-	-	-	-	-	-
Descriptive norms	18	0.35	12	0.27	-	-	-	-	-	-
Self-efficacy	2	0.33	1	0.22	37	0.65	50	0.51	90	0.47
Perceived behavioral control	68	0.46	61	0.27	26	0.26	-	-	-	-
Control beliefs	19	0.41	17	0.26	1	0.68				
Capacity	7	0.60	7	0.39	-	-	-	-	-	-
Autonomy	7	0.27	7	0.19	-	-	-	-	-	-
Intentions	n/a	n/a	69	0.40	47	0.66	n/a	n/a	47	0.36
Implicit influences	n/a	n/a	-	-	87	<0.30	-	-	-	-
Implicit Associations Test	n/a	n/a	15	0.27	-	-	-	-	-	-

Data taken from Brewer et al., 2016; Ellis et al., 2018; Forscher et al., 2019; Gardner et al., 2011; Greenwald et al., 2006; McEachan et al., 2011, 2016; Milne et al., 2000; Rhodes et al., 2019; Sheeran et al., 2014, 2016; Steinmetz et al., 2016; Webb & Sheeran, 2006. Note N is in 1000's. For r+ small, medium, large effect sizes equate to .1, .3 and .5, respectively; for d+ small, medium, large effect sizes equate to .2, .5 and .8, respectively (based on Cohen, 1992).

correlations were broadly similar across different health behaviors for intentions, but for behavior they tended to be higher for physical activity and speeding/unsafe driving compared to vaccination, cancer screening, smoking and safe sex/condom use. However, the most striking difference was for action versus inaction regret. Action regret is about regretting doing something like taking up smoking. More anticipated action regret about doing or starting a behavior is positively correlated with not starting that behavior. This usually applies to risk behaviors like smoking. Inaction regret is about regretting not doing something. Anticipated inaction regret about not doing or starting a behavior is negatively correlated with engaging in that behavior and usually applies to protection (e.g., physical activity) and detection (e.g., attending screening) behaviors. The Brewer et al. (2016) review showed that although the correlations for inaction regret with behavior was positive and the correlations for action regret with behavior were negative, they were of approximately the same magnitude.

There has been relatively little research on the factors that might make deliberative or affective risk perceptions more or less predictive of engaging in health behavior (i.e., validity moderation). Future research could usefully explore the moderating factors that do influence these relationships (see Burning Issue Box 7.2).

CHANGING RISK PERCEPTIONS

Given affective risk perceptions could be more strongly related with health behaviors than deliberative risk perceptions, changing affective risk perceptions may be a particularly important way to change health behaviors. That's not to say that being able to change deliberative risk perceptions is not important. Indeed interventions that target both types of risk perceptions (affective and deliberative) could lead to larger changes in health behaviors than interventions that target just one. As such, we consider ways to change each type of risk perceptions.

Many studies have attempted to change risk perceptions to produce changes in intentions and behavior. Sheeran et al.'s (2014) meta-analysis showed changes in risk appraisal were associated with small to medium sized effects on intentions ($d_+ = 0.31$) and behavior ($d_+ = 0.23$). These effect sizes were similar for deliberative risk perceptions and affective risk perceptions (Table 7.1). These effects were also in the small to medium sized range for anticipatory emotions like fear and worry (intention: $d_+ = 0.31$; behavior: $d_+ = 0.21$) and perceived severity (intention: $d_+ = 0.32$; behavior: $d_+ = 0.34$). There was no strong evidence of differences between protection/risk versus detection behaviors in any of these relationships (i.e., moderation effects; see Burning Issue Box 7.2 on engagement moderation).

A more focused review by Ellis et al. (2018) looked at interventions reported in 37 publications that focused on changing affective forecasting (i.e., predictions about how a decision/behavior will make you feel; this maps onto affective risk perceptions). These studies mainly examined anticipated regret. They reported a small but significant effect size across these studies on anticipated regret (d_+ = .24), intention (d_+ = .19) and behavior (d_+ = .29). The included studies either tried to change anticipated affect using messages and narrative text or the salience of anticipated affect by asking questions about anticipated regret or not. Ellis et al. (2018) reported that these approaches led to similar sized changes in behavior.

Persuasive messages to promote health behavior change through targeting deliberative risk perceptions are one common approach to change risk perceptions. Health promotion leaflets that promote the benefits of health promotion behaviors (e.g., physical activity) or detection behaviors (e.g., bowel screening) or detail the costs associated with health risk behaviors (e.g., smoking) are common. In this section, we look at the ways in which messages are best "framed" to change protection, risk or detection health behaviors. In addition, because some individuals might easily dismiss information about health risk behaviors because they are seen as threatening to the individual (e.g., "that cholesterol test indicating I've got high cholesterol is faulty and it's not important!"), we cover self-affirmation as an approach to reduce defensiveness and the tendency to dismiss health messages about health risk behaviors.

Message framing

Prospect theory states that presenting the same information about an outcome or risk in different ways alters people's perspectives, preferences and actions (Kahnkeman & Tversky, 1979; see Burning Issue Box 2.1). This work has not, in general, distinguished between affective or deliberative risk perceptions. People tend to avoid risks when they are considering gains (e.g., how many people saved) and prefer risks when considering losses (e.g., how many people died).

Rothman and Salovey developed a **message framing** approach built on prospect theory and reasoned that within the health domain, the influence of gain and loss framed messages is contingent on the perceived function of the health behavior and its associated risk (Rothman & Salovey, 1997; Rothman et al., 1999). Health detection behaviors (such as screening) carry the risk that a disease or abnormality will be found and therefore are perceived as risky, whereas health promotion behaviors (such as eating healthily) or reducing health risk behaviors (such as quitting smoking) are perceived as being relatively risk free as they are performed to avoid future health problems. They suggest that detection behaviors will be encouraged when health information is framed in terms of losses ("If you do not do X you will not achieve Y"; e.g., "Failing to attend for screening will mean you miss out on the chance to get treatment for any problems") and promotion/risk behaviors will be encouraged when gain framed messages are employed ("If you do X you will achieve Y"; e.g., "Quitting smoking can lead to improved health and living a longer life").

Although some studies have shown gain-framed messages are more effective than loss-framed messages for promotion/risk behaviors, such as sunscreen use (Detweiler et al., 1999), psoriasis symptom reduction (Keyworth et al., 2018), regular physical exercise (Robberson & Rogers, 1988) and loss-framed messages are more effective than gain-framed messages for detection behaviors like mammography screening (Banks et al., 1995) and HIV testing (Kalichman & Coley, 1995), the evidence base is somewhat complicated. For instance, more recently loss-framed messages were found to be more effective in promoting colorectal cancer screening but only when culturally targeted (Lucas et al., 2021). Moreover, a meta-analysis of the persuasive impact of message framing on attitudes, intentions and behaviors concluded that loss frame appeals were not particularly effective for increasing detection behaviors, but were more effective for increasing promotion behaviors (Gallagher & Updegraff, 2012).

Self-affirmation

Self-affirming involves reflecting on one's cherished values, actions or attributes. The result of this self-reflection is to restore or reinforce the person's sense of who they are and what they stand for in the face of perceived threats to their identity. **Self-affirmation** theory calls this sense of who they are "self-integrity," which is defined as the experience of the self as "adaptively and morally adequate" (Steele, 1988, p. 262). The theory suggests that people are strongly motivated to maintain self-integrity. As health messages are often perceived as threatening to self-integrity because they focus attention on one's negative behaviors, individuals may be motivated to play down the importance of such messages. So, for example, a smoker exposed to a health message about the risks of smoking may protect his/her self-integrity in one of two ways, either denigrate the potential risks of smoking set out in the message or make renewed efforts to quit smoking. Unfortunately from the point of view of the originator of the message it is often the former response that is adopted. Self-affirmation theory offers a useful way round this problem.

It is suggested that self-integrity can be restored or reinforced by affirming sources of self-worth that are important to the person's identity but unrelated to the threat. For example, a smoker may remind herself of her strengths as a mother leading to the self-concept of being a smoker becoming less threatening to her self-integrity. The key consequence from the point of view of intervention is that salient, self-affirming thoughts can reduce the pressure to diminish the threat in other self-threatening information and thereby promote the ability to think objectively (Steele, 1988, p. 290). Someone who self-affirms in this way then has available to them the perspective and resources to better confront a self-threat (Sherman & Cohen, 2006). The idea that self-affirming can promote more objective appraisal of threatening material is appealing to researchers interested in using health messages to change behavior. This is because such messages typically contain important yet unwelcome information and resistance to them is common, particularly among high risk groups (Freeman, Hennessy & Marzullo, 2001).

Epton et al. (2015) reviewed 144 studies and concluded that self-affirming promotes greater general and personal acceptance of health risk information, and less message derogation. For example, Jessop et al. (2009) reported that self-affirmation led to sunbathing women rating a leaflet about skin cancer and sun safety as less overblown, exaggerated, manipulative and straining the truth. Several studies also show that self-affirmation can increase intentions to change health risk behaviors (e.g., Harris & Napper, 2005) and even health-relevant behaviors. For example, Sherman et al. (2000, study 2) showed that, compared to non-self-affirmed, the self-affirmed took more leaflets about HIV and purchased more condoms. Recent research has shown that self-affirming via an explicit focus on values or self-generation of affirming thoughts through essay writing are two of the most effective forms of self-affirmation to change health behavior intentions (Iles et al., 2021). Future research could usefully address whether self-affirmation can have effects on behavior change that is sustained over time.

_____

ATTITUDES/OUTCOME EXPECTANCIES AND HEALTH BEHAVIOR

Attitudes are an individual's overall evaluation of an attitude object which here is usually a behavior (e.g., "My smoking is…bad/good"). Such attitudes towards behaviors are important predictors of intentions in the Theory of Planned Behavior (TPB) and Reasoned Action Approach (RAA). The assumption is that we tend to intend and then engage in behaviors we evaluate positively and intend not to perform and not engage in behaviors we evaluate negatively. In the TPB, attitudes are treated as overall evaluations, while in the RAA they are split into cognitive/instrumental attitudes and affective/experiential attitudes. **Cognitive attitudes** tend to be tapped by semantic differentials such as harmful-beneficial or negative-positive (e.g., "My smoking would be… harmful-beneficial"). In contrast **affective attitudes** tend to be tapped by semantic differentials such as unpleasant-pleasant or not enjoyable-enjoyable e.g., "My smoking would be… unpleasant/pleasant"). Attitudes are not the same as outcome expectancies (beliefs about the outcome of a behavior). However, models like the TPB and RAA assume that attitudes are based on outcome expectancies about the result of performing a behavior (see below).

In both the TPB and RAA, attitudes are assumed to be based on judgements about the likelihood of various consequences of engaging in the behavior (referred to as behavioral beliefs). These expectancies or likelihoods are weighted by the evaluation of each outcome as positive or negative. Attitudes are assumed to be based on the sum of these expectancy-values, i.e., if you think mainly negative outcomes will follow smoking you are likely to evaluate your smoking negatively, while if you think that mainly positive outcomes will follow you eating healthily you are likely to evaluate your healthy eating positively. It is assumed that an individual will have a limited number of consequences or outcomes in mind when considering performing a behavior or not (i.e., only a few outcomes will be salient). This expectancy-value framework is based on Fishbein's (1967) summative model of attitudes.

CORRELATIONAL STUDIES ON ATTITUDES/OUTCOME EXPECTANCIES

McEachan et al.'s (2011) meta-analysis of TPB studies indicated that attitudes and behavioral beliefs both show medium to large sized correlations with intentions and small to medium sized correlations with behavior (Table 7.1). Behavioral beliefs only showed small to medium sized correlations with attitudes ($r_+ = 0.38$) suggesting that other factors may influence attitudes. McEachan et al. (2011) also reported similar sized correlations across different health behaviors. In summary, attitudes and outcome expectancies might be useful targets for interventions designed to change a broad range of health behaviors.

A similar review on applications of the RAA to health behaviors (McEachan et al., 2016) indicated affective attitudes to have large sized correlations with intentions and medium sized correlations with behavior, while cognitive attitudes had medium to large sized correlation effects with intentions and small to medium sized correlation effects with behavior (Table 7.1). For example, Conner and Norman (2021) showed that it was affective rather than cognitive attitudes that predicted long-term healthy eating over periods of up to 10 years. Conner et al. (2022) recently showed that when such affective attitudes were stable over time they were particularly predictive of later health behavior. The larger effects for affective compared to cognitive attitudes is notable given that interventions in the health domain have typically targeted cognitive (e.g., health) over affective (e.g., pleasantness) aspects of health behaviors. The stronger effects for affective attitudes over cognitive attitudes suggest the former might be particularly useful targets for changing health behaviors (see further discussion in a later section). However, interventions targeting both cognitive and affective attitudes might yield greater changes in health behavior and more research should test this possibility.

CHANGING ATTITUDES/OUTCOME EXPECTANCIES

It is worth distinguishing between studies that focus on changing attitudes and those that focus on changing outcome expectancies. In the TPB/RAA attitudes are assumed to be based on outcome expectancies about the behavior. The TPB and RAA assume that the best way to change attitude (and intentions plus behavior) is to target behavioral beliefs about outcomes of engaging in the behavior (Ajzen & Schmidt, 2020). Persuasive messages are typically used to target expectancy (e.g., making perceived likelihood of positive outcomes appear more likely or making perceived likelihood of negative outcomes appear less likely), evaluation (e.g., making positive outcomes appear more positive or making negative outcomes appear more negative) or the salience of beliefs (e.g., introducing new positive outcomes). Steinmetz et al. (2016) indicated that across 14 tests of such interventions a small to medium sized change in (behavioral) outcome expectancies was produced (Table 7.1), although this was not statistically significant. The subsequent effects on intentions and behavior were not reported.

There is a much larger body of literature that has focused on directly changing attitudes, typically using persuasive messages (see Hamilton & Johnson, 2020 for a review). Sheeran et al. (2016) provide a useful meta-analysis of studies focusing on health behaviors using interventions to change attitudes and examining effects on intentions and behavior. Across 87 tests, Sheeran et al. (2016) reported that interventions produced a small–medium sized change in attitudes (Table 7.1). This change in attitude was associated with small to medium sized changes in intentions (59 tests) and behavior (67 tests) (Table 7.1). Similar sized effects were observed for frequently or infrequently performed prevention (i.e., protection and risk) behaviors and disease management behaviors. Burning Issue Box 7.4 on changing sedentary behaviors notes that persuasion was suggested to be a promising means of changing this behavior.

BURNING ISSUE BOX 7.4

CHANGING SEDENTARY BEHAVIOR

Sedentary behaviors include sitting and lying down, for example, when reading this textbook, watching television or using the internet. Research has shown that excessive sedentary behavior is a risk factor for various health outcomes. This includes becoming overweight and getting heart disease but also impacts on frailty in older adults. Interestingly the risk seems to remain even when controlling for physical activity – so don't think that going for a run means you can have a well-earned rest (well, not too much of a rest, anyway!). Reducing the duration and frequency of sedentary periods can be useful ways to reduce these risks.

Gardner et al. (2016) took the approach of reviewing the literature to identify interventions that might be effective in reducing sedentary behavior in adults. Out of 38 interventions, promising interventions mainly targeted sedentary behavior (versus physical activity) and used behavior change techniques (BCTs) such as environmental restructuring, persuasion, or education. Self-monitoring, problem solving and restructuring the social or physical environment were particularly promising BCTs and persuasion was rated as promising too. Gardner et al. (2017) suggested that effective sedentary reduction interventions might usefully incorporate environmental modification (e.g., standing desks) and self-regulatory skills training (e.g., self-monitoring of sedentary behavior and setting goals to reduce sedentary behavior).

In the next sections we look at interventions that focus on three topics. First, we explore research on outcome expectancies as a means to change health behavior. Second, we consider how the Elaboration Likelihood Model provides a means to understand work on attitude change. And third, we review recent research focusing on changing affective attitudes.

Changing outcome expectancies

Models like the Theory of Planned Behavior (TPB) and Social Cognitive Theory (SCT) emphasize the importance of expectancies as determining individual's decisions about how to act. They suggest that behavior and decisions are based upon an elaborate, but subjective, cost/benefit analysis of the likely outcomes of differing courses of action. As such they have roots going back to Expectancy-Value Theory (Peak, 1955) and Subjective Expected Utility Theory (SEU; Edwards, 1954). It is assumed that individuals generally aim to maximize utility and so prefer behaviors with lots of benefits and few costs. The overall utility or desirability of a behavior is assumed to be based upon the summed products of the probability (expectancy) and utility (value) of specific, salient outcomes or consequences.

As an example, imagine that Liam and Amy both perceive the key outcomes of taking up smoking to be effects on their health and whether smoking will make them look cool. We can assess the utility of taking up smoking to Liam and Amy by getting them to rate each outcome in terms of likelihood (e.g., Taking up smoking will damage my health, very unlikely -2 -1 0 +1 +2 very likely) and value (Damaging my health is…, very bad -2 -1 0 +1 +2 very good). Liam thinks taking up smoking is slightly likely to damage his health (rated +1) and slightly likely to look cool (rated +1) but rates damaging his health as very bad (rated -2) and being cool as slightly good (rated +1). His overall utility for taking up smoking will be -1 (i.e., [+1 × -2] + [+1 × +1]). Amy is not sure taking up smoking will really damage her health (rated 0) but will definitely look cool (rated +2) and rates damaging her health as slightly bad (rated -1) and being cool as really good (rated +2). Her overall utility for taking up smoking will be +4 (i.e., [0 × -1] + [+2 × +2]). In this case we might expect Amy to be more likely to take up smoking than Liam because she rates the behavior more positively (i.e., her utility for smoking is higher) and is likely to have a more positive attitude towards smoking.

While such considerations may well provide good predictions of which behaviors are selected, it has been noted by several authors that they do not provide an adequate description of the way in which individuals actually make decisions (e.g., Frisch & Clemen, 1994). For example, except for the most important decisions, it is unlikely that individuals integrate information in this way because it requires a lot of mental energy to achieve this. Nevertheless considerable research emphasizes the power of outcome expectancies to predict intentions and behavior. They provide an important insight into why individuals perform behaviors and also useful targets for interventions to change behaviors.

Research in recent years has looked at different dimensions on which such beliefs might fall. In SCT, outcome expectancies are split into physical, social and self-evaluative depending on the nature of the outcomes considered. More recently, Rhodes et al. (2010) suggested three dimensions along which outcome expectancies might be placed. First, beliefs may be distinguished along positive (e.g., physical activity makes me feel good) versus negative (e.g., physical activity is painful) valences. This approach is central to assessment of **attitudinal ambivalence** and a focus of belief structure in models like the transtheoretical model and the Health Belief Model. It has also been argued that it is the positive-negative dimension that value judgements tap in traditional applications of the TPB/RAA (Conner &

Sparks, 2015). Second, beliefs may be distinguished across an affective (e.g., physical activity is fun) versus instrumental (physical activity prevents disease). Third, beliefs may be distinguished by the temporal proximity of the expected outcome. That is, physical activity has proximal (e.g., stress management) and distal (e.g., weight control, disease prevention) temporal outcomes.

Rhodes et al.'s (2010) 2 × 2 × 2 model of beliefs suggests eight different types of beliefs that might be distinguished (Figure 7.1). Future research might usefully assess whether specific types of beliefs are key for particular behaviors. For example, Rhodes et al. (2010) present data suggesting that interventions targeting proximal positive affective beliefs (fun, accomplishment, stress relief) may yield greater intentions to be physically active, and a secondary focus on overcoming proximal negative affective beliefs (muscle soreness, pain) may also have merit. This would be in contrast to typical health promotion messages that might target distal negative instrumental beliefs (physical activity will help you live longer). Studies support the focus on affective compared to instrumental beliefs when changing behaviors such as physical activity (Conner et al., 2011c) or fruit and vegetable consumption (Carfora et al., 2016).

Health risk behaviors like binge drinking may also be particularly influenced by proximal positive affective beliefs (fun, stress relief). A number of studies use parts of this classification of beliefs or outcomes in relation to understanding health risk behaviors. For example, Goldberg et al. (2002) noted the importance of positive beliefs (e.g., There is an x% chance that I'll have a better time at the party if I drink alcohol than if I don't drink) in relation to predicting drinking in young people. Research also suggests that people tend, in general, to emphasize proximal over distal outcomes. For example, Hall and Fong's (2007) temporal self-regulation theory emphasizes the importance of proximal over distal outcomes in determining behavior (see Burning Issue Box 7.5 on discounting).

Grogan et al. (2011) used an interesting intervention focusing on the proximity of the outcome to reduce smoking in a sample of young women. In this research a computerized facial age-progression technique was used to show how the individual's face "aged" differently if they continued to smoke or not (Figure 7.2). This technique made the distal negative outcome of smoking on how the face looks more immediate and proximal and reduced self-reported smoking (although only over limited periods of time). Research has shown this technique to also be effective in reducing sun exposure (Williams et al., 2013).

	Positive outcomes		Negative outcomes	
	Proximal outcomes	Distal outcomes	Proximal outcomes	Distal outcomes
Affective outcomes	Feeling good about self for stopping smoking	Feeling pride in being a non-smoker	Missing the pleasure of smoking	Regretting never being able to have a cigarette
Instrumental outcomes	Saving money by not Buying cigarettes	Being healthier as a non-smoker	Not knowing what to do with your hands	Not wanting to be around people smoking

FIGURE 7.1 A 2 × 2 × 2 structure for behavioral beliefs as applied to smoking cessation.

BURNING ISSUE BOX 7.5

DISCOUNTING OF OUTCOMES

Discounting of outcomes refers to the idea that temporally proximal outcomes (e.g., doing physical activity leads to be being tired and sweaty) influence behavior more strongly than do distal consequences (doing physical activity leads to better health and a longer life).

Temporal self-regulation theory (TST; Hall & Fong, 2007) provides one account of why risk behaviors (e.g., excessive drinking) are adopted even though the long-term negative consequences seem to vastly outweigh the short-term positive consequences. TST, like several other models, suggests that intentions are key determinants of behavior. However, TST also suggests that behavioral prepotency and self-regulatory capacity are additional key determinants of behavior. Behavioral prepotency refers to the frequency of past performance of the behavior and the presence of cues to action in the environment (i.e., the fact that we tend to act in similar ways to which we have in the past, especially when in similar environments). Self-regulatory capacity refers to the individual's capacity to effortfully regulate their own behavior (this may be determined by executive function, energy levels or conscientiousness). It is usually measured by the personality construct of self-control. So even when the long term negative consequences of a behavior outweigh the short term benefits, risk behaviors can occur when the behavior is habitual or cued in certain environments and when self-regulatory capacity is limited (such as when drinking alcohol).

Changing attitudes via systematic processing and heuristics

Attitude change in response to a persuasive message is something we are all familiar with. But what factors influence the amount and duration of attitude change? In general, research focusing on changing health behaviors through changing attitudes has tended to focus on developing strong messages to change behavior. Petty and Cacioppo (1986) define strong messages as those that produce mainly favorable thoughts about the message. So, if after reading a message about the benefits of eating five portions of fruit and vegetables a day you have mainly positive thoughts, then your attitude towards eating five portions of fruit and vegetables a day is likely to become more positive. If your reactions are negative or quite mixed then little or no attitude change will occur.

Models of attitude change suggest there are two distinct routes to attitude change. In one route, the information in the persuasive message is systematically and carefully considered and attitude change is determined by the extent

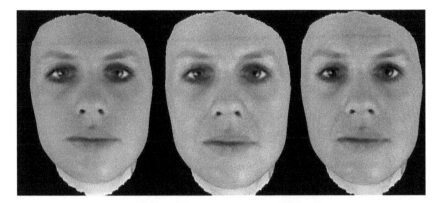

FIGURE 7.2 Effects of smoking on aging – baseline photo; photo aged to 50 years without smoking; photo aged to 50 years with smoking (see Grogan et al., 2011).

that the message produces mainly favorable thoughts about the message. This route to persuasion is called the ***central or systematic route***. It is what we traditionally think of as persuasion and requires quite a bit of mental effort. The second route to persuasion does not require careful scrutiny of the message or detailed thought and is labelled the ***peripheral or heuristic route***. Here, persuasion depends on the presence of peripheral cues that prompt the use of **heuristics** (i.e., simple rules like experts have more reliable information and so produce more attitude change than the same message from a non-expert). Figure 7.3 sets out the two routes, the factors influencing which route dominates and the consequences of each route for attitude change.

Petty and Cacioppo (1986) argue that because we receive so many messages each day, we do not have the motivation or ability to carefully process each one. They refer to the amount of systematic processing devoted to a message as "cognitive elaboration" and, consequently, their model is known as the *Elaboration Likelihood Model* (ELM). High elaboration is associated with central route (effortful) processing of messages while low elaboration is associated with peripheral route (effortless) processing. The ELM suggests that both central processing and peripheral processing occur simultaneously for all messages but that usually one or other will dominate.

Elaboration and central route processing are more likely when we are highly motivated because the message is about an issue of interest to us. The strength of the arguments in the message are then critical to the amount of persuasion that occurs. This is consistent with traditional views of how persuasion works: strong arguments will persuade us to change our views; weak arguments will be dismissed and have little impact on attitude change.

Ability to think about a message also influences the amount of elaboration. Having time pressure or being distracted (e.g., when messages are presented

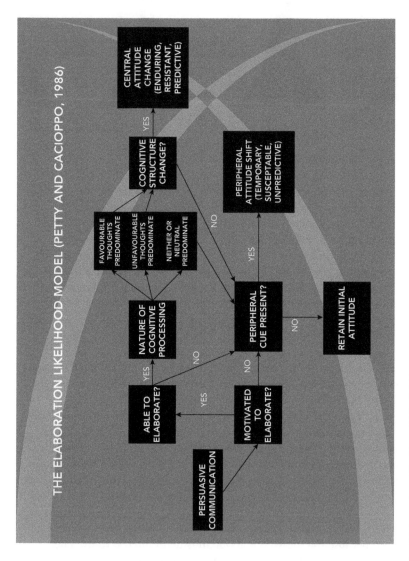

FIGURE 7.3 The Elaboration Likelihood Model (Petty & Cacioppo, 1986).

quickly amid distractions as is the case in many television or radio advertisements), for example, can reduce elaboration and persuasion will be more likely via the peripheral route. This route involves little systematic processing (low cognitive elaboration) and other characteristics of the message are more likely to determine whether or not it is persuasive. For example, people use simple rules or decision-making heuristics to evaluate messages (Chaiken, 1980). These include "expertise = accuracy" ("she's an expert so what she says must be right") or "consensus = correctness" ("if so many people agree they must be right") and "length = strength" ("there are lots of arguments so it must be true").

In general, research using the ELM has focused on both developing strong messages to change behavior and using peripheral cues to change behavior. Attitude change resulting from systematic (central route) processing is generally more likely to be stable and more likely to influence subsequent behavior. However, as a persuader if you do *not* have strong arguments then you are better discouraging systematic processing and relying instead on peripheral cues like numerous arguments, consensus and perceived expertise. So, if your health product or service has a number of features that are likely to be valued by consumers that are different from similar products then developing a strong message about those features may be the best way to win new customers. This sort of persuasive message is common in paper adverts for high cost items like cars and computers where customers have the motivation and opportunity to carefully consider arguments. In contrast, if your product is very similar to other products then using peripheral cues may be a better approach. This sort of persuasive message is common in television adverts for low cost items like washing powder or food products where customers do not have the motivation or opportunity to carefully consider the product. Peripheral cues like associating the product with a happy tune or getting celebrity endorsements are more common here.

BURNING ISSUE BOX 7.6

HEALTH BEHAVIORS AND NET ZERO: THE CASE OF REDUCING MEAT CONSUMPTION

The focus of this book is on health behaviors; behaviors engaged in because of their impacts on health. Many of the lessons learned in relation to predicting and changing health behaviors may generalize to other sorts of behaviors such as behaviors that help protect the environment and contribute towards achieving net zero (i.e., balancing the carbon we put into and take out of the environment in response to the climate emergency). Reducing car use and increasing recycling are good examples that individuals try to engage in. However, some behaviors can have both health and environmental effects. For example, replacing car use with walking can have both health and environmental impacts. One behavior that may be particularly important in this regard is reducing meat (particularly red meat) consumption. Reducing red meat consumption is associated with reduced risk of cancer and a positive impact on the environment (reduced biodiversity loss and greenhouse gas emissions as farm production switches away from meat production).

Carfora et al. (2017) showed that a daily text message focused on self-monitoring of red meat consumption (e.g., "Remember to monitor your red meat consumption for not exceeding two medium servings per week using the daily food diary") significantly reduced red meat consumption one week later compared to a group not receiving messages. Interestingly the intervention appeared to have its effects through changing identities (e.g., as a healthy eater) and intentions. In particular, the message group reported stronger healthy eating and weaker meat-eating identities and intentions. The changes in identities may lead to longer term effects on meat eating. Carfora et al. (2019) also used a daily text message intervention to see if messages focused on health (e.g., "If you eat little red and processed meat, you will protect your health from colon cancer/heart disease/respiratory disease") versus environmental (e.g., "If you eat little red and processed meat, you will protect the environment from the release of harmful greenhouse gases/soil acidification/climate change") outcomes was more successful. Both interventions reduced red meat consumption one month later and appeared to do so through changing attitudes towards red meat consumption. Interestingly a combined condition with health and environmental messages was not successful in changing meat eating (perhaps there was just too much information to absorb in the combined condition).

Future research could usefully explore a broader range of interventions to reduce meat consumption and the value of focusing on health versus environmental reasons (or both) for long-term behavior change.

Impact of changing affective attitudes

It is possible that changing affective attitudes leads to larger changes in health behaviors than changing other types of attitudes. For example, Conner et al. (2011c) demonstrated that participants exposed to messages focusing on the affective benefits of exercise (makes you feel good, enjoyable) backed up with citations to scientific articles (to imply an expert

INSTRUMENTAL CONDITION:

It is well-known that regular physical activity can have a tremendous effect on your health. Experts say that adults should engage in approximately 30-60 minutes of accumulated physical activity per day (where each separate bout is a minimum of ten minutes)[1]. Another position stand is for adults is defined as a daily energy expenditure of 1.5 kilocalories/kilogram of body weight/day or more; roughly equivalent to brisk walking one half hour every day or more)[2,4]. Research has shown that regular moderate-vigorous physical activity is associated with the following health benefits: [1,2,3,4,5]

- Weight control and decreased risk of obesity.
- Reduces the risk of dying prematurely.
- Reduces the risk of heart disease.
- Reduces the risk of developing diabetes.
- Reduces the risk of developing high blood pressure.
- Helps reduce blood pressure in people who already have high blood pressure.
- Reduces the risk of developing colon and breast cancer.
- Helps build and maintain healthy bones, muscles, and joints.
- There is a linear relationship between increased activity and health benefits (↑PA =↑benefits).

Some Statistics[4]:

- Globally, there are more than 1 billion overweight adults, at least 300 million of them obese.
- An estimated 16.7 million - or 29.2% of total global deaths - result from the various forms of cardiovascular disease (CVD), many of which are preventable by action on the major primary risk factors: unhealthy diet, physical inactivity, and smoking. Inactivity greatly contributes to medical costs - by an estimated $75 billion in the USA in 2000 alone.
- At least 60% of the global population fails to achieve the minimum recommendation of 30 minutes moderate intensity physical activity daily.
- Physical inactivity is estimated to cause 2 million deaths worldwide annually. Globally, it is estimated to cause about 10-16% of cases each of breast cancer, colon cancers, and diabetes, and about 22% of ischaemic heart disease.
- The risk of getting a cardiovascular disease increases by 1.5 times in people who do not follow minimum physical activity recommendations.
- In Canada, physical inactivity accounts for about 6% of total health care costs.

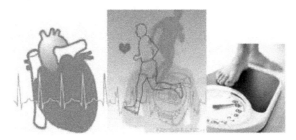

1. Public Health Agency of Canada. *Physical Activity Unit*, retrieved October 31, 2006 from: http://www.phac-aspc.gc.ca/pau-uap/paguide/why.html
2. CFLRI. Surveys Statistics Summaries, retrieved October 31, 2006 from: http://cflri.ca/eng/statistics/index.php
3. Centers for Disease Control and Prevention. *Physical Activity and Health*, retrieved October 31, 2006 from: http://www.cdc.gov/nccdphp/sgr/contents.htm
4. World Health Organization. *Physical Activity*, retrieved October 31, 2006 from: http://www.who.int/dietphysicalactivity/publications/facts/pa/en/index.html
5. Warburton, D., Nicol, C., & Bredin, S. (2006). Health benefits of physical activity: the evidence. *Canadian Medical Association Journal*, *174*, 801-809.

FIGURE 7.4 A &B: Messages used in Conner et al. (2011c).

(Continued)

AFFECTIVE CONDITION:

It is well-known that regular physical activity can have a tremendous effect on your immediate well-being. Experts say that adults should engage in approximately 30-60 minutes of accumulated physical activity per day (where each separate bout is a minimum of ten minutes)[1]. Another position stand is Activity for adults is defined as a daily energy expenditure of 1.5 kilocalories/kilogram of body weight/day or more; roughly equivalent to brisk walking one half hour every day or more)[2]. Read on for some of the ways physical activity can improve your daily life:

- Regular physical activity has been shown to reduce anxiety, depression, and stress which can improve how you feel, your mood, and increase your sense of wellbeing.
- Research has shown that regular activity improves general reports of quality of life.
- Physical activity can be associated with increased energy levels and reduced fatigue, giving you more energy and vitality to enjoy your day.
- Physical activity is an outlet for socializing with friends and creating new social connections for many people through sports, fitness clubs, as well as with exercise partners and groups.
- Many types of physical activity provide a fun, enjoyable activity to do in your leisure time.
- Physical activity often improves the way one feels about their body/appearance, through more positive body image and self-esteem.

Some Specifics From the Research:

- 85% of studies looking at the acute affects of physical activity on mood showed some degree of improved mood following exercise.[3]
- Some studies suggest that physical activity can raise endorphin levels, thus decreasing feelings of depression, and elevating mood.[4]
- After only 20 minutes of moderate to vigorous physical activity, anxiety symptoms have been shown to decrease.[5]
- 60% of studies report a positive association between physical activity and self-esteem.[6]

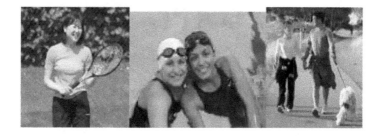

1. Public Health Agency of Canada. *Physical Activity Unit*, retrieved October 31, 2006 from: http://www.phac-aspc.gc.ca/pau-uap/paguide/why.html
2. World Health Organization. *Physical Activity*, retrieved October 31, 2006 from : http://www.who.int/dietphysicalactivity/publications/facts/pa/en/index.html
3. Yeung, R. (1996). The acute affects of exercise on mood state. *Journal of Psychosomatic Research*, 40, 123-141.
4. O'Neal, H., Dunn, A., & Martinsen, E. (2000). Depression and exercise. *Journal of Sport Psychology*, 31, 110-135.
5. O'Connor, P., Raglin, J., & Martinsen, E. (2000). Physical activity, anxiety, and anxiety disorders. *Journal of Sport Psychology*, 31, 136-155.

FIGURE 7.4 (Continued)

source, see Figure 7.4) reported doing several more exercise sessions at three-week follow-up compared to individuals exposed to an equivalent cognitive message focusing on health benefits (again which citations to scientific articles) or those in a control group (see Figure 7.5). Additional analyses showed that changes in behavior were explained or mediated by

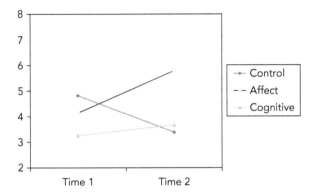

FIGURE 7.5 Frequency of moderate/vigorous exercise of at least 30 minutes duration.

(From Conner et al., 2011c).

changes in affective attitudes (see Chapter 6 regarding mediation analyses). The authors argue that the data show the value of targeting affective attitudes as one means to achieve behavior change. It may also be the case that the affective messages were more novel to respondents compared to the cognitive messages that stressed general health messages about the benefits of exercising. This greater novelty might have led to more systematic (i.e., careful) processing of the affective messages resulting in more positive affective attitudes and greater impacts on behavior. Carfora et al. (2016) showed similar effects in relation to eating fruit and vegetables. Conner et al. (2020) provide a review of the impact of changing affective attitude on behavior change.

NORMS AND HEALTH BEHAVIOR

Norms are included in the TPB and RAA as predictors of intentions (referred to as subjective norms in the TPB and social norms in the RAA). Norms are a person's beliefs about whether significant others think he/she should engage in the behavior (i.e., normative beliefs). Norms are based on beliefs about salient others' approval or disapproval of whether one should engage in a behavior (e.g., "Would my best friend want me to do this?") weighted by the *motivation to comply* with each salient other on this issue (e.g., "Do I want to do what my best friend wants me to do?"). It is assumed that an individual will only have a limited number of individuals or groups (often referred to as referents) in mind when considering performing a behavior. The RAA distinguishes between injunctive norms (concerning the social approval of others) and descriptive norms (perceptions of what others do). It is assumed that the more an individual perceives that salient others want them to perform a behavior and they engage in the behavior that the more the individual will intend to engage in the behavior.

CORRELATIONAL STUDIES ON NORMS/NORMATIVE BELIEFS

McEachan et al.'s (2011) meta-analysis indicated norms and normative beliefs both show medium to large sized correlations with intentions and small to medium sized correlations with behavior (Table 7.1). Normative beliefs only showed small to medium sized correlations with overall norms ($r_+ = 0.32$) suggesting that other factors may influence overall norms. They also reported norms showed slightly stronger correlations with intentions for risk and safer sex ($r_+ = 0.40$; $r_+ = 0.45$, respectively) than for detection, physical activity, diet and abstinence ($r_+ = 0.33$; $r_+ = 0.32$; $r_+ = 0.35$; $r_+ = 0.33$, respectively) health behaviors, with a similar pattern (albeit weaker) for the correlations between norms and behavior for risk, safe sex and abstinence ($r_+ = 0.26$; $r_+ = 0.21$; $r_+ = 0.21$, respectively) than for detection, physical activity and diet ($r_+ = 0.19$; $r_+ = 0.18$; $r_+ = 0.15$, respectively) health behaviors. The fact that the magnitude of these relationships for norms is smaller than that for attitudes might suggest that it would be more effective to target attitudes than norms, although this may vary from one health behavior to another.

A similar review on applications of the RAA to health behaviors (McEachan et al., 2016) indicated injunctive and descriptive norms each have medium to large sized correlations with intentions and small to medium sized correlations with behavior (Table 7.1). Hence, both might be targets for interventions, although it is not clear if there is any advantage in targeting both simultaneously in attempts to change behavior.

CHANGING NORMS/NORMATIVE BELIEFS

Sheeran et al. (2016), in a meta-analysis, reported that interventions produced a medium-large sized change in norms which were associated with small to medium sized changes in intentions (16 tests) and small-medium sized changes in behavior (17 tests) (Table 7.1).

There are not published reviews on the effectiveness of interventions to independently change injunctive or descriptive norms (or indeed both) and the consequences for intentions and behavior. However, Prestwich et al. (2016) did show that studies that targeted descriptive norms versus other types of norms in relation to drinking alcohol produced slightly stronger effects on behavior.

In the next section we look at interventions that have used the social norms approach.

Social norms approach (SNA) to changing norms

The SNA (Perkins, 2003; Berkowitz, 2004) suggests that the correction of misperceptions about social norms is an important mechanism for changing behavior. For example, believing that most other people like you regularly binge drink alcohol can promote your own alcohol use. Via the SNA, which provides accurate feedback about what other people like you think and do in relation to a behavior, learning that many fewer people (than you thought) actually engage in binge drinking may change your own norms and lead to a change in your binge drinking. However, Prestwich et al.'s (2016) review suggested that even when large changes in normative beliefs about alcohol consumption are achieved, there is only a small reduction in alcohol intake. The SNA has also been used in relation to changing detection behaviors such as bowel screening. Wilding et al. (2020, see Figure 7.6 for the messages used) showed SNA messages combined with implementation intentions (see Chapters 3 and 7) increased bowel screening rates. In using the SNA it is important that the normative information is perceived as accurate and that it refers to a social group very similar to you.

WHO takes part in screening?

Most people aged between 60-74 in the **North East of England** are choosing to take part in bowel cancer screening.

Around

70%

of people in the UK have already taken part in some form of cancer screening

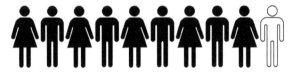

Around **9 in 10** people believe that cancer screening is almost <u>always</u> a good idea

Every day, over 110 people in the UK find out that they have bowel cancer.
Using the test can make sure you are diagnosed early **before signs of cancer show.**
Nearly **everyone** (over 90%) who is diagnosed early will survive bowel cancer.

These are some of the many reasons why most people take part in screening.

Choose to protect yourself, use your screening kit

FIGURE 7.6 Social norms approach (SNA) message use in relation to bowel screening (Wilding et al., 2020).

SELF-EFFICACY, PERCEIVED BEHAVIORAL CONTROL AND HEALTH BEHAVIOR

Self-efficacy is the belief that a behavior is or is not within an individual's control and is usually assessed as the degree of confidence the individual has that they could still perform the behavior in the face of various obstacles (e.g., "I am confident I can eat healthily even when out with friends"). It is a key component of Social Cognitive Theory (SCT) where it is assumed to directly influence behavior and also indirectly influence behavior through intentions.

Perceived behavioral control (PBC) is a person's expectancy that performance of the behavior is within their control and confidence that they can perform the behavior and is similar to Bandura's (1982) concept of self-efficacy (as in the SCT and Protection Motivation Theory, see Chapter 2 for overviews). In the Theory of Planned Behavior and Reasoned Action Approach, perceived behavioral control is assumed to influence behavior via intentions and also to moderate the intention-behavior relationship, meaning you are more likely to enact that intention of going for a run if you're confident you're able to go for a run.

PBC is assumed to be based on control beliefs concerning whether one has access to the necessary resources and opportunities to perform the behavior successfully (e.g., "How often does this facilitator/inhibitor occur?"; "How often are you with friends when they are smoking?, never/frequently"), weighted by the perceived power or importance of each factor to facilitate or inhibit the action (e.g., "How much does this facilitator/inhibitor make it easier or more difficult to perform this behavior?"; "How much does being with friends when they are smoking make it more or less difficult to resist smoking?"). These factors include both internal control factors (information, personal deficiencies, skills, abilities, emotions) and external control factors (opportunities, dependence on others, barriers). It is assumed that an individual will only consider a limited number of control factors when considering performing a behavior.

The RAA splits PBC into capacity (the perceived ease/difficulty of performing the behavior and people's confidence in performing the behavior should they wish) and autonomy (people's belief that they have control over the behavior and its performance is up to them). Capacity is very similar to most definitions of self-efficacy.

BURNING ISSUE BOX 7.7

PREDICTING AND CHANGING COVID-19 PROTECTION BEHAVIORS

Perhaps unsurprisingly the last few years have seen a great deal of attention focused on reducing risks associated with COVID-19 by altering behaviors that might reduce the spread of the virus. Studies in this area largely fall into three categories: identifying predictors of COVID-19 behaviors, intervening to change proxies of behavior (e.g., intentions) and intervening to change COVID-19 behaviors using various designs (with relatively few randomized trials). Here, we illustrate these approaches with reference to different behaviors: quarantining, vaccinations, mask wearing, hand-hygiene and composite measures (comprising of these and other relevant behaviors such as social distancing). For other behaviors such as face touching and panic buying (anybody remember concerns about running out of toilet paper?), there are relatively few high quality studies suggesting these are gaps that require particular attention in the future (Lunn, 2020).

Predictors of behaviors

In a rapid review of the evidence during the COVID-19 outbreak, Webster et al. (2021) identified that to promote quarantine adherence, clear knowledge of the disease and quarantine procedures, perceived quarantine benefits and disease risk, and social norms were all important. In addition, more practical issues (that could affect self-efficacy) like running out of supplies and being able to afford to not go to work also played a role. Several of these factors, along with minimizing the duration of quarantine, were also highlighted as being important for limiting the psychological impact of quarantine including anger and post-traumatic stress symptoms (Brooks et al., 2020).

Further evidence hints at the joint, and possibly interacting, roles of cognitions and external factors. For example, Schüz et al. (2021) showed that the power of different components of the Reasoned Action Approach to predict engaging in various COVID-19 protection behaviors (e.g., keeping at least 2 meters away from other people when outside, washing hands when returning home) varied between different demographic groups. In particular, intentions were weaker predictors and autonomy was a stronger predictor in more compared to less deprived groups. This would suggest the need for targeted interventions in different groups (see Schüz & Webb Hooper, 2020). In relation to the operating conditions framework (Rothman & Sheeran, 2021) this would represent a specification of the operating conditions under which intentions versus autonomy influence COVID-19 protection behaviors.

Changing determinants

Other research has focused on how best to change targets in order to change behavior. For example, in an intervention study, Capasso et al. (2021) showed that messages targeting cognitive attitudes and positive anticipated affective reactions (i.e., feeling pride) led to stronger COVID-19 vaccination intentions in an Italian sample.

In another example, vignettes suggesting higher mask use in others and explaining how face masks protect others (but not how face masks protect the wearer) increased intentions to wear face masks (Bokemper et al., 2021) suggesting the importance of social elements to such behaviors.

Changing behaviors

At a broad level, based on a review of the evidence, Lunn et al. (2020) argue that calls for collective action can be effective in national emergencies (like the COVID-19 outbreak) and these are aided by good communication (calls from leaders for collective action that clearly indicate how such actions are in the best interests of the group can enhance trust, social norms and commitment), enhancing group identity and using just punishment (e.g., social disapproval for non-compliance).

Environmental-based interventions have had mixed success in changing COVID-19 behaviors. Sometimes, effective interventions need to enable accessibility. Pre-COVID, it was estimated that only 15% of people in sub-Saharan Africa had access to soap and water to enable handwashing. It has been noted that since the start of COVID-19, access to such facilities, and subsequently handwashing, has greatly increased (Amegah, 2020).

In places where there is wide access to facilities that aid hand hygiene, increasing frequency of such practices beyond national awareness campaigns might be more difficult. For instance, Weijers and de Koning (2021) reported similar rates of hand sanitizer use in a field experiment that compared three conditions with different messages/ prompts to use hand sanitizer positioned on a stand at the entrance to three department stores (condition 1 (control): "You can disinfect your hands here"; condition 2 (salience): the same message as condition 1 but with blue arrows on the floor pointing to the sanitizer; condition 3 (nudge): "Disinfect your hands, to reduce the likelihood you or someone close to you becomes ill!"). However, it should be noted that just making hand sanitizer available and in a visible location is likely to have increased use in itself (Cure & van Enk, 2015).

Rather than try to increase hand-hygiene *frequency*, an alternative approach is to improve *quality*. For instance, smart handwashing stations that use UV light and digital cameras to highlight to users areas on their hands that they have missed have shown promise (Herbert et al., 2020).

A recent review of seven studies that tested the effect of intervention strategies on actual COVID-19 vaccination uptake or bookings (Batteux et al., 2022) suggested that reminders/personal invitations help increase rates though comparing different types of communication messages (social norm messages, communicating personal and social benefits etc.) did not identify a clear winner. Monetary incentives also produced mixed results.

CORRELATIONAL STUDIES ON SELF-EFFICACY/PERCEIVED BEHAVIORAL CONTROL (PBC)/CONTROL BELIEFS

Does self-efficacy and PBC correlate with different types of health behaviors and intentions to engage in these behaviors? The evidence points to a strong yes to this question.

McEachan et al.'s (2011) meta-analysis indicates that self-efficacy, PBC and control beliefs each have medium to large sized correlations with intentions and small to medium sized correlations with behavior (Table 7.1). Control beliefs only showed medium–large sized correlations with PBC ($r_+ = 0.38$) suggesting that other factors may influence overall PBC. They reported PBC showed slightly stronger correlations with behavior for physical activity and diet ($r_+ = 0.31$; $r_+ = 0.30$, respectively) than for risk, detection, safe sex and abstinence ($r_+ = 0.22$; $r_+ = 0.20$; $r_+ = 0.21$; $r_+ = 0.26$, respectively) health behaviors. It is also notable that the magnitude of these relationships is similar to attitudes but larger than norms (Table 7.1). Therefore both self-efficacy and PBC appear to be appropriate targets for interventions designed to change a range of health behaviors. Future research could usefully address the operating conditions that make self-efficacy a weaker or stronger predictor of health behaviors (i.e., validity moderation; see Burning Issue Box 7.2).

A similar review on applications of the RAA to health behaviors (McEachan et al., 2016) indicated that capacity has large relationships with intentions and medium to large sized relationships with behavior, while autonomy has small to medium sized relationships with intentions and behavior (Table 7.1). This suggests that capacity may be a better target for interventions to change health behavior than autonomy.

CHANGING SELF-EFFICACY/PERCEIVED BEHAVIORAL CONTROL (PBC)/CONTROL BELIEFS

Sheeran et al.'s (2016) meta-analysis indicated that interventions produced a medium-large sized change in self-efficacy which were associated with medium to large sized changes in intentions (50 tests) and small-medium sized changes in behavior (90 tests) (Table 7.1).

Steinmetz et al. (2016) indicated that across six tests interventions produced a large sized change in control beliefs, while 80 tests interventions produced a small sized change in perceived behavioral control (Table 7.1). The subsequent effects on intentions and behavior were not reported. There are no published reviews on the effectiveness of interventions to change capacity versus autonomy or the consequences for intentions and behavior. Nevertheless given the overlap between capacity and self-efficacy then we might expect similar effects for those two. Overall this research suggests that we can change self-efficacy towards particular health behaviors effectively and this will produce changes in the associated intentions and behavior.

Bandura (1997) has shown that self-efficacy over performing a behavior can be enhanced in four distinct ways (in decreasing order of effectiveness): through mastery experiences, vicarious experience, verbal persuasion or changing perception of physiological and affective states (see Chapter 2 for further details about these strategies). Warner and French (2020) provide a review of targeting self-efficacy to change behavior and highlight the targeting of mastery experiences, vicarious experience, verbal persuasion and reducing anxiety as effective ways to change self-efficacy.

The operating conditions that make these different manipulations have stronger or weaker effects on self-efficacy (i.e., engagement moderation; see Burning Issue Box 7.2) would be a useful focus for future research.

_____

INTENTIONS AND HEALTH BEHAVIOR

Intentions represent a person's motivation or conscious plan or decision to exert effort to perform the behavior. They are a key proximal determinant of behavior in the TPB, RAA, PMT (labelled protection motivation) and in SCT (labelled goals). It is worth emphasizing that a number of other influences on behavior (e.g., attitudes in the TPB) are mediated through intentions in this model, in other words, attitudes predict intentions which, in turn, predict behavior.

An interesting question in relation to intentions and health behaviors is the extent to which risk behaviors are "planned" in the way that models such as the TPB, RAA, PMT and SCT would suggest. Let's take the example of smoking initiation in adolescents. Is it the case that the key determinant of smoking initiation in adolescents is the plan or intention to take up smoking? Alternatively, is it the lack of a sufficiently strong plan not to smoke that leads to adolescents starting smoking? Although models like the TPB have typically considered doing intentions and not doing intentions as simple opposites, other research has taken alternative approaches. Some research has suggested that we might usefully consider both doing and not doing cognitions as potentially independent predictors of behavior (see Burning Issue Box 7.8). It is still unclear whether these effects for doing versus not doing cognitions are stronger for risk compared to protection and detection health behaviors. Other research has suggested the need to focus on alternative predictors of these risk behaviors such as affect.

BURNING ISSUE BOX 7.8

ARE DOING AND NOT DOING HEALTH COGNITIONS OPPOSITES?

Models such as the Theory of Planned Behavior (TPB) tend to focus on predicting behavior based on knowledge of individual's cognitions (intentions, attitudes, norms, PBC) about doing that behavior. So, for example, in predicting quitting smoking we might look at intentions to quit, attitudes to quitting, norms about quitting and PBC about quitting. But what about cognitions about *not* quitting and continuing to smoke? The traditional assumption is that these two sets of cognitions (about doing and not doing) are essentially opposites and therefore we don't need to consider both. Richetin et al. (2011) present data from three different health behaviors to suggest this is not always the case. For eating meat (a health risk behavior), doing vigorous physical activity and breastfeeding (both health promotion behaviors) they show that cognitions about doing and not doing these behaviors both predict intentions and behavior. More importantly both types of cognition were simultaneously predictive. This research suggests the value of considering both doing and not doing cognitions in predicting why someone engages in a behavior. More recent research has examined doing and not doing cognitions in relation to engaging in cosmetic surgery (Richetin et al., 2020) and the environmental behavior of reducing resource use (e.g., using less water when brushing teeth) (Richetin et al., 2012).

Richetin et al. (2011) also suggest that doing and not doing cognitions may be based on conflicting goals. So doing vigorous physical activity might be performed to achieve goals such as staying fit and slim and eliminating stress. In contrast, not doing vigorous physical activity might serve the goals of having time for other activities, avoiding tiredness and getting rest. In terms of changing behaviors, this would imply that we need to be careful about which goals we activate!

CORRELATIONAL STUDIES ON INTENTIONS

McEachan et al.'s (2011) meta-analysis indicated that, across 237 tests, intentions show medium to large sized correlations with behavior (Table 7.1) with stronger correlations for physical activity ($r_+ = 0.45$) than for risk, detection, diet, safe sex and abstinence ($r_+ = 0.37$; $r_+ = 0.37$; $r_+ = 0.38$; $r_+ = 0.34$; $r_+ = 0.35$, respectively) health behaviors (see also, McEachan et al., 2016). These findings point to intentions being a key target for interventions to change health behavior.

It is notable that intention is the strongest correlate of health behavior in Table 7.1. This supports the view taken in models like the TPB/RAA/PMT that intention is the key proximal determinant of behavior that mediates the effects of other variables. However, intentions do not show a perfect relationship with behavior (see Chapter 2 on the intention-behavior gap) and considerable research has focused on moderators of the intention-behavior relationship (see validity moderation in Burning Issue Box 7.2). For example, Rhodes et al. (2022) review a large number of moderators of the intention–physical activity relationship. Moderators tested included 19 different sociodemographic and/or medical variables, seven personality variables, five physical capability variables, 10 psychological capability variables, five social opportunity variables, nine environmental opportunity variables, six automatic motivation variables and 17 reflective motivation variables. One such key moderator that may help explain when intentions are stronger predictors of behavior is intention stability (one of the more consistent moderators identified in the Rhodes et al., 2022 review; significant in 9/12 [75%] tests). More stable intentions can predict health behaviors over considerable periods of time (Conner et al., 2002). Conner and Norman (2022) provide a review of work on moderators of the intention–health behavior relationship and focus on intention stability as a key explanatory variable (see also Chapter 2).

Some of this work on moderators has suggested intentions may be weaker predictors of behavior in more versus less deprived groups (see Burning Issue Box 7.9). This might suggest that despite the strong correlation between intentions and behavior that it will not be sufficient to just target intentions and expect health behavior change in some groups. Similarly, other research has suggested intentions may be weaker predictors of behavior in individuals who are low on the personality trait conscientiousness (see Burning Issue Box 7.10). This might suggest that, at least in individuals low in conscientiousness, targeting intentions may not be sufficient to change health behavior.

BURNING ISSUE BOX 7.9

ARE DIFFERENCES IN HEALTH BEHAVIORS ACROSS SOCIO-ECONOMIC STATUS GROUPS REFLECTED IN STUDIES TESTING SOCIAL/HEALTH COGNITION MODELS?

A variety of studies have found higher levels of engagement with health protective behaviors such as physical activity and healthy eating in higher socio-economic status groups. This could be because of weaker intentions to engage in such behaviors in lower socio-economic status groups, although there is not strong evidence to support this view. An alternative possibility is that lack of resources available to lower socio-economic status individuals interferes with their ability to translate healthy intentions into healthy behaviors. Such a moderating effect of socio-economic status on the intention-behavior gap has been shown for promotion behaviors such as breastfeeding and physical activity and risk behaviors such as smoking initiation (Conner et al., 2013b). In each case, the relationship between intentions and behavior was weaker in lower compared to higher socio-economic status groups. This finding could help explain why those from lower socio-economic status groups engage in less health promotion behaviors. Similar findings have been reported in studies of multiple health behaviors (Schüz et al., 2020) and COVID-19 protection behaviors (Schüz et al., 2021).

Schüz et al. (2021) also observed an interaction between autonomy and deprivation, such that more deprived individuals were less likely to do protection behaviors at lower levels of autonomy. At higher levels of autonomy, there was no difference in COVID protection behaviors between most and least deprived. Enhancing autonomy (e.g., through offering choice etc.) could be a way of minimizing these differences.

BURNING ISSUE BOX 7.10

HOW CAN BEING CONSCIENTIOUS IMPROVE HEALTH?

It pays to be conscientious! Conscientiousness refers to the ability to control one's behavior and to complete tasks. Highly conscientious individuals are more organized, careful, dependable, self-disciplined and achievement-oriented than those low in conscientiousness (McCrae & Costa, 1987).

A growing body of research shows conscientiousness to have positive impacts on health behaviors, health outcomes, and even longevity. For example, Friedman et al. (1993) showed that those high in conscientiousness at age 11 were likely to live longer (by about two years) compared to those low in conscientiousness.

An important mechanism by which conscientiousness may influence health is through health behaviors. Friedman et al. (1995) showed that the impact of conscientiousness on longevity was partly accounted for by its effect on reducing smoking and alcohol use. A review of work on the relationship between conscientiousness and behavior (Bogg & Roberts, 2004) showed conscientiousness to be positively related to a range of protective health behaviors (e.g., exercise) but negatively related to a range of risky health behaviors (e.g., smoking). Other studies have shown this effect of conscientiousness on health behaviors such as physical activity to be explained by impacts on intentions. In some studies, intentions have been shown to mediate the impact of conscientiousness on behavior. For example, Conner and Abraham (2001) showed that those with higher levels of conscientiousness also had stronger intentions to exercise and this helped explain the effects of conscientiousness on exercise behavior. Other studies have shown moderation effects. For example, Conner et al. (2007b) showed that intentions were better predictors of exercise behavior among those with high compared to low levels of conscientiousness suggesting highly conscientious individuals are more likely to fulfil their intentions. In a review of moderators of the intention-physical activity relationship, Rhodes et al. (2022) reported that in 80% (4/5 tests) of studies testing the relationship, higher levels of conscientiousness were significantly associated with stronger intention-physical activity relationships.

CHANGING INTENTIONS

Across 47 tests, Webb and Sheeran (2006) reported that interventions produced a medium-large sized change in intentions which were associated with small to medium sized changes in behavior (47 tests) (Table 7.1). They noted that interventions using incentives and social encouragement had the largest effects on behavior ($d_+ = 0.56$) compared to other techniques (provided information, used persuasive communication or risk information: $d_+ = 0.26$; used planning, experiential tasks and rehearsal of relevant skills: $d_+ = 0.20$; used self-monitoring: $d_+ = 0.12$; used personal experiments: $d_+ = 0.06$). In their review, Steinmetz et al. (2016) indicated that across 72 tests of interventions, a medium-large sized change in intentions ($d_+ = 0.34$) was observed. The subsequent effects on behavior were not reported.

Sheeran et al.'s (2016) review suggests that we can change intentions by targeting attitudes, norms or self-efficacy/perceived behavioral control (PBC) consistent with the TPB. The size of effects on intention change were similar for changing attitudes, norms and self-efficacy/PBC ($d_+ = 0.48$, 0.49, 0.51, respectively), suggesting that it perhaps does not matter which of these three are targeted. This would suggest that the interventions discussed earlier in relation to changing attitudes, norms and self-efficacy/PBC could be usefully employed to change intentions. However, we need to know more about when targeting attitudes, norms or self-efficacy/PBC leads to large versus small changes in intentions (i.e., engagement moderation; Burning Issue Box 7.2) and it has also been argued that intentions based on attitudes (particularly affective attitudes) rather than norms leads to intentions that are more likely to lead to behavior (Sheeran & Webb, 2016).

In the next sections we look at interventions that focus on two topics in relation to intentions. The focus is on research that draws on simple techniques to help promote behavior change in those individuals who are generally positively disposed (i.e., motivated or have a positive intention) towards performing the behavior but do not seem to get round to doing it. This contrasts with the techniques reviewed by Webb and Sheeran (2006) that are more useful in getting individuals more motivated to perform a behavior. We consider first, the question-behavior effect, and second implementation intentions (see also Chapter 3).

BURNING ISSUE BOX 7.11

HOW DOES SELF-CONTROL INFLUENCE HEALTH BEHAVIOR?

Self-control refers to the capacity to override impulses, resist temptations, overturn dominant responses and to advance long-term over short-term goals. It is all about ways to control yourself in order to help achieve the things that are important to you. The personality trait of self-control is stable over time, mainly inherited and difficult to change through training. It is also consistently related to engaging in various health promotion behaviors like healthy eating, physical activity and avoiding health risk behaviors like smoking with a small to medium sized effect (r_+ = .26; De Ridder et al., 2012). How does this personality trait have these effects?

In a recent study, Conner et al. (2023) explored and provided support for five different pathways. One reason why self-control promotes health behaviors is that increased self-control leads people to see health actions as both desirable and feasible which, in turn, means that people set goals to undertake health-protection behaviors and avoid health risk behaviors and enact those goals (*valuation pathway*). A second reason is that self-control promotes habit formation (see Burning Issue Box 3.3) which leads to higher rates of attainment of health goals (*habituation pathway*). A third reason is that self-control moderates intention-behavior consistency (i.e., act as a moderator) such that intentions are more effectively translated into action at higher levels of self-control (*translation pathway*). A fourth reason is that self-control influences the basis of intention formation (*prioritization pathway*). The intentions of people with high self-control are more strongly based on the instrumental consequences of health behaviors (cognitive attitudes) and the feasibility of acting (PBC) and less on habits and injunctive norms during intention formation compared to those with low self-control. Finally, self-control moderates associations between affective attitudes, habits and behavior (*inhibition pathway*). In particular, high self-control enables people to overcome affective and habitual influences that could threaten health behavior performance.

Future research could usefully exploit understanding of how these different pathways explain the effects of self-control on health behaviors to generate interventions to change health behaviors in different groups. For example, implementation intentions could be used to alter the weight attached to different considerations during intention formation (e.g., focusing on health reasons for acting in some and normative reasons in others).

Question-behavior effect

Research has indicated that merely asking questions about a behavior may be sufficient to produce changes in that or related behaviors (for reviews see Wilding et al., 2016; Wood et al., 2016). This has come to be known as the **question–behavior effect** (QBE). Use of the QBE in relation to changing health behavior is illustrated by Godin et al. (2008). This study showed that receiving a questionnaire containing questions about intentions to donate blood (along with a range of other questions from the TPB) resulted in increased blood donation at six months (donation rates of 54% vs. 49%, respectively) and 12 months (70% vs. 65%, respectively) compared to a group not receiving a questionnaire. The QBE has subsequently been tested across a range of health behaviors including screening attendance (Sandberg & Conner, 2009) and influenza vaccination (Conner et al., 2011a, Study 2). It has also been shown to be useful in promoting change in multiple health behaviors simultaneously (Wilding et al., 2019).

The most common explanation of the QBE is that asking behavioral intention questions heightens the accessibility of the person's attitude towards that behavior (**attitude accessibility**) which in turn increases the likelihood that attitude consistent behavior will be performed. For example, Morwitz and Fitzsimons (2004) showed that completing purchase intention questions increased the activation level of pre-existing brand attitudes (towards different brands of car). When the brand attitude was both highly accessible and positively valenced, participants were more likely to choose that brand, whereas when the activated attitude was both highly accessible and negatively valenced participants were less likely to choose that brand. Wood et al. (2014) showed that changes in the accessibility of attitudes mediated or explained the effects of asking intention questions on behavior. An interesting consequence of this suggested mechanism is that the QBE can decrease performance of the behavior among those with negative reactions to the behavior. For example, Conner et al. (2011a) showed that screening attendance and influenza vaccination rates among those with negative attitudes and intentions to these behaviors were actually lower for those who completed a questionnaire about these behaviors compared to those who did not receive a questionnaire.

Putting these findings together (i.e., QBE increases behavior when the underlying cognitions are positive and the QBE decreases behavior when the underlying cognitions are negative), Ayres et al. (2013) showed that measuring intentions compared to not measuring intentions only resulted in an increase in the behavior (requesting a personalized health plan) when motivation to protect one's health was also high (based on receiving feedback or not on one's risk factors).

The findings from these and other QBE studies suggest that a relatively simple and cost effective way to promote various health protection behaviors and health detection behaviors is to get individuals to complete intention questions focused on that behavior. However, such effects are only likely to be effective if the underlying cognitions are positive; this makes sense in that it seems unlikely that by simply asking questions we can make someone do something they do not want to do.

Implementation intentions

Another way in which we can increase the performance of health promotion behaviors is through the use of **implementation intentions** or simple if-then plans. Prestwich et al. (2015), note that "to form an implementation intention, the person must first identify a response that will lead to goal attainment and, second, anticipate a suitable opportunity to initiate that response." For example, in order to enact the goal intention to exercise, the person might specify the behavior "go jogging for 20 minutes" and specify a suitable opportunity as "tomorrow morning before work" (p. 324). Mark uses implementation intentions to try to help him exercise at least once per week. Mark's implementation intention is that if it is 5pm on a Wednesday he will get ready to do some exercise. Usually this involves putting his sports gear in a bag to play squash, going to the gym or the climbing wall, although if he is at home it might mean putting his gear on to go out on his mountain bike. Gollwitzer (1993) argues that by forming implementation intentions individuals pass control of intention enactment to the environment. The specified environmental cue prompts the action so that the person does not have to remember the goal intention or decide when to act.

An increasing number of studies have shown the power of implementation intentions to promote both health detection and health promotion behaviors. In relation to the former, Orbell et al. (1997) was one of the first studies to demonstrate an effect of implementation intentions for a health detection behavior. They found that 64% of women asked to form an implementation intention to perform a breast self-exam did so compared to only 16% in the control condition. Wilding et al. (2020) used implementation intentions combined with a motivation intervention to increase bowel screening attendance. Studies have shown similar effects in relation to health protection behaviors like exercise (e.g., by combining a motivation enhancing technique with implementation intentions, Prestwich et al., 2003) and in reducing health risk behaviors like smoking (e.g., by combining anti-smoking motivational messages with forming an implementation intention about how to refuse the offer of a first cigarette, Conner et al., 2019).

Implementation intentions have been shown to increase the performance of a range of health behaviors with, on average, a medium effect size (see Gollwitzer & Sheeran, 2006, for a meta-analysis; for a more detailed evaluation of their impact on behavior, see Chapter 2). Prestwich et al. (2015) provide an in-depth review of both basic and applied research with implementation intentions along with a taxonomy of implementation intentions to change behavior (see Figure 7.7). It is notable that the application of implementation intentions to changing health protection behaviors usually requires the individual to identify appropriate opportunities to perform the behavior. In contrast, the application of implementation intentions to changing health risk behaviors usually requires the individual to identify appropriate alternative ways to act or other strategies when faced with the temptation to perform the health risk behavior (see Figure 7.7).

An interesting recent development has been the idea of collaborative implementation intentions (Prestwich et al., 2005). This is where a pair of individuals form an implementation intention to perform the behavior together. Prestwich et al. (2012) showed such collaborative implementation intentions to be more effective than individual implementation intentions, partner support or a control condition in promoting physical activity, on some but not all measures taken at one-, three- and six-month periods. Carr et al. (2021) have since indicated some promise of the technique for promoting physical activity in postpartum mothers. Studies have also shown such collaborative implementation intentions to be effective for promoting breast self-examination (Prestwich et al., 2005). Effects on healthy eating are less clear cut (Prestwich et al., 2014) though there is some promising evidence in support of reducing salt-intake in heart failure patients (Teoli Nunciaroni et al., 2021).

A variation of collaborative implementations, dyadic planning (Burkert et al., 2011), has emerged which involves an individual being helped in the formation of the plan by their partner but not requiring the partner and individual to perform the behavior together. This approach is sometimes viable when collaborative implementation intentions are not, for example, when the behavior does not apply to the partner (e.g., they do not smoke) or the partner has no interest in performing the target behavior themselves. In terms of risk behaviors, stop smoking dyadic plans for an individual, who cohabits and is in a romantic relationship with a non-smoker, were similarly effective to individual implementation intentions (Buitenhuis et al., 2021).

In comparisons of all three planning types (collaborative, dyadic, individual), evidence suggests collaborative could be best for reducing sedentary behavior, collaborative and individual might be better for increasing exercise habits relative to control, while dyadic might be best for promoting physical activity behavior (see Kulis et al., 2022). Further research is needed to compare and contrast these forms of planning, identify when and for whom each type of plan works best and to contrast these strategies against other types of dyadic interventions that have been applied successful to change health promotion and risk behaviors (see Carr et al., 2019, for a review).

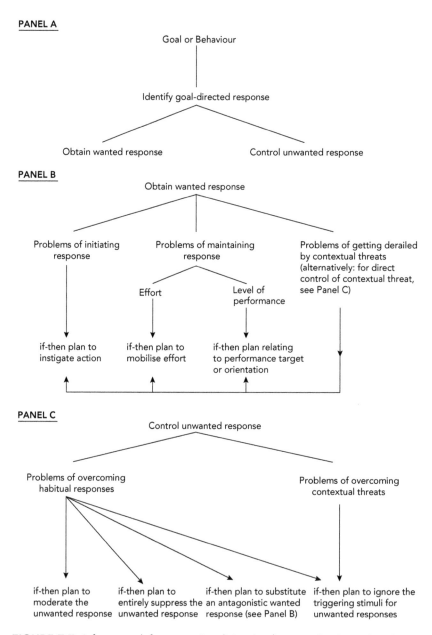

FIGURE 7.7 A framework for operationalizing implementation intentions in relation to particular volitional problems (redrawn from Prestwich et al., 2015). Note panel B applies to using implementation intentions to promote health promotion behaviors, and panel C applies to using implementation intentions to reduce health risk behaviors.

IMPLICIT INFLUENCES AND HEALTH BEHAVIOR

The influences on health behavior described in models like the TPB, PMT and SCT focus on more deliberative (or thoughtful) influences without considering more implicit or impulsive influences that may also drive health behavior. Such implicit influences are those factors that influence behavior but are not based on careful thought and may also be important for health risk behaviors. The Reflective-Impulsive Model (RIM; see Chapter 2) developed by Strack and Deutsch (2004) distinguishes two separate but interacting systems that together guide behavior: the reflective and the impulsive. The **reflective system** is seen as reasoned, conscious and intentional and covers many of the models such as the TPB, PMT and SCT. In contrast, an **impulsive system** consists of associative clusters that have been learned through experience. These learned associations can then trigger a behavior in response to a simple stimuli. For example, for Mark the smell of coffee can be enough to automatically direct attention to cake (attentional bias), thoughts of cake (implicit attitudes: automatic positive or negative evaluations) and to his buying and eating cake if available.

CORRELATIONAL STUDIES ON IMPLICIT INFLUENCES

A number of impulsive system factors have been explored in relation to health behaviors. For example, attentional bias and implicit associations have both been associated with health behaviors.

Attentional bias refers to a bias in attention either toward or away from particular objects. Calitri et al. (2010) reported that greater attentional bias for health food words and less attentional bias for non-food words both predicted reductions in body mass index over a period of a year.

Implicit associations have been argued to reflect associations between objects and evaluations (e.g., between smoking and positive evaluations) and are often assessed using reaction time-based measures such as the Implicit Association Test (IAT). Implicit associations have been found to be associated with health behaviors such as condom use (Stacy et al., 2006), smoking (Payne et al., 2007) and snack consumption (Conner et al., 2007a). Various reviews also suggest that implicit associations are predictive of behavior even after taking account of explicit attitude measures (Hofmann et al., 2008; Rooke et al., 2008) or other explicit cognitions such as outcomes expectancies, self-efficacy and intention (Conroy et al., 2010). However, there is continuing debate about the power of implicit associations to predict behavior after controlling for self-report measures (e.g., Buttrick et al.,

2020) including affective attitudes (Ayres et al., 2012; Conner et al., 2011b), suggesting that some explicit measures like affective attitudes may also tap these impulsive influences.

In one of the limited number of reviews in this area, Greenwald et al. (2009) reported that IAT scores were associated with a small to medium sized correlation with behavior (Table 7.1). It is worth noting that only a limited number of these tests involved health behaviors and that more recent reviews that better account for measurement error suggest the association between scores on the IAT and behavior may be weaker and less consistent (Buttrick et al., 2020). Nevertheless there is some limited evidence that implicit associations may be useful targets for interventions to change health behaviors. However, it may be that such implicit influences are more important for some behaviors than others (see Burning Issue Box 7.2).

CHANGING IMPLICIT INFLUENCES

Deutsch and Strack (2020) provide a review of using the RIM to change behavior. Implicit influences on health behaviors may be more difficult to change given they are often based on prolonged periods of learning. However, learning approaches have been used to try to reduce risk behaviors via changes in implicit cognition (attentional biases, automatic approach tendencies, implicit attitudes), and priming has been used to change health behaviors more directly.

Training to reduce attentional bias to alcohol stimuli has been shown to promote reduction in alcohol consumption and delayed relapse over a three-month period among those with alcohol dependence (Schoenmakers et al., 2010). The formation of implementation intentions has also been shown to reduce attentional bias and impact on habitual behaviors like high fat food consumption (Achtziger et al., 2008).

Automatic approach tendencies have been manipulated using the "go-no-go" paradigm. For example, pictures of unhealthy foods may be paired with cues that the recipient is asked to respond to, for example, by touching a screen ("go"), or refrain from responding to, for example, by not touching a screen ("no-go"). If recipients are conditioned not to touch the unhealthy but desirable food images over many pairings this may help inhibit automatic approach responses in the real world (e.g., Veling et al., 2013). Being trained not to respond to pictures of doughnuts or chocolate may make it easier to ignore or refuse these foods subsequently. A meta-analysis of 19 experimental studies, conducted mainly with undergraduates, suggested that inhibition training of this kind may be effective in changing health behavior patterns (Allom, Mullen & Hagger, 2016). The effect size was small ($d_+ = 0.38$) and varied depending on how long the training lasted (longer training worked better). With an alternative approach, Wiers et al. (2011) used a computer task to train alcohol-dependent patients to make an avoidance movement (i.e., push) to pictures of alcohol and an approach movement (i.e., pull) to non-alcoholic drinks. They showed this reduced alcohol relapse rates compared to a control condition from 59–43% over a one-year period.

Interventions to change implicit attitudes have used evaluative conditioning (EC) which attempts to change the valence of an evaluation of a target by pairing the target with another positive or negative stimulus. In one of the few studies on health behaviors, Hollands et al. (2011) measured implicit and explicit attitudes to snacks and then paired images of snacks with aversive images of obesity and heart disease. The EC procedure reduced the favorability of implicit attitudes to snacks without changing explicit attitudes and also reduced the likelihood of choosing a snack as a reward. Mediation analyses showed the change in implicit attitude partially explained the impact of EC on behavior.

Research on goal-priming has shown that mental representations of goals can be activated without the individual knowing about or intending it. This can be achieved through subliminal presentation of goal-relevant stimuli or through subtle and unobtrusive supraliminal presentation. For example, Stroebe et al. (2008) showed that subliminally priming the goal of eating enjoyment inhibited the goal of controlling one's weight in restrained eaters. In a field study, Papies and Hamstra (2010) showed that priming the goal of dieting via a subtle exposure to a poster led to a reduced number of snacks being consumed by restrained eaters.

A meta-analysis of procedures to change implicit measures (Forscher et el., 2019) reported the effects of a whole raft of techniques including pairing of concepts, activating mindsets, mood/emotion manipulation and introducing goals. The effects were generally small (Table 7.1). The effects of changing scores on implicit measures on behavior were also generally small and varied depending on technique used (range g_+/d_+ = -0.29 to 0.39) with threat being the only manipulation showing a significant average effect on behavior (range g_+/d_+ = 0.39) across six tests. It would appear that the impact of changing implicit influences on behavior is generally quite modest and may be quite short-lived.

Given some mixed evidence, future research needs to identify the operating conditions (Rothman & Sheeran, 2021; see Burning Issue Box 7.2) for when implicit influences on health behavior are to be expected. For example, perhaps it is only some health behaviors (e.g., sedentary behaviors) where such implicit influences are predictive (i.e., a validation moderator).

_____

CONCLUSIONS

It is worth reviewing the information in Table 7.1 on the key determinants highlighted in this chapter. In terms of predictors, it is notable that affective risk perceptions and affective attitudes were the strongest correlates on intentions, while intentions and capacity were the strongest predictors of behavior. It is also worth noting that mainly the correlations with intentions were from cross-sectional studies while the correlations with behavior were from mainly prospective studies (although often with a relatively short time delay). Experimental studies show that interventions produce the strongest effects on deliberative risk perceptions, control beliefs, self-efficacy and intentions. Manipulations of attitude, norms and self-efficacy produce the greatest impact on intention and manipulations of self-efficacy produce the greatest change in health behaviors. Similar to the correlational studies, the experimental studies mainly measured the impacts on the construct and on intentions very shortly after the intervention (usually in the same session), although the effects on behavior were measured later. In general, all this evidence could benefit from studies with follow-up tests beyond 6-months.

BURNING ISSUE BOX 7.12

Q&A ON PSYCHOLOGICAL APPROACHES TO CHANGING HEALTH BEHAVIORS

Question 1: Are particular health behaviors easier to predict than others?

The most common way to measure how easy it is to predict behaviors is in terms of how much variance in behavior key predictors account for. So, for example, McEachan et al. (2011) reviewed the use of the Theory of Planed Behavior (TPB) to predict various health behaviors. They found that the TPB explained the most variance in physical activity and the least variance in safer sex behaviors. That would suggest that physical activity is easier to predict than safer sex! However, we must remember that studies will vary in other ways than just the behavior they measure. For example, many physical activity studies now report objective measures of behavior while safer sex studies are usually reliant on self-reported behavior.

Question 2: Could particular theories work better for certain health behaviors?

The social/health cognition models we have examined were developed to work for a broad range of health behaviors rather than being specific to particular theories work better for some types of health behavior and other theories work better for other types of health behaviors. However, directly comparing theories in this way can be difficult because different numbers and types of predictors are involved. It is easier to compare particular components of theories across different behaviors. For example, McEachan et al. (2011) showed that intentions were stronger predictors of physical activity than abstinence (risk) behaviors like reducing drinking.

Question 3: How can intentions be made more stable?

To increase the performance of health promotion behaviors and detection behaviors (or avoidance of risk behaviors) getting individuals to have positive and stable intentions to perform them may lead to long term performance. For example, Conner et al. (2002) showed that stable intentions to eat healthily was associated with healthy eating six years later. However, to date we know relatively little about what promotes stable intentions. Conner et al. (2016) suggest that if we can get individuals to prioritize their intentions to perform health promotion behaviors this may lead to more stable intentions. They also showed that simple messages suggesting the importance of such prioritization could be effective. Nevertheless future studies identifying effective interventions to promote stable intentions would be a useful development in this area (see Conner & Norman, 2022, for a review).

Question 4: What's more important in predicting behavior: an individual's personality or their cognitions?

Personality traits like conscientiousness show only small to medium sized effects on health behaviors while cognitions like intentions show medium to large sized effects. So cognitions are the more important predictors (see Conner & Abraham, 2001).

Question 5: Given the effects of the Question-Behavior Effect (QBE) on behavior change tend to be small, is it an important behavior change technique?

In selecting a behavior change technique to apply, the associated effect size is a key consideration. However, cost of implementing the intervention is often another consideration. While the QBE is associated with a small effect size it would be a cheap intervention to implement. It may well therefore be a useful intervention in certain circumstances. For example, various screening programs that require individuals to be sent invitations could very cheaply add a questionnaire about the screening behavior to produce a valuable increase in participation rates.

Question 6: Are health risk behaviors more difficult to *predict* than health promotion behaviors?

There is no definitive answer to this question. The data from McEachan et al. (2011) suggest that the key predictors of behavior in the Theory of Planned Behavior (TPB) do similarly well in predicting health promotion and health risk behaviors. When we examine the overall amount of variance explained together by intentions and perceived behavioral control from the TPB then less variance in risk behaviors is explained compared to that explained for physical activity and dietary behaviors. However, the amounts of variance explained for risk behaviors is similar to that explained for detection, safer sex and abstinence behaviors. Conner et al. (2017) provide a more detailed test of differences for protection versus risk health behaviors in the same sample of individuals and did observe some differences.

Question 7: Are health risk behaviors more difficult to *change* than health promotion behaviors?

The simple answer is yes. Health risk behaviors tend to be more ingrained and based on past behavior or the formation of bad habits. For example, McEachan et al. (2011) showed that past behavior was considerably more important in predicting risk behaviors than physical activity, dietary or abstinence behaviors. This may mean we need to do more to change health risk behaviors particularly where there is an addictive element such as in smoking. Nevertheless interventions like implementation intentions can be effective in changing even health risk behaviors.

Question 8: What's the best model of health risk behavior?

There is no simple answer to this question. Very few studies have attempted to directly compare models for the same sample of individuals either for health promotion or health risk behaviors. Models like the Theory of Planned Behavior appear to do quite well although models such as the Prototype Willingness Model (Gibbons & Gerrard, 1995) that were specifically developed for such behaviors might be expected to work best.

Question 9: What's the single biggest determinant of engaging in health risk behaviors?

Aside from past behavior (and habits), intentions and self-efficacy are probably the strongest determinants of health risk behaviors as they are for health promotion behaviors and detection behaviors (see Table 7.1).

SCIENCE OF HEALTH BEHAVIOR CHANGE: IN ACTION

In the first section of the book, you learned about how to take a scientific approach to health behavior change (broadly overviewed in Chapter 1). In particular, you learned about different theories (Chapter 2) and behavior change techniques (Chapter 3) and how to apply them to develop theory-based interventions (Chapter 4). In addition, you learned about how to design studies adopting different methodological approaches (Chapter 5) and to statistically test whether a particular intervention was effective in changing behavior (Chapter 6). Along the way, you encountered examples of different critical thinking skills to help you to evaluate the quality of health behavior change studies. Next, we present our first *Science of Health Behavior Change: In Action Box*, with subsequent boxes in Chapters 8 and 9. These boxes take a published individual study that attempted to change a health behavior and critically evaluates it against what we have learned.

Box 7.1 considers the study of Milne et al. (2002) who tested the impact of implementation intentions on exercise participation (a health promotion behavior). In particular, they aimed to assess the effects of an implementation intention plus a motivational intervention compared to a motivational intervention alone or a control condition. Theory would suggest that implementation intentions are particularly effective when individuals are

SCIENCE OF HEALTH BEHAVIOR CHANGE IN ACTION BOX 7.1: MILNE ET AL. (2002)

Study: *Milne et al. (2002). Combining motivational and volitional interventions to promote exercise participation: Protection motivation theory and implementation intentions*
Aim: To increase exercise in undergraduate students. Method: Participants were randomized to one of three conditions: a combined motivational and volitional intervention (based on Protection Motivation Theory (PMT) & implementation intentions), a motivational intervention only (the same PMT-based intervention) or a control. Results: The PMT-manipulation changed PMT constructs related to threat and appraisal but it did not influence exercise behavior. Those in the combined group increased their exercise significantly more than those in the motivational intervention group or control group. Authors' conclusion: Both motivation and volition are needed for goal attainment.

THEORY & TECHNIQUES OF HEALTH BEHAVIOR CHANGE		
BCTs	INTERVENTION: Based on Michie et al.'s (2013) taxonomy:Combined intervention: 1.1 Goal setting (behavior); 1.4 Action planning; 5.1 Information about health consequences; 5.2 Salience of consequences; 15.1 Persuasion of ability; 15.2 Mental rehearsal of successful performance. Motivational intervention only: 5.1 Information about health consequences; 5.2 Salience of consequences; 15.1 Persuasion of ability; 15.2 Mental rehearsal of successful performance.	
	CONTROL: None	
Critical Skills Toolkit		
3.1	Does the design enable the identification of which BCTs are effective?	*No. Adding an implementation intention-only condition would ensure a 2 (implementation intention: yes/no) × 2 (PMT: yes/no) full-factorial design. Without this condition, it is unclear whether both implementation intentions and the motivational intervention are needed or whether implementation intentions only are sufficient for behavior change.*
4.1	Is the intervention based on one theory or a combination of theories (if any at all)?	*Combined intervention: Protection Motivation Theory (PMT) with implementation intentions (a BCT rather than a theory) added to it. While adding implementation intentions to PMT risks undermining the established theory (by modifying PMT), the modification is in keeping with the Model of Action Phases which specifies behavior is determined through a combination of motivational and volitional elements. PMT-only intervention: based only on PMT.*

	Are all constructs specified within a theory targeted by the intervention?	*The main determinants of protection motivation: threat appraisal (via perceived severity & perceived vulnerability) and coping appraisal (via self-efficacy, response efficacy and response costs) were targeted by specific BCTs in the PMT conditions. The only element of the theory that was not explicitly targeted by the PMT-interventions was rewards (intrinsic & extrinsic) that increase the likelihood of a maladaptive response.*
	Are all behavior change techniques explicitly targeting at least one theory-relevant construct?	*Yes. Linking each BCT to a particular construct provides justification for the inclusion of that BCT – i.e., it is being used in a theoretically consistent way – often some BCTs are added as "extras" and not linked to a specific theory-relevant construct so it is theoretically unclear why it is included.*
	Do the authors test why the intervention was effective or ineffective (consistent with the underlying theory)?	*No. Mediation analyses were not conducted. Although the PMT variables changed as a result of the PMT manipulation, it is not clear whether changes in the PMT variables mediated the effect of the PMT-based messages on intentions.*
	Does the study tailor the intervention based on the underlying theory?	*No. All participants within a study condition received the same materials. However, given the brevity and likely low cost of the intervention, the lack of tailoring is unlikely to represent a major issue.*

2.2 and TC 2.4	What are the strengths/ limitations of the underlying theory?	*See Theory Critique Box 2.4. See Critical Skills Toolkit 2.2 (general criticisms of social cognition models). The most relevant point here is that most social cognition models including PMT view motivation as the direct precursor to behavior. Evidence suggests a gap. A strength of the current study is it tried to bridge this gap by targeting motivation plus volition using implementation intentions.*
THE METHODOLOGY OF HEALTH BEHAVIOR CHANGE		
5.1, 5.2, 5.4, 5.6,	Methodological approach	*The study adopted an experimental (see Critical Skills Toolkit 5.4), parallel groups design though with gradual build-up of intervention content (see Critical Skills Toolkit 5.6) and used questionnaires (see Critical Skills Toolkit 5.1, 5.2).*
6.1	For experimental designs: Is the study between-subjects, within-subjects or mixed?	*Mixed design because participants were allocated to one of three conditions (between-subjects) and completed measures at multiple time-points (within-subjects). For advantages & disadvantages of this design, see Critical Skills Toolkit 6.1.*
5.2, 5.5,BIB 5.2	Are the measures reliable & valid?	*The main outcome variable – exercise – was measured by a single item with no known reliability or validity (see Burning Issue Box 5.2). The measures of PMT variables were, in some cases, not internally reliable (though these were appropriately analyzed as single items) and these measures had not been previously validated.*

5.5	May other variables have been manipulated other than the independent variable?	*Low risk of bias. The manipulations appeared appropriate. Thus, the internal validity of the experiment was not threatened by the risk of confounds.*
	Non-random allocation of participants to condition	*Unclear risk. Participants were randomized to condition but it is not clear how this randomization took place (hence, an inappropriate method of randomization could have been used). Although there were no reported differences across the groups at baseline (suggesting randomization was successful), differences between the groups (arising from potentially inappropriate randomization methods) could be present on unmeasured variables.*
	Blinding & Allocation Concealment	*Unclear risk. The authors note that the "participants were anonymous to the experimenter" but this does not necessarily mean that the experimenter was blinded to condition. There was no other evidence of blinding or allocation concealment and this may be more problematic given exercise was measured by self-report rather than objectively. There was also risk of demand effects given the text used in the implementation intention condition may have led participants to believe that their behavior should change: "It has been found that if you form a definite plan of exactly when and where you will carry out an intended behavior you are more likely to actually do so (p. 170)"*

ANALYZING HEALTH BEHAVIOR CHANGE DATA		
6.2	Was the sample size calculated a-priori?	*The sample size was not calculated a-priori. However, given the effects of the combined intervention was large, this is unlikely to be a major issue.*
Fig. 6.1	Was the hypothesis tested with an appropriate statistical test?	*Yes.*
5.5, 6.4	Incomplete outcome data	*It is unclear whether attrition rates differed across the three study conditions. It is a possibility, therefore, that attrition may have been higher in the experimental groups which would suggest an issue with acceptability. Moreover, the analyses were not conducted on an intention-to-treat basis. However, the attrition rates were reasonably low (of the 273 participants who completed the questionnaire at baseline, 250 participants completed the questionnaires at both follow-ups). In addition, given the effects of the combined intervention were large, it is unlikely that the results would suggest different conclusions if they were analyzed on an intention-to-treat basis. The participants who dropped out were similar on the measured variables compared to those who completed the study, suggesting that the results are generalizable to the types of participants recruited (i.e., other undergraduate students).*

5.5	Selective outcome reporting	*Unclear given the trial protocol was not pre-published, however, all of the measures reported in the Method section were analyzed and reported in the Results section.*
4.2	Lack of variability (non-sig. effects only)	*Not applicable. The participants in the combined intervention exercised more during the follow-up period compared to those in the PMT-only and control groups. Those in the PMT-based conditions increased their PMT-relevant cognitions as predicted.*
6.3	Non-linear relationship (non-sig. effects only)	*Not applicable – effects significant.*
REPLICABILITY: Are the effects likely replicable?		
BIB 5.4	The case for	*The key effect (the effect of adding implementation intentions on behavior) was large in size.*
BIB 5.4	The case against	*No preregistration or data avail-ability/sharing statement; no a-priori sample size calculation; has a between-subjects design ele-ment; risk of selective outcome reporting, blinding and allocation concealment were unclear; two participants dropped from analyses for medical reasons despite completing all measures (although 2 out of 250 participants will unlikely have a major impact on the key finding with a large effect size). Some of the smaller effects (e.g., on fear, $p < .05$) may be less likely to replicate.*

motivated to perform the behavior. Therefore it was expected that the combined implementation intention plus motivational intervention would be particularly effective in increasing exercise participation.

SUMMARY

This chapter examined psychology-based approaches to health behavior change. Research on six key determinants of health behavior (risk perceptions, attitudes/outcome expectancies, norms, self-efficacy, intentions and implicit influences) from important models/theories of health behavior was reviewed. For each key determinant we reviewed literature on how well each determinant was related to intentions and behavior and also on how to change that determinant in order to produce changes in intentions and behavior. The focus was on a range of different health behaviors including promotion, risk and detection health behaviors.

FURTHER READING

Norman, P., & Conner, M. (2015). Predicting and changing health behaviour: Future directions. In M. Conner and P. Norman (Eds.), *Predicting and changing health behaviour: Research and practice with social cognition models* (3rd Ed.; pp. 390–430). Maidenhead: Open University Press. This chapter looks at future directions for research on social cognition models and health behaviors.

McEachan, R.R.C., Conner, M., Taylor, N.J., & Lawton, R.J. (2011). Prospective prediction of health-related behaviors with the Theory of Planned Behavior: A meta-analysis. *Health Psychology Review, 5*, 97–144. A comprehensive review of the application of prospective tests of the TPB to health behaviors that draws attention to differences across behaviors.

Sheeran, P., Bosch, J.A., Crombez, G., Hall, P.A., Harris, J.L., Papies, E.K., & Wiers, R.W. (2016). Implicit processes in health psychology: Diversity and promise. *Health Psychology, 35*, 761–766. This introduction to a special issue of the journal on implicit processes and health behaviors overviews and summarizes the range of approaches taken in recent research.

GLOSSARY

Affective attitudes: Attitudes tapped by semantic differentials such as unpleasant-pleasant or not enjoyable-enjoyable (e.g., My using ecstasy would be… boring/exciting).

Affective risk perceptions: Affective risk perceptions refer to the affect associated with risk. For example, affective reactions such as worry, anxiety or anticipated regret may be associated with thinking about engaging in a health behavior.

Anticipated affect: Attitudes tapped by semantic differentials such as no regret-regret or not guilty-guilty and referring to how one might feel after performing the behavior (e.g., If I used ecstasy I would feel regret, strongly disagree/strongly agree).

Attitude accessibility: Refers to how quickly an attitude can be brought to mind.

Attitudinal ambivalence: Ambivalence refers to having mixed evaluations of an attitude object (e.g., Evaluating a cream cake as positive because of the taste, but simultaneously evaluating it as negative because of it being perceived to be unhealthy).

Central or systematic route to persuasion: Refers to the careful consideration of persuasive messages where strong messages with good arguments will have bigger effects on attitude change than weak messages. Attitude change by this route leads to strong attitudes that predict behavior, are stable over time and resistant to persuasion.

Cognitive attitudes: Attitudes tapped by semantic differentials such as harmful-beneficial or negative-positive (e.g., My using ecstasy would be… harmful/beneficial).

Deliberative risk perceptions: Deliberative risk perceptions are systematic, logical and rule-based and emphasize the idea that individuals rely on a number of reason-based strategies to derive an estimated likelihood that a negative or positive outcome will occur.

Health detection behaviors: Behaviors that help detect potential

problems that when treated early can lead to better health outcomes. These include various self-examination behaviors (e.g., breast self-examination) plus various forms of screening attendance (e.g., cervical screening).

Health promotion behaviors: Behaviors that help protect or maintain health when engaged in. These include things such as exercise and compliance with medical regimens.

Health risk behaviors: Behaviors that damage or risk health. These include behaviors such as smoking and alcohol consumption.

Heuristics: Simple rules about messages (e.g., messages from experts are more reliable).

Implementation intentions: Simple if-then plans about what to do in response to a cue. For example, in pursuit of the goal of exercising more the implementation intention to go jogging on a Friday at noon may be helpful.

Impulsive system: Part of the reflective-impulsive model. Refers to the way in which a variety of less reasoned influences can impact on behavior. Many of these influences are based on earlier learning processes.

Message framing: Whether the persuasive message focuses on losses or gains. For example, in relation to quitting smoking, messages could focus on the losses associated with continuing (e.g., Smoking can lead to worse health and dying younger) or the gains associated with quitting (i.e., Quitting smoking can lead to improved health and living a longer life).

Peripheral or heuristic route to persuasion: Refers to non-careful consideration of persuasive messages where persuasion is mainly driven by simple cues or heuristics such as longer messages are stronger. Attitude change by this route leads to weak attitudes that are less predictive of behavior, less stable over time and more open to persuasion.

Question-Behavior Effect: Relates to findings showing that merely asking questions about a behavior (e.g., Do you intend to eat a low fat diet?) may be sufficient to produce changes in that (e.g., eating a low fat diet) or related (e.g., eating healthily in other ways) behaviors.

Reflective system: Part of the reflective-impulsive model. Refers to the way in which a variety of more reasoned influences can impact on behavior.

Self-affirmation: Self-integrity (experience of the self as "adaptively and morally adequate") can be restored or reinforced by affirming sources of self-worth that are important to the person's identity.

Social/health cognition models: Theories that specify the important thoughts and feelings (jointly referred to as social or health cognitions) that differentiate those performing and not performing a behavior.

REFERENCES

Achtziger, A., Gollwitzer, P.M., & Sheeran, P. (2008). Implementation intentions and shielding goal striving from unwanted thoughts and feelings. *Personality and Social Psychology Bulletin, 34*, 381–393.

Ajzen, I., & Schmidt, P. (2020). Changing behavior using the theory of planned behavior. In M. S. Hagger, L. D. Cameron, K. Hamilton, N. Hankonen & T. Lintunen (Eds.), *Handbook of behavior change* (pp. 17–31). Cambridge University Press.

Allom, V., Mullen, B., & Hagger, M. (2016). Does inhibitory control training improve health behaviour? A meta-analysis. *Health Psychology Review, 10*, 168–186.

Amegah, A.K. (2020). Improving handwashing habits and household air quality in Africa after COVID-19. *The Lancet Global Health, 8*, e1110–e1111.

Ayres, K., Conner, M.T., Prestwich, A., & Smith, P. (2012). Do implicit measures of attitudes incrementally predict snacking behaviour over explicit affect-related measures? *Appetite, 58*, 835–841.

Ayres, K., Conner, M.T., Prestwich, A. et al. (2013). Exploring the question-behaviour effect: Randomized controlled trial of motivational and question-behaviour interventions. *British Journal of Health Psychology, 18*, 31–44.

Bandura, A. (1982). Self-efficacy mechanism in human agency. *American Psychologist, 37*, 122–147.

Bandura, A. (1997). *Self-Efficacy: The Exercise of Control.* New York: Freeman.

Banks, S.M., Salovey, P., Greener, S., et al. (1995). The effects of message framing on mammography utilization. *Health Psychology, 14,* 178–184.

Batteux, E., Mills, F., Jones, L.F., Symons, C., & Weston, D. (2022). The effectiveness of interventions for increasing COVID-19 vaccine uptake: a systematic review. *Vaccines, 10,* 386.

Berkowitz, A. (2004). The Social Norms Approach: Theory, Research and Annotated Bibliography. Retrieved from http://www.alanberkowitz.com/articles/social_norms.pdf.

Bogg, T., & Roberts, B.W. (2004). Conscientiousness and health-related behaviors: A meta-analysis of the leading behavioral contributors to mortality. *Psychological Bulletin, 130,* 887–919.

Bokemper, S.E., Cucciniello, M., Rotesi, T. et al. (2021). Experimental evidence that changing beliefs about mask efficacy and social norms increase mask wearing for COVID-19 risk reduction: Results from the United States and Italy. *PLoS ONE, 16,* e0258282.

Brewer, N.T., DeFrank, J.T., & Gilkey, M.B. (2016). Anticipated regret and health behavior: A meta-analysis. *Health Psychology, 35,* 1264–1275.

Brooks, S.K., Webster, R.K., Smith, L.E. et al. (2020). The psychological impact of quarantine and how to reduce it: rapid review of the evidence. *Lancet, 395,* 912–920.

Buitenhuis, A.H., Tuinman, M.A., & Hagedoorn, M. (2021). A planning intervention to quit smoking in single-smoking couples: does partner involvement improve effectiveness? *Psychology & Health, 36*(1), 1–15

Burkert, S., Scholz, U., Gralla, O., Roigas, J., & Knoll, N. (2011). Dyadic planning of health-behavior change after prostatectomy: a randomized-controlled planning intervention. *Social Science & Medicine, 73,* 783–792.

Buttrick, N., Axt, J., Ebersole, C.R., & Huband, J. (2020). Re-assessing the incremental predictive validity of implicit association tests. *Journal of Experimental Social Psychology, 88,* 103941.

Calitri, R., Pothos, E.M., Tapper, K., Brunstrom, J.M., & Rogers, P.J. (2010). Cognitive biases to healthy and unhealthy foods words predict change in BMI. *Obesity, 18,* 2282–2287.

Capasso, M., Caso, D., & Conner, M. (2021). Anticipating pride or regret? Effects of anticipated affect focused persuasive messages on intention to get vaccinated against COVID-19. *Social Science and Medicine, 289,* 114416.

Carfora, V., Caso, D., & Conner, M. (2016). Randomized controlled trial of "messaging intervention" to increase fruit and vegetable intake in adolescents: Affective versus instrumental messages. *British Journal of Health Psychology, 21,* 937–955.

Carfora, V., Caso, C., & Conner, M. (2017). Correlational study and randomised controlled trial for understanding and changing red meat consumption: The role of eating identities. *Social Science and Medicine, 175,* 244–252.

Carfora, V., Catellani, P., Caso, D., & Conner, M. (2019). How to reduce red and processed meat consumption by daily text messages targeting environment or health benefits. *Journal of Environmental Psychology, 65,* 101319.

Carr, R., Prestwich, A., Kwasnicka, D. et al. (2019). Dyadic interventions to promote physical activity and reduce sedentary behaviour: Systematic review and meta-analysis. *Health Psychology Review, 13,* 91–109.

Carr, R., Quested, E., Stenling, A. et al. (2021). Postnatal Exercise Partners Study (PEEPS): A pilot randomised trial of a dyadic physical activity intervention for postpartum mothers and a significant other. *Health Psychology and Behavioral Medicine, 9*, 251–284.

Caso, D., Carfora, V., & Conner, M. (2016). Predicting intentions and consumption of fruit and vegetables in Italian adolescents. Effects of anticipated regret and self-identity. *Psicologia Sociale, 3*, 319–326.

Chaiken, S. (1980). Heuristic versus systematic information processing and the use of source versus message cues in persuasion. *Journal of Personality and Social Psychology, 37*, 1397–1397.

Cohen, J. (1992). A power primer. *Psychological Bulletin, 112*, 155–159.

Conner, M., & Abraham, C. (2001). Conscientiousness and the Theory of Planned Behavior: Towards a more complete model of the antecedents of intentions and behavior. *Personality and Social Psychology Bulletin, 27*, 1547–1561.

Conner, M., Abraham, C., Prestwich, A. et al. (2016). Impact of goal priority and goal conflict on the intention-health behavior relationship: Tests on physical activity and other health behaviors. *Health Psychology, 35*, 1017–1026.

Conner, M., & Norman, P. (2019). Editorial. Health behaviour: Cancer screening, blood and organ donation, and opioid (mis)use. *Psychology & Health, 34*, 1029–1035.

Conner, M., & Norman, P. (2021). Predicting long-term healthy eating behaviour: Understanding the role of cognitive and affective attitudes. *Psychology & Health, 36*, 1165–1181.

Conner, M., & Norman, P. (2022). Understanding the intention-behavior gap: The role of intention strength. *Frontiers in Psychology, 13*, 923464.

Conner, M., Godin, G., Norman, P., & Sheeran, P. (2011a). Using the question-behavior effect to promote disease prevention behaviors: Two randomized controlled trials. *Health Psychology, 30*, 300–309.

Conner, M., Godin, G., Sheeran, P., & Germain, M. (2013a). Some feelings are more important: Cognitive attitudes, affective attitudes, anticipated affect and blood donation. *Health Psychology, 32*, 264–272.

Conner, M., Grogan, S., Simms-Ellis, R. et al. (2018). Do electronic cigarettes increase cigarette smoking in UK adolescents? Evidence from a 12-month prospective study. *Tobacco Control, 27*, 365–372.

Conner, M., Grogan, S., West, R. et al. (2019). Effectiveness and cost-effectiveness of repeated implementation intention formation plus anti-smoking messages on adolescent smoking initiation: A cluster randomized controlled trial. *Journal of Consulting and Clinical Psychology, 87*, 422–432.

Conner, M., McEachan, R., Jackson, C. et al. (2013b). Moderating effect of socioeconomic status on the relationship between health cognitions and behaviors. *Annals of Behavioral Medicine, 46*, 19–30.

Conner, M., Norman, P., & Bell, R. (2002). The Theory of Planned Behavior and healthy eating. *Health Psychology, 21*, 194–201.

Conner, M., Perugini, M., O'Gorman, R., Ayres, K., & Prestwich, A. (2007a). Relations between implicit and explicit measures of attitudes and measures of behavior: Evidence of moderation by individual difference variables. *Personality and Social Psychology Bulletin, 33*, 1727–1740.

Conner, M., Prestwich, A., & Ayres, K. (2011b). Using explicit affective attitudes to tap impulsive influences on health behavior: A commentary on Hofmann et al. (2008). *Health Psychology Review, 5*, 145–149.

Conner, M., Rhodes, R., Morris, B., McEachan, R., & Lawton, R. (2011c). Changing exercise through targeting affective or cognitive attitudes. *Psychology & Health, 26*, 133–149.

Conner, M., Rodgers, W., & Murray, T. (2007b). Conscientiousness and the intention-behavior relationship: Predicting exercise behavior. *Journal of Sports and Exercise Psychology, 29*, 518–533.

Conner, M., Sandberg, T., McMillan, B., & Higgins, A. (2006). Role of anticipated regret in adolescent smoking initiation. *British Journal of Health Psychology, 11*, 85–101.

Conner, M., & Sparks, P. (2015). The theory of planned behaviour and the reasoned action approach. In M. Conner & P. Norman (Eds.), *Predicting and changing health behaviour: Research and practice with social cognition models* (3rd Ed.; pp. 142–188). Maidenhead: Open University Press.

Conner, M., van Harreveld, F., & Norman, P. (2022). Attitude stability as a moderator of the relationships between cognitive and affective attitudes and behaviour. *British Journal of Social Psychology, 61*, 121–142.

Conner, M., Wilding, S., Wright, C.A., & Sheeran, P. (in press). How does self-control promote health behaviors? A multi-behavior test of five potential pathways. *Annals of Behavioral Medicine.*

Conner, M.T., Williams, D.M., & Rhodes, R.E. (2020). Affect-based interventions. In M.S. Hagger, L.D. Cameron, K. Hamilton, N. Hankonen & T. Lintunen (Eds.), *Handbook of behavior change* (pp. 495–509). New York, NY: Cambridge University Press.

Conroy, D.E., Hyde, A.L., Doerksen, S.E., & Ribiero, N.F. (2010). Implicit attitudes and explicit motivation prospectively predict physical activity. *Annals of Behavioral Medicine, 39*, 112–118.

Cure, L., & Van Enk, R. (2015). Effect of hand sanitizer location on hand hygiene compliance. *American Journal of Infection Control, 43*, 917–921.

Davidson, K.W., Mogavero, J.N., & Rothman, A.J. (2020). Using early phase studies to advance intervention research: The science of behavior change. *Health Psychology, 39*(9), 731–735.

De Ridder, D.T.D., Lensvelt-Mulders, G., Finkenauer, C., Stok, F.M., & Baumeister, R.F. (2012). Taking stock of self-control: A meta-analysis of how trait self-control relates to a wide range of behaviors. *Personality and Social Psychology Review, 16*, 76–99.

Detweiler, J.B., Bedell, B.T., Salovey, P., Pronin, E., & Rothan, A.J. (1999). Message framing and sunscreen use: Gain-framed messages motivate beach-goers. *Health Psychology, 18*, 189–196.

Deutsch, R., & Strack, F. (2020). Changing behavior using the reflective-impulsive model. In Hagger, M.S., Cameron, L.D., Hamilton, K., Hankonen, N., & Lintunen, T. Eds. *Handbook of behavior change* (pp. 164–177). Cambridge University Press.

Edwards, W. (1954). The theory of decision making. *Psychological Bulletin, 51*, 380–417.

Ellis, E.M., Elwyn, G., Nelson, W.L. et al. (2018). Interventions to engage affective forecasting in health-related decision making: A meta-analysis. *Annals of Behavioral Medicine, 52*, 157–174.

Epton, T., Harris, P.R., Kane, R., van Koningsbruggen, G.M., & Sheeran, P. (2015). The impact of self-affirmation on health-behavior change: A meta-analysis. *Health Psychology, 34*, 187–196.

Ferrer, R. A., & Klein, W.M.P. (2015). Risk perceptions and health behavior. *Current Opinion in Psychology*, *5*, 85–89.

Fishbein, M. (1967). Attitude and the prediction of behavior. In M. Fishbein (Ed.), *Readings in Attitude Theory and Measurement* (pp. 477–492*)*. New York: Wiley.

Forscher, P.S. et al. (2019). A meta-analysis of procedures to change implicit measures. *Journal of Personality and Social Psychology*, *117*, 522–559.

Freeman, M.A., Hennessy, E.V., & Marzullo, D.M. (2001). Defensive evaluation of antismoking messages among college-age smokers: The role of possible selves. *Health Psychology*, *20*, 424–433.

Friedman, H.S., Tucker, J.S., Schwartz, J.E. et al. (1995). Childhood conscientiousness and longevity: Health behaviors and cause of death. *Journal of Personality and Social Psychology*, *68*, 696–703.

Friedman, H.S., Tucker, J.S., Tomlinson-Keasay, C. et al. (1993). Does childhood personality predict longevity? *Journal of Personality and Social Psychology*, *65*, 176–185.

Frisch, D., & Clemen, R.T. (1994). Beyond expected utility: rethinking behavioral decision making. *Psychological Bulletin*, *116*, 46–54.

Gallagher, K., & Updegraff, J.A. (2012). Health message framing effects on attitudes, intentions, and behaviour: A meta-analytic review. *Annals of Behavioral Medicine*, *43*, 101–116.

Gardner, B., de Bruijn, G.-J., & Lally, P. (2011). A systematic review and meta-analysis of applications of the Self-Report Habit Index to nutrition and physical activity behaviors. *Annals of Behavioral Medicine*, *42*, 174–187.

Gardner, B., Smith, L., Lorencatto, F., Hamer, M., & Biddle, S.J.H. (2016). How to reduce sitting time? A review of behaviour change strategies used in sedentary behaviour reduction interventions among adults. *Health Psychology Review*, *10*, 89–112.

Godin, G., Conner, M., Sheeran, P. et al. (2010). Social structure, social cognition, and physical activity: A test of four models. *British Journal of Health Psychology*, *15*, 79–95.

Godin, G., Germain, M., Conner, M., Delage, G., & Sheeran, P. (2014). Promoting the return of lapsed blood donors: A 7-arm randomized controlled trial of the question-behavior effect. *Health Psychology*, *33*, 646–655.

Goldberg, J.H., Halpern-Felsher, B.L., & Millstein, S.G. (2002). Beyond invulnerability: The importance of benefits in adolescents' decision to drink alcohol. *Health Psychology*, *21*, 477–484.

Gollwitzer, P.M. (1993). Goal achievement: the role of intentions. *European Review of Social Psychology*, *4*, 142–185.

Gollwitzer, P.M., & Sheeran, P. (2006). Implementation intentions and goal achievement: A meta-analysis of effects and processes. *Advances in Experimental Social Psychology*, *38*, 69–119.

Greenwald, A.G., Poehlman, T.A., Uhlmann, E.L., & Banaji, M.R. (2009). Understanding and using the Implicit Association Test: III. Meta-Analysis of predictive validity. *Journal of Personality and Social Psychology*, *97*, 17–41.

Grogan, S., Flett, K., Clark-Carter, D. et al. (2011). Brief Report: A randomized controlled trial of an appearance-related smoking intervention. *Health Psychology*, *30*, 805–809.

Hall, P.A., & Fong, G.T. (2007). Temporal self-regulation theory: A model for individual health behaviour. *Health Psychology Review*, *1*, 6–52.

Hamilton, K., & Johnson, B.T. (2020). Attitudes and persuasive communication interventions. In M. S. Hagger, L. D. Cameron, K. Hamilton, N. Hankonen, & T. Lintunen (Eds.), *The handbook of behavior change* (pp. 445–460). Cambridge University Press.

Harkin, B., Webb, T., Chang, B. et al. (2016). Does monitoring goal progress promote goal attainment? A meta-analysis of the experimental evidence. *Psychological Bulletin, 142*, 198–229.

Harris, P.R., & Napper, L. (2005). Self-affirmation and the biased processing of health-risk information. *Personality and Social Psychology Bulletin, 31*, 1250–1263.

Herbert, J., Horsham, C., Ford, H. et al. (2020). Development of a smart hand-washing station in a school setting during the COVID-19 pandemic: Field study. *JMIR Public Health and Surveillance, 6*, e22305.

Hofmann, W., Friese, M., & Wiers, R.W. (2008). Impulsive versus reflective influences on health behavior: A theoretical framework and empirical review. *Health Psychology Review, 2*, 111–137.

Hollands, G.J., Prestwich, A., & Marteau, T.M. (2011). Using aversive images to enhance healthy eating food choices and implicit attitudes: An experimental test of evaluative conditioning. *Health Psychology, 30*, 195–203.

Iles, I.A., Gillman, A.S., Ferrer, R.A., & Klein, W.M.P. (2021). Self-affirmation inductions to reduce defensive processing of threatening health risk information. *Psychology & Health, 36*, 1–22.

Jessop, D.C., Simmonds, L.V. & Sparks, P. (2009). Motivational and behavioural consequences of self-affirmation interventions: A study of sunscreen use among women. *Psychology & Health, 24*, 529–544.

Kahnkeman, D., & Tversky, A. (1979). Prospect theory: An analysis of decision under risk. *Econometrica, 47*, 263–291.

Kalichman, S.C., & Coley, B. (1995). Context framing to enhance HIV-antibody testing messages targeted to African American women. *Health Psychology, 14*, 247–254.

Keyworth, C., Nelson, P.A., Bundy, C. et al. (2018). Does message framing affect changes in behavioural intentions in people with psoriasis? A randomized exploratory study examining health risk communication. *Psychology, Health & Medicine, 23*, 763–776.

Kulis, E., Szczuka, Z., Banik, A. et al. (2022). Insights into effects of individual, dyadic, and collaborative planning interventions on automatic, conscious, and social process variables. *Social Science & Medicine, 314*, 115477.

Larsen, K.R., Ramsay, L.J., Godinho, C.A. et al. (2019). *ICF Behave V1.0: Towards an interdisciplinary taxonomy of behaviors.* PLoS One.

Lucas, T., Thompson, H. S., Blessman, J. et al. (2021). Effects of culturally targeted message framing on colorectal cancer screening among African Americans. *Health Psychology, 40*(5), 305–315.

Lunn, P. et al. (2020). Using behavioural science to help fight the coronavirus, ESRI Working Paper, No. 656, The Economic and Social Research Institute (ESRI), Dublin.

McCrae, R.R., & Costa, P.T. (1987). Validation of the five-factor model of personality across instruments and observers. *Journal of Personality and Social Psychology, 54*, 81 90.

McEachan, R.R.C., Conner, M., Taylor, N.J., & Lawton, R.J. (2011). Prospective prediction of health-related behaviors with the Theory of Planned Behavior: A meta-analysis. *Health Psychology Review, 5*, 97–144.

McEachan, R.R.C., Lawton, R.J., & Conner, M. (2010). Classifying health-related behaviours: Exploring similarities and differences amongst behaviours. *British Journal of Health Psychology*, *15*, 347–366.

McEachan, R., Taylor, N., Harrison, R. et al. (2016). Meta-analysis of the Reasoned Action Approach (RAA) to understanding health behaviors. *Annals of Behavioral Medicine*, *50*, 592–612.

Milne, S., Orbell, S., & Sheeran, P. (2002). Combining motivational and volitional interventions to promote exercise participation: Protection motivation theory and implementation intentions. *British Journal of Health Psychology*, 7, 163–184.

Milne, S., Sheeran, P., & Orbell, S. (2000). Prediction and intervention in health-related behavior: A meta-analytic review. *Journal of Applied Social Health Psychology*, *30*, 106–143.

Morwitz, V.G., & Fitzsimons, G.J. (2004). The mere measurement effect: Why does measuring intentions change actual behavior? *Journal of Consumer Psychology*, *14*, 566–572.

Orbell, S., Hodgkins, S., & Sheeran, P. (1997). Implementation intentions and the theory of planned behavior. *Personality and Social Psychology Bulletin*, *23*, 945–954.

Papies, E.K., & Hamstra, P. (2010). Goal priming and eating behavior: Enhancing self-regulation by environmental cues. *Health Psychology*, *29*, 384–388.

Payne, B.K., McClernon, F.J., & Dobbins, I.G. (2007). Automatic affective responses to smoking cues. *Experimental and Clinical Psychopharmacology*, *15*, 400–409.

Peak, H. (1955). Attitude and motivation. In M.R. Jones (Ed.), *Nebraska symposium on motivation* (Vol. 3, pp. 149–188). Lincoln: University of Nebraska Press.

Perkins, H.W. (2003). *The social norms approach to preventing school and college age substance abuse: A handbook for educators, counsellors, and clinicians*. San Francisco: Jossey-Bass.

Petty, R.E., & Cacioppo, J.T. (1986). The elaboration likelihood model of persuasion. In: L. Berkowitz (Ed.), *Advances in Experimental Social Psychology*, *19*, 123–205.

Prestwich, A., Conner, M., Lawton, R. et al. (2005). Individual and collaborative implementation intentions and the promotion of breast self-examination. *Psychology & Health*, 20, 743–760.

Prestwich, A., Conner, M., Lawton, R. et al. (2012). Randomized controlled trial of collaborative implementation intentions targeting working adults' physical activity. *Health Psychology*, *31*, 486–495.

Prestwich, A., Conner, M., Lawton, R. et al. (2014). Partner and planning-based interventions to reduce fat consumption: Randomized controlled trial. *British Journal of Health Psychology*, *19*, 132–148.

Prestwich, A., Kellar, I., Conner, M. et al. (2016). Does changing social influence engender changes in alcohol intake? A meta-analysis. *Journal of Consulting and Clinical Psychology*, *84*, 845–860.

Prestwich, A., Lawton, R., & Conner, M. (2003). The use of implementation intentions and a decision balance sheet in promoting exercise behaviour. *Psychology & Health*, *18*, 707–721.

Prestwich, A., Sheeran, P., Webb, T.L., & Gollwitzer, P.M. (2015). Implementation intentions and health behaviours. In M. Conner & P. Norman (Eds.), *Predicting health behaviour: Research and practice with social cognition models* (2nd Ed.; pp. 321–357). Maidenhead: Open University Press.

Renner, B., Spivak, Y., Kwon, S., & Schwarzer, R. (2007). Age and health behaviour change: Differences in predicting physical activity of South Korean adults. *Psychology & Aging, 22*, 482–493.

Rhodes, R., & Conner, M. (2010). Comparison of behavioral belief structures in the physical activity domain. *Journal of Applied Social Psychology, 40*, 2105–2120.

Rhodes, R.E., Cox, A., & Reza Sayar, M.A. (2022). What Predicts the Physical Activity Intention–Behavior Gap? A Systematic Review. *Annals of Behavioral Medicine, 56(1)*, 1–20.

Richetin, J., Conner, M., & Perugini, M. (2011). Not doing is not the opposite of doing: Implications for attitudinal models of behavioral prediction. *Personality and Social Psychology Bulletin, 37*, 40–54.

Richetin, J., Perugini, M., Conner, M. et al. (2012). To reduce and not to reduce resources consumption? That is two questions. *Journal of Environmental Psychology, 32*, 112–122.

Richetin, J., Osterini, D., & Conner, M. (2020). Predicting engaging in cosmetic surgery: A test of the role of doing and not doing cognitions. *Journal of Applied Social Psychology, 50*, 53–62.

Robberson, M.R., & Rogers, R.W. (1988). Beyond fear appeals: Negative and positive persuasive appeals to health and self-esteem. *Journal of Applied Social Psychology, 13*, 277–287.

Rooke, S.E., Hine, D.W., & Thorsteinsson, E.B. (2008). Implicit cognition and substance use: A meta analysis. *Addictive Behaviors, 33*, 1314–1328.

Rothman, A.J., & Sheeran, P. (2021). The operating conditions framework: Integrating mechanisms and moderators in health behavior interventions. *Health Psychology, 40*, 845–857.

Rothman, A.J., & Salovey, P. (1997). Shaping perceptions to motivate healthy behaviour: The role of message framing. *Psychological Bulletin, 121*, 3–19.

Rothman, A.J., Martino, S.C., Bedell, B., Detweiler, J., & Salovey, P. (1999). The systematic influence of gain- and loss-framed messages on interest in different types of health behaviour. *Personality and Social Psychology Bulletin, 25*, 1357–1371.

Sandberg, T., & Conner, M. (2008). Anticipated regret as an additional predictor in the theory of planned behaviour: A meta-analysis. *British Journal of Social Psychology, 47*, 589–606.

Sandberg, T., & Conner, M. (2009). A mere measurement effect for anticipated regret: Impacts on cervical screening attendance. *British Journal of Social Psychology, 48*, 221–236.

Schoenmakers, T.M., de Bruin, M., Lux, I.F.M. et al. (2010). Clinical effectiveness of attentional bias modification in abstinent alcoholic patients. *Drug and Alcohol Dependence, 109*, 30–36.

Schüz, B., Brick, C., Wilding, S., & Conner, M. (2020). Socioeconomic status moderates the effects of health cognitions on health behaviors: Two multi-behavior studies. *Annals of Behavioral Medicine, 54*, 36–48.

Schüz, B., Conner, M., Wilding, S. et al. (2021). Do socio structural factors moderate the effects of health cognitions on COVID-19 protection behaviours? *Social Science and Medicine, 285*, 114261.

Schüz, B., & Webb Hooper, M.F. (2020). Addressing underserved populations and disparities in behavior change. In Hagger, M.S., Cameron, L.D., Hamilton, K., Hankonen, N., & Lintunen, T. Eds. *Handbook of behavior change* (pp. 385–400). Cambridge University Press.

Sheeran, P., Harris, P.R., & Epton, T. (2014). Does heightening risk appraisals change people's intentions and behavior? A meta-analysis of experimental studies. *Psychological Bulletin, 140*, 511–43.

Sheeran, P., Klein, W.M.P., & Rothman, A.J. (2017). Health behavior change: Moving from observation to intervention. *Annual Review of Psychology, 68*, 573–600.

Sheeran, P., Maki, A., Montanaro, E. et al. (2016). The impact of changing attitudes, norms, and self-efficacy on health-related intentions and behavior: A meta-analysis. *Health Psychology*, 35, 1178–1188.

Sheeran, P., & Webb, T. (2016). The intention-behavior gap. *Social and Personality Psychology Compass, 10*, 503–518.

Sherman, D.A.K., Nelson, L.D., & Steele, C.M. (2000). Do messages about health risks threaten the self? Increasing the acceptance of threatening health messages via self-affirmation. *Personality and Social Psychology Bulletin, 26*, 1046–1058.

Sherman, D.K., & Cohen, G.L. (2006). The psychology of self-defense: Self affirmation theory. *Advances in Experimental Social Psychology, 38*, 183–242.

Stacy, A.W., Ames, S.L., Ullman, J.B., Zogg, J.B., & Leigh, B.C. (2006). Spontaneous cognition and HIV risk behavior. *Psychology of Addictive Behaviors, 20*, 196–206.

Steele, C.M. (1988). The psychology of self-affirmation: Sustaining the integrity of the self. In L. Berkowitz (Ed.), *Advances in Experimental Social Psychology, 21*, 261–302.

Steinmetz, H., Knappstein, M., Ajzen, I., Schmidt, P., & Kabst, R. (2016). How effective are behavior change interventions based on the theory of planned behavior? A three-level meta-analysis. *Zeitschrift für Psychologie, 224(3)*, 216–233.

Strack, F., & Deutsch, R. (2004). Reflective and impulsive determinants of social behaviour. *Personality and Social Psychology Review, 8*, 220–247.

Stroebe, W., Mensink, W., Aarts, H., Schut, H., & Kruglanski, A.W. (2008). Why dieters fail: Testing the goal conflict model of eating. *Journal of Experimental Social Psychology, 44*, 26–36.

Teoli Nunciaroni, A., de Freitas Agondi, R., Ceretta Oliveira, H. et al. (2021). Implementation intention strategy to reduce salt intake among heart failure patients: a randomized controlled trial. *Science of Nursing and Health Practices / Science infirmière et pratiques en santé, 4*, 30–46

Veling, H., Aarts, H., & Stroebe, W. (2013). Using stop signals to reduce impulsive choices for palatable unhealthy foods. *British Journal of Health Psychology, 18*, 354–368.

Webb, T.L., & Sheeran, P. (2006). Does changing behavioral intentions engender behavior change? A meta-analysis of the experimental evidence. *Psychological Bulletin, 132*, 249–268.

Webster, R.K., Brooks, S.K., Smith, L.E. et al. (2021). How to improve adherence with quarantine: rapid review of the evidence. *Public Health, 182*, 163–169.

Weijers, R.J., & de Koning, B.B. (2021). Nudging to increase hand hygiene during the COVID-19 pandemic: A field experiment. *Canadian Journal of Behavioural Science, 53*, 353–357.

Wiers, R.W., Eberl, C., Rinck, M., Becker, E., & Lindenmeyer, J. (2011). Retraining automatic action tendencies changes alcoholic patients' approach bias for alcohol and improves treatment outcome. *Psychological Science, 22,* 290–297.

Wilding, S., Conner, M., Prestwich, A., Lawton, R., & Sheeran, P. (2019). Using the question-behavior effect to change multiple health behaviors: An exploratory randomized controlled trial. *Journal of Experimental Social Psychology, 81,* 53–60.

Wilding, S., Conner, M., Sandberg, T. et al. (2016). The Question-Behaviour Effect: A theoretical and methodological review and meta-analysis. *European Review of Social Psychology, 27,* 196–230.

Wilding, S., Tsipa, A., Branley-Bell, D. et al. (2020). Cluster randomized controlled trial of volitional and motivational interventions to improve bowel cancer screening uptake: A population level study. *Social Science and Medicine, 265,* 113496.

Williams, A.L., Grogan, S., Clark-Carter, D., & Buckley, E. (2013). Impact of a facial-aging intervention versus and health literature intervention on women's sun protection attitudes and intentions. *Psychology & Health, 28,* 993–1008.

Wood, C., Conner, M., Sandberg, T., Godin, G., & Sheeran, P. (2014). Why does asking questions change health behaviours? The mediating role of attitude accessibility. *Psychology & Health, 29,* 390–404.

Wood, C., Conner, M., Sandberg, T., et al. (2016). The impact of asking intention or self-prediction questions on subsequent behavior: A meta-analysis. *Personality and Social Psychology Review, 20,* 245–268.

8

CHAPTER 8
ENVIRONMENT- AND POLICY-BASED APPROACHES TO HEALTH BEHAVIOR CHANGE

OVERVIEW

In this chapter we examine the role of environmental factors and policies that influence health behaviors. Various aspects of the environment might be expected to influence our behavior. For example, a lack of suitable exercise facilities in the local area can impact even the most fervent exerciser. Similarly, a lack of financial resources can prevent individuals from buying healthier but more expensive foods and consumer products. However, these influences of the environment can have effects on behavior either directly (where a mediating variable is not proposed, is automatic/unconscious, or there is no evidence of a mediating variable), indirectly (mediated effects), or by interacting with cognitions (moderation effects). In this chapter we consider these direct, mediated and moderated effects by which environmental factors may influence our behavior. Under direct paths, we explore and examine nudge theory and choice architecture as a research area that has tested how adapting the environment (broadly defined) might change behavior. Under mediated paths, we consider how changing the environment might change cognitions, such as social norms or intentions, and consequently behavior. Under moderated paths, we examine how aspects of the environment may interact with cognitions to produce behavior. We then overview the effects of public policy-based solutions and social marketing approaches in changing behavior.

DOI: 10.4324/9781003302414-9

USING CLASSIC AND SOCIAL/HEALTH COGNITION MODELS

The behaviorist approach considered in Chapter 2 has always focused on external, environmental reinforcement contingencies as primary explanations for behavior and behavior change. The simple formula is: change the reinforcement schedule or behavioral cost, and you will see a change in the behavior. This approach is direct in nature and is similar to nudging behavior (which we overview later in this chapter), which impacts behavior via non-conscious processes, because deliberative or reflective cognitive processes need not be invoked or involved in changing behavior. By changing the accessibility, availability, desirability or cost of performing certain behavioral alternatives, corresponding changes in the behaviors should be observed.

In support of this behavioral approach, Faith et al. (2006) brought sets of five-year-old twins into the laboratory for two visits during which lunch eating behaviors occurred. On the first visit, there was no intervention; baseline eating behaviors were observed. On the second visit, twins were randomly assigned to a treatment or control condition, one twin in each condition. In the contingent rewards condition, children were told that, for each serving of fruits or vegetables that they selected in their lunch, they would receive a voucher that could be exchanged for prizes at a later time. In the non-contingent rewards (control) condition, the children were told that they would receive a set of vouchers for prizes during lunch, but were not told that they were based on selecting certain types of food. Compared to their baseline eating behavior, twins in the contingent rewards group significantly increased their consumption of vegetables and fruits, and decreased their consumption of total energy and fat. Children in the control condition did not change their eating behavior compared to baseline levels. Also, because in such a co-twin research design, the children are matched for their genotypes, the outcomes are much more likely due to the reward contingency rather than any genetic predisposition. Findings such as these illustrate the power of positive reinforcement as an environmental variable that can increase healthier eating behaviors and other positive health behaviors.

The environment has also played a prominent role in some social/health cognition models, albeit in different ways. For instance, in the major theorist model (Fishbein et al., 2001, see Chapter 2), the environment is assumed to have a **direct effect** on behavior, facilitating behavior or preventing action even when the individual has the necessary skills and intentions. In contrast, in the Social Cognitive Theory (see Chapter 2), environmental factors are assumed to only influence behavior indirectly through changing goals or intentions, which in turn influence behavior (i.e., an **indirect/mediated effect**).

_____

DIRECT ENVIRONMENTAL IMPACTS ON BEHAVIOR

NUDGE THEORY AND CHOICE ARCHITECTURE

Thaler and Sunstein are behavioral economists whose books *"Nudge: Improving decisions about health, wealth and happiness"* (2008) and *"Nudge: The final edition"* (2021) have been influential in attempts to change behavior by changing aspects of the environment. They focus on the impact of the environment on decisions and behaviors. They suggest that we do not make choices in a vacuum but in an environment where many features of that environment influence our decisions. It is assumed that many of these environmental features are designed to influence behavior directly, outside of conscious awareness. Others are more transparent and require more cognitive and behavioral effort to have their effect.

Thaler and Sunstein use the term **choice architecture** to describe the creation or modification of aspects of the environment that influence choices. *Nudge* attempts to show how choice architecture can be used to influence people into making certain choices. Their approach describes various strategies under headings such as defaults, expecting error, giving feedback and creating incentives. For example, the idea of changing defaults from an "opt in" default to an "opt out" default has been successful in changing different types of behavior. One famous example by Johnson and Goldstein (2003) shows that by making organ donation consent the default option (compared to the requirement that potential donors exert the effort to opt in to the donation program), donation rates increase dramatically. To cite some specific cases, *opt-out* countries such as Sweden and Austria reported significantly higher numbers of donors (85.9% and 99.98%, respectively), compared to *opt-in* countries such as Denmark, the Netherlands and the UK (4.25%, 27.5% and 17.17%, respectively).

Since the publication of *Nudge* and related work, there have been several attempts to test the ideas in socially important contexts. For example, Thorndike et al. (2014) reported long-term effects of nudge and choice architecture interventions to decrease the likelihood of employees purchasing high-calorie foods and to increase the likelihood of their purchasing healthier foods. After a baseline period, they introduced food labels with a traffic light signal theme. Foods were labelled as "green" (healthy), "yellow/amber" (neutral) or "red" (unhealthy/high calorie). Three months after the traffic light scheme had been introduced, they then used choice architecture to make "green" choices more available and accessible, and to make the "red" choices less available and accessible. Following their interventions, they found significant reductions in "red" choices and increases in "green

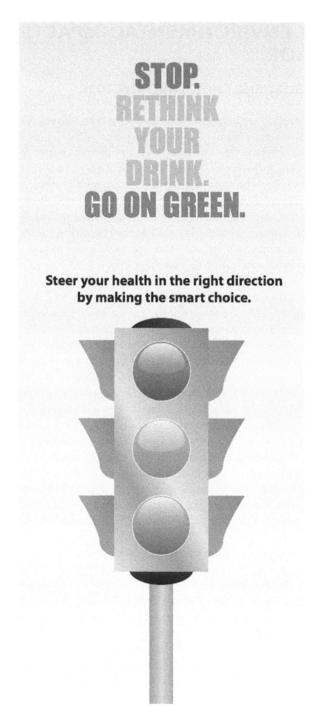

FIGURE 8.1 Images such as this one are used to nudge people in the direction of healthy food and drink choices.

choices." The biggest change was for "red" (high calorie) beverages, which were reduced by 39%. In addition, most of their changes were sustained over two years post-baseline.

More recent research builds on this approach in innovative ways. Potter et al. (2022) introduced participants to a virtual supermarket and were given a shopping list consisting of ten categories (e.g., ready meals, cheese, pizza, bar of chocolate, etc.). They were then asked to select an item from each of those categories for their shopping cart/basket (with no budget limit). Across experimental conditions, the products only differed in how they were presented and labeled. In some conditions, the products had environmental impact scores ranging from A–E, where A (in dark green) indicated a low environmental impact scores and E (in dark red) indicated a high environmental impact score. The environmental impact scores were described as reflecting a product's impact on things like water usage, biodiversity loss and greenhouse gas emissions. Those in the control condition saw the same products, but without environmental impact score labels. Across two experiments, with some variation on the design of the labels between studies, the environmental impact score of products selected was significantly lower in the experimental conditions (ecolabels) compared to in the control conditions. Using a similar experimental supermarket methodology, Potter et al. (2023) presented food products to participants with either environmental impact score labels (ecolabels), healthiness/nutrition labels, both or neither. Compared to control conditions, those who saw ecolabels selected products with significantly lower environmental impact scores; this occurred whether or not a nutrition label was also present.

In a different type of informational intervention (not using food labels), Miller et al. (2016) compared two interventions to a control condition in a Florida, USA, public school lunch program. The first intervention required that students use an online pre-ordering system for their lunches, whereas the second intervention used the same pre-ordering system along with behavioral nudges, which helped students to order a balanced and healthy meal. Specifically, students were prompted to order one element of each from among fruits, vegetables, whole grains, dairy and a main entrée. The second intervention yielded the best outcomes overall, compared to both other conditions. Specifically, students using the program with behavioral nudges for ordering more balanced meals did in fact select more fruits, vegetables and low-fat milk with their lunches.

Different types of informational intervention have been applied in the wider environment rather than on the product itself (e.g., with food labels) to change different types of health behavior. For example, Grant and Hofmann

(2011) used a very simple manipulation of a sign about hand hygiene to change behavior among health professionals in a hospital. In Study 1, one of three messages was randomly assigned to be displayed next to hand-sanitizing gel dispensers around the hospital. The control sign read, "Gel in, wash out"; the personal consequences sign read, "Hand hygiene prevents you from catching diseases"; the patient-consequences sign read, "Hand hygiene prevents patients from catching diseases." Based on measuring the amount of gel used, the rates of dispenser use were 40.1, 34.0 and 54.2%, respectively, for the three groups showing that the message emphasizing patient consequences and presumably cueing professional behavior was most effective. In a second study, the personal consequences and patient consequences signs were compared using covert, independent observation. The rates of hand-hygiene adherence in the two groups were almost identical at baseline but 9.5% higher in the patient compared to personal consequences condition (89.2% vs. 79.7% adherence) at follow-up. These findings are a striking demonstration of how a simple manipulation (in this case changing one word) can produce significant changes in behavior (but see Chapter 7, Burning Issue Box 7.7, for a failed attempt to promote hand-sanitizer use during the COVID-19 outbreak).

Using a different type of environment-based approach, this time altering availability, position and presentation, Piernas et al. (2022) recruited 185 UK grocery stores owned by the same retailer and assigned them to an intervention or not during an approximately seven-week period leading up to Easter. The intervention consisted of the removal of prominent free-standing confectionary stands in the store (the products were still available elsewhere in the store, in their normal locations); control stores kept those promotional stands in place. Although the control and intervention stores did not differ in the key outcomes at baseline, the increase in confectionary sales during the intervention period was 18% for control stores, but only 5% for intervention stores. The average weight (in grams) of confectionary sales increased 31% for controls, but only 12% for intervention stores. Finally, the monetary value of confectionary sales (in GBP/£) increased 10% in control stores, but actually decreased 3% in the intervention stores. Similarly, Pechey et al. (2022) showed that by decreasing the number of meat-free options on a menu, a significant decrease in meat-free choices was observed.

Metcalfe et al. (2020) conducted a review of intervention studies that used nudge-like methods in school meal settings. Such methods include increasing the variety of healthy food options, altering the placement and availability of health options, and using "stop light"-type labels on food choices, among others. They found that nudge interventions tend to have a positive relationship with healthy food selection. However, the results are more mixed when examining actual food consumption; some findings are positive and some are negative. Also, although healthy food selection increases, it can lead to an increase in throwing that selected food out.

In their typology of interventions in proximal physical micro-environments (TIPPME), Hollands et al. (2017) provide a framework to describe and classify approaches to influence the selection, purchase and consumption of food, alcohol and tobacco products. These approaches include manipulations of information (e.g., labels), availability, presentation and position, such as those described already in this section. Another approach is to manipulate functionality; changing how things work or influence how people interact with products. Illustrating the role of functionality manipulations, Hanks et al. (2012) tested the idea of a "convenience line" in addition to standard cafeteria lines in a school. In the convenience line students could only purchase healthy items (e.g., salads, sandwiches, fruits and vegetables). This additional convenience line resulted in a significant reduction in the purchase of unhealthy foods. A final category in Hollands et al.'s (2017) typology relates to size. We turn to manipulations relating to size next.

There are various approaches to manipulating environmental aspects related to size to nudge people to behave in healthier or less unhealthy ways. For example, cigarette manufacturers could change the number of cigarettes per pack, and alcohol producers could change the amount of alcohol per can or bottle. Servings in pubs and restaurants could alter the amount of beer or wine served by changing the size of the glass.

There is some correlational data supporting the idea that packages with more cigarettes are associated with more smoking (e.g., Hill et al., 1998), but good RCT designs and findings are generally lacking. However, Lee et al. (2023) randomized 252 smokers to smoke their usual brand of cigarette in either 20-cigarette packs or 25-cigarette packs. Those in the 20-cigarette packs condition smoked significantly fewer (7.6%) cigarettes per day, compared to the 25-cigarette packs condition.

Researchers have examined the effects of alcohol container and serving glass sizes on alcohol consumption (see Mantzari & Marteau, 2022, for a brief review). For example, Codling et al. (2020) randomly assigned 166 UK households to ordering wine purchases in two different sizes across the intervention period. They either bought 75cl bottles then 50cl bottles, or they bought 50cl bottles then 75cl bottles. Significantly more wine was consumed per day when households had the 75cl vs. 50cl bottles, and they consumed 1.5l of wine significantly faster when the bottles came in 75cl amounts vs. 50cl amounts. Pilling et al. (2020) examined wine purchases over three years in five UK bars and restaurants, varying the serving glasses between 250ml, 300ml, 370ml, 450ml and 510ml. The serving glass sizes did not seem to affect wine purchases in bars, but there was some effect in restaurants. Specifically, compared to the standard 300ml glass, when using the smaller glasses (250ml) there was no difference, whereas using the 370ml glasses led to a significant (7.3%) increase in wine sales. There was no difference when using the 450ml glasses (510ml glasses are not used in restaurants).

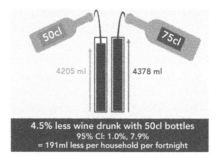

FIGURE 8.2 Visual representation of the results of Codling et al.'s (2020) findings comparing overall wine consumption between 50cl bottles and 75cl bottles.

Image from Mantzari & Marteau's (2022) review.

Mantzari, E. and Marteau, T. M. (2022). Impact of sizes of servings, glasses and bottles on alcohol consumption: A narrative review. *Nutrients, 14*(20): 4244. https://doi.org/10.3390/nu14204244

While the interventions considered so far relate primarily to the immediate, micro-environment in which the behavior occurs, another way of changing the environment to (hopefully) affect behavior is to reduce the amount of public advertising for unhealthy food, cigarettes or alcohol. For example, since the 1970s there have been several federal laws passed in the US against tobacco advertising, including prohibiting advertisements of tobacco products on TV and the radio, on transport and billboards, of paid product placements and in sporting sponsorships, among others. The marketing of alcohol products is also heavily regulated in the US. In the UK, regulations were passed in 2007 limiting children's exposure to advertisements for high fat, salt and sugar (HFSS). In 2018, the Mayor of London announced new restrictions against the outdoor advertisements for HFSS across all of Transport for London. Yau et al. (2022) compared the HFSS purchases of the London area to the same categories of food purchased in the comparison area (North England), and reported a significant drop in calories purchased: about 1,000 kcal fewer per week per household in the intervention areas compared to controls. Significant relative purchase decreases were found in the categories of fat, saturated fat and sugar, but not salt.

Across these different types of nudges and choice architectures, these studies illustrate the power of choice architecture in often influencing health behaviors and the selection of more environmentally responsible food products. Future research might systematically examine the degree to which nudges work across a broader range of protection, risk and detection of health behaviors.

HOW DO PEOPLE FEEL ABOUT NUDGES?

As we noted above, some of the environmental cues or nudges that influence behavior are largely outside of our awareness, whereas others are more visible and require more conscious, deliberate decision-making. Some researchers (e.g., Jung & Mellers, 2016; Kahneman, 2011) have used the terms **System 1 thinking** and **System 2 thinking** to refer to these types of nudges, respectively (see also Strack & Deutsch, 2004, for a discussion of a similar model, called the *Reflective-Impulsive* Model also covered in Chapters 2 and 7). That is, System 1 nudges tend to have more of an automatic or impulsive influence on behavior. Examples of this type of nudge include automatic enrollment into an organ donation program, smaller portions of food and changes in the visibility and accessibility of food items in shops or cafeterias. System 2 nudges, by comparison, require more effort, deliberation and reflection. For example, System 2 nudges might include food labels, nutritional information charts and overt prompts to make different food selections. These types of nudges can provide education and information enabling individuals to make more informed choices. So, when consumers are made aware of these different types of nudges influencing their behavior, how do they feel about them? One hypothesis is that people may feel that nudges are an attempt to control or manipulate their behavior, reacting negatively (called **psychological reactance**; see Brehm, 1966; Sunstein, 2017) and resisting the nudge attempt, especially if those nudges are of the System 1 type.

In a US sample of adults, Jung and Mellers (2016) explored the role of individual differences in support for different types of nudges, and found some interesting patterns. First, there was general support for nudges to increase the likelihood of positive behaviors, but stronger support was obtained for System 2 (informational) nudges than for System 1 (automatic/default) nudges. Concerning individual differences, or preferences based on dispositional variables, empathetic people showed support for both types of nudges, especially when they were framed as have societal benefits. People scoring high on individualism and politically conservative respondents were unfavorable toward both types of nudges. Participants with high scores on a scale of reactance (e.g., "I become frustrated when I am unable to make free and independent decisions" and "When someone forces me to do something, I feel like doing the opposite") and who reported a strong desire for control were primarily against System 1 nudges, and mediation models showed that the key determining factors in their resistance to such nudges were feelings that their autonomy was threatened by such nudges, and that such nudges were too paternalistic.

In samples of adults in both the UK and the US, Petrescu et al. (2016) asked respondents about the acceptability of a variety of interventions, based on nudging or choice architecture, to reduce obesity. These interventions, such as reducing portion sizes, changing the size and shape of containers and making foods differentially accessible to consumers, included both System 1 and System 2 type nudges. In both the UK and US samples, respondents showed a preference for educational interventions (System 2 nudges) to policy-based interventions, such as taxation on sugary beverages. Attitudes toward interventions based on choice architecture were also assessed in their study. In this case, respondents preferred interventions that were presented as effective in solving the problem, even when told about the automatic or "System 1" nature of them. That is, generally speaking, as long as an intervention works, respondents rated them as acceptable even knowing that it works largely non-consciously.

BURNING ISSUE BOX 8.1

ARE NUDGES ETHICAL?

Some people might be uncomfortable with or even explicitly oppose nudges and choice architecture, especially if they are perceived as reducing personal autonomy and freedom, or if they are seen as "sneaky" and being used outside of our awareness or consent. This issue is something that several researchers and economists (e.g., Fischer & Lotz, 2014) have discussed, under the broader consideration of the ethical implications of applying these principles, even if it is presumably for the "greater good" of society.

One ethical concern with nudges is that nudging programs may actually exacerbate or contribute to health inequalities and disparities. Some communities simply have limited or no access to more optimal choices, like adequate health care and healthy food choices. This latter point is a concern in many parts of the world, including even in the US, where many rural regions are referred to as "food deserts" because people in such regions – numbering about 23 million Americans – have no transportation and no supermarkets with fresh, healthy food within a mile. In the UK, food deserts (defined in the UK as being more than 500 meters from adequate food provisions) tend to be concentrated instead in urban areas (Wrigley, 2002). Choice architecture interventions are moot for such communities because the healthier options are not available in the first place. From this perspective, nudges and choice architecture can be seen as partially instrumental in perpetuating inequalities, such that those with privilege and access benefit from such interventions, and those without privilege and access cannot benefit from them in the first place.

Another ethical concern is that if nudging and choice architecture techniques are assumed to be effective and low-cost interventions, then other strategies (like economic and policy-based solutions, discussed below) might be abandoned. For example, instead of raising the price of tobacco or alcohol (economic policies which are known to be effective), it may be a mistake to rely solely on nudges to change behavior, even if such nudges are perceived as being less paternalistic.

Sunstein (2015), one of the original co-authors of *Nudge*, has discussed the ethics of nudges in the light of several critiques, some of which are discussed above. Ethical arguments against nudges (see Rachlin, 2015) are typically captured by the sentiment that our tendency to behave in certain default ways should not be used against us, such as increasing organ donation rates. This is especially true if such techniques are outside of our awareness or threaten our autonomy or our freedom to choose. Sunstein argues that nudges and choice architecture are everywhere already, and that they do not necessarily constrain human agency, but instead promote or facilitate it.

SOCIAL NORMS AS ENVIRONMENTAL GUIDES TO BEHAVIOR

There are two general types of social norms that guide behavior: descriptive and injunctive social norms. Descriptive norms refer simply to who is doing what, or to how many others are engaged in a certain behavior or hold a particular attitude position. For example, a perceived descriptive norm might include the percentage of university students that a particular person believes drinks lots of alcohol on regular occasions. These kinds of norms signal to us what is generally typical of those around us. For example, Burger et al. (2010) randomly assigned undergraduate women to one of three experimental conditions. In the healthy norms condition, they came to the laboratory and saw an empty Nutrigrain wrapper on the table and were asked to throw it in the trash bin nearby, where there were several other Nutrigrain wrappers, indicating that prior participants had chosen healthy snacks. In the unhealthy norms condition, the set-up was identical except that the participants encountered only Snickers bar wrappers. For those in the control condition, both the table and the trash bin were empty. The experimenter brought out two cups and filled one with cold water and one with hot water, and introduced the study as a taste test involving the effects of temperature. Then four snack bars were brought out: a Snickers bar, a Milky Way bar and two Nutrigrain bars of different flavors. Following this first part, a second experimenter came in who was unaware of the condition (i.e., could not see the trash bin). She re-iterated the cover story about the effects of temperature and noted in passing that the wrappers in the trash bin were from the previous women who had participated in the study, thus making the norms salient for similar, undergraduate women as a reference group. They were then asked to select a snack while she (the experimenter) went to prepare some other study materials, turning her back for privacy during snack selection. Once a choice was made, the three unchosen snacks were removed and the study proceeded. Snack selections were consistent with a descriptive norm theory prediction, such that 67.5% of those in the healthy norms condition (Nutrigrain) chose the healthy snack, whereas only 40% of those in the unhealthy norms condition (Snickers) chose the healthy snack. Control participants chose the healthy snack 55% of the time.

Injunctive norms, on the other hand, refer to what others consider to be acceptable or unacceptable behavior. Perceived injunctive norms guide behavior by signaling what is acceptable, appropriate or valid behavior (Cialdini et al., 1990). They may also include sanctions or consequences for engaging in or refraining from certain behaviors. Descriptive and injunctive norms sometimes pull us in different directions. Jared, one of the authors of this book, may see many of his peers smoking cigarettes (descriptive norm), but he knows that his family and close friends would strongly disapprove (injunctive norm) if they were to discover him smoking. Sometimes injunctive norms can backfire as well, because we sometimes perceive them as overtly moralistic, or attempting to restrict our personal freedom (*reactance*; see Silvia, 2006). Stok et al. (2014) compared the relative strength of descriptive versus injunctive norms on intentions to eat more fruit, as well as actual fruit consumption, in high school students. In the descriptive norms condition, participants were told (along with a standard health message) that most high school students try to eat a good amount of fruit themselves. In the injunctive norms condition, they were told that most high school students think that other students should eat a good amount of fruit. Those in the descriptive norms condition had significantly greater fruit eating intentions as well as consumption (over the next two days) compared to the injunctive norms condition, which actually decreased in intentions (but not behavior) even compared to the no–norms control condition. Descriptive norms represent an important component of the Reasoned Action Approach (see Chapter 2).

In the UK in the last few years, there has been an embracing of the ideas about the role of social norms by government in an attempt to address various public health behaviors that have social consequences. A Behavioural Insights Team was set up by the government in 2010 with the aim of using influence techniques like social norms and related concepts to design simple interventions to change important behaviors. Concerning social norms, the Behavioural Insights Team has focused on the ways that healthy behaviors can spread contagiously through social networks.

They cite a large study of American smokers and their families over three generations beginning in the late 1940s (Christakis & Fowler, 2008). In this study, people in close social networks exerted influence on each other, and it was observed that spouses and friends tended to quit smoking together. This is an example of how the behavior of other people can impact our own behavior.

INDIRECT IMPACTS ON BEHAVIOR: HOW CHANGING THE ENVIRONMENT MAY CHANGE COGNITIONS

While the social norms-type approach has features of direct environmental effects on behavior (i.e., that the effects are likely to work to a large extent relatively automatically), it is probable that this approach changes norms which in turn explains subsequent changes in behavior (i.e., a mediated approach).

The *social norms* approach has been used in attempts to change various behaviors, such as the misuse of alcohol and smoking initiation in young people (Haines et al., 2003). The key feature of this approach as a research tool is that individuals first provide information about their own behavior and attitudes. Later, the same individuals make estimates of the numbers of others in their local environment who perform the behavior or approve of the behavior. Feedback is then provided on the actual behaviors and attitudes of others based on the earlier survey. So, for example, an individual might estimate that about half the members of their school would approve of smoking and that about one-quarter are actual smokers. Based on the survey they can then be provided with information to debunk these ideas by showing the actual numbers are quite a lot lower (e.g., showing that only 1 in 5 approve of smoking and only 1 in 10 actually smoke). The assumption is that this more accurate information concerning prevalent social norms will prompt the individuals to decide not to smoke and to be less likely to take up smoking in the future. There is evidence for the success of this approach, particularly in relation to reducing drinking (see Prestwich et al., 2016, for a review). Other researchers (e.g., Chung et al., 2015; see also Smith & Delgado, 2015) have also shown that exposure to others making either risky or safer decisions in domains like gambling or food choices influence the degree to which we make similar risky or safe decisions.

Burger and Shelton (2011) used a similar technique to change the use of stairs over the lift in order to promote physical activity. They found that a sign emphasizing the benefits of using the stairs only produced a modest increase in use of the stairs, while a sign emphasizing that most people used the stairs showed a significant increase in stair use (from 85% to 92% comparing before and after the sign).

In a meta-analytic review of several experimental tests of the effect of social norms on eating behavior, Robinson et al. (2014) found clear evidence that informational social norms have an impact. When study participants were given a "high intake norm," or information about others consuming a lot of food, it increased the amount of food consumed, compared to control conditions. Likewise, the studies that manipulated a "low intake norm" also found a significant effect such that, compared to controls, low intake norms reduced food consumption in study participants. In addition to impacting the quantity of food consumed, social norms can also impact the type of food chosen (healthy snacks versus junk food). It is worth nothing that in most of these studies (e.g., Cruwys et al., 2012), participants are given free access to food such as popcorn, pizza or fruits and vegetables, so the dependent variables are objective, observable behaviors.

One caveat to the social norms approach, especially when considering *perceived* social norms, is that people often display a heuristic thinking pattern known as the False Consensus Effect, which means that they generally overestimate the prevalence of support for their attitudes, traits or behaviors (see Kenworthy & Miller, 2001; Krueger & Clement, 1994). In addition, there is evidence for a selective exposure effect in estimating agreement for our behavioral and attitudinal positions (e.g., Bosveld et al., 1994). This means that, when estimating the number of people who behave like us or share our opinions, we typically refer cognitively to those who are already similar to us to begin with. We might therefore believe that our unhealthy behaviors are more acceptable because of a perceived social norm that is artificially inflated due to heuristic thinking.

BURNING ISSUE BOX 8.2

HOW CAN INDIVIDUALS FOREGO PERSONAL GAINS FOR THE GREATER GOOD?

What's the issue?

In 1968, Garrett Hardin published a paper in *Science* titled "The Tragedy of the Commons." This describes the story of how herdsmen add extra cows to their own herds for personal gains. Unfortunately, this ultimately destroys the communal land that the cows graze leading to hardship for all. Many environmental and health problems have a similar profile. In the short term, each individual wanting to travel in the city may gain by taking their car rather than using the bus (more convenience, comfort, etc.). However, if everyone uses a car to travel, then in the longer term everyone will suffer due to poor air quality and increased traffic. In terms of public health, widespread immunization can help to break the chain of infection. However, in a population where a lot of people are immune there is a relatively low risk of infection anyway and there are drawbacks to the individual of being immunized (e.g., some people perceive certain immunizations to contain harmful ingredients, they have side effects, etc.). By deciding to not vaccinate based on these assumptions, individuals risk the status of public immunity (as well as increasing their own risk for contracting harmful, infectious diseases); as the proportion of non-immune individuals increases in a population, the likelihood of disease outbreaks also increases (see Fu et al., 2011).

Such a discussion is not just an academic exercise. Obviously the COVID-19 outbreak is one prominent example. However, there are other examples. In 2014, the Philippines had a severe outbreak of measles, and this disease was subsequently introduced to the US population. In that year, the US experienced 23 different measles outbreaks, infecting hundreds of people. The vast majority of those infected during these measles outbreaks were unvaccinated (Centers for Disease Control and Prevention, 2016). Mandatory immunization would help to protect the status of public immunity and solve the social dilemma, but there are some obvious ethical concerns with forced immunization. The good news is that general vaccination programs do work. Recently, the Americas were declared free of measles by the Pan American Health Organization, meaning that transmission of measles does not occur for local strains of the disease. The bad news is that strains from the outside can still be introduced to the Americas and infect non-vaccinated or susceptible people, and that decisions to not vaccinate are potentially a threat to public health.

Commons dilemmas can be difficult to resolve because the problem is not strongly influenced one way or another by a single individual taking action. One more person using the car rather than the bus will not markedly effect air pollution or congestion. Similarly, one person switching from using the car to the bus will have little impact in general. Indeed, for that individual, switching to travelling by bus in the city may not be in their interest (i.e., less comfort and flexibility). However, across a range of individual health behaviors, many individuals do choose to act in ways that might benefit the good of all to the potential detriment of their own perceived self-interests because individuals often consider the *right* or *moral* thing to do. According to the **Norm Activation Model** (NAM; Schwartz, 1977; Schwartz & Howard, 1984), a given behavior is adopted not because of the expected outcomes of performance, but for more internalized feelings that can be captured by the concept of moral or personal norm. Personal norms are activated when individuals are aware of the potential adverse consequences of their actions on others or on the environment, and when they believe they can reverse or prevent those consequences. Both sets of beliefs need to be made salient or applied for behavior consistent with the moral norm to occur and to actively influence behavior.

Returning to our example of car use contributing to air pollution, an individual needs to believe their car use is contributing to air pollution and that their reducing car use will help reduce air pollution before the moral norm will be activated (i.e., for the individual to decide it is the right thing to do to reduce use of their car and to take action). Schwartz (1977) proposed that these personal norms are not experienced as intentions, but as feelings of moral obligation and so can directly influence behavior rather than indirectly through changing intentions. A number of studies have shown the NAM to provide good levels of prediction of low-cost environmental behaviors like using public transport over personal cars. Others have argued that moral norms may also moderate the relationship between intentions and behavior by strengthening the relationship between intentions and behaviors perceived to have moral consequences (e.g., Godin et al., 2005).

One other aspect of the environment that has received quite a lot of research attention in terms of how its effects on behavior are mediated by other variables is *level of deprivation*. Deprivation can be measured in a number of ways including income, education and material deprivation (e.g., the extent to which the area you live in is materially deprived). Analyses of neighborhood-level indices of deprivation show that increasing deprivation is associated with lower levels of physical activity (Cubbin et al., 2006).

In a sample of nearly 1,500 Canadian adults, Godin et al. (2010) examined level of education, family income, material deprivation and social deprivation as predictors of physical activity. Importantly, they also measured intention and perceived behavioral control over physical activity in the same sample. This was done to allow for tests of mediation effects on subsequent physical activity. In their data, simple correlations showed education, income and material deprivation to be significantly associated with physical activity levels (social deprivation was not significantly associated with physical activity levels). As you might guess, physical activity was higher among those who were better educated, had higher income and were less deprived. However, these effects were modest compared to the effects for intention and perceived behavioral control. Specifically, the effect sizes for the environmental variables were small, but the effect sizes for intentions and perceived behavioral control were of medium magnitude. Interestingly, the effects of both education and income were partially mediated by intention and perceived behavioral control (there were no significant effects for material deprivation). These findings suggest that part, but not all, of the effect of education and income on physical activity is explained by education and income also yielding lower levels of intention and perceived behavioral control over physical activity. The fact that mediation is partial in this case suggests there are likely other mechanisms by which education and income impact on physical activity levels.

Earlier in this chapter we discussed some research on the effectiveness of ecolabels to influence healthy and environmentally-responsible food selection (Potter et al., 2023). Riskos et al. (2021) examined this kind of relationship with a goal of examining the mediating pathways involved. In their study, the perceived credibility and information value of ecolabels was related to "green" product purchase behaviors via the mediation of both effortful cognitive elaboration (i.e., System 2 thinking) about ecolabel information as well as increased positive attitudes toward purchasing "green" products.

Getting a better understanding of when cognitions do not mediate, partially mediate or completely mediate the effects of changes in the environment on behavior might help us design more effective interventions. For example, where the effects of the environment are mediated by cognitions, it may be useful to consider combining interventions that target environmental changes (e.g., providing more sports centers) with ones that target different cognition changes (e.g., strengthening intentions to be physically active).

HOW THE ENVIRONMENT INTERACTS WITH COGNITIONS IN DETERMINING BEHAVIOR

In addition to mediated effects, we may also find **moderated effects**, or interaction effects, between aspects of the environment and cognitions about the behavior itself, in determining behavior. In general, an interaction effect means that the direct effect of one variable, such as the environment, is different for different groups of people. These groups may be based on experimental conditions, created by random assignment or they may be formed by self-selection, such as when people prefer to live in one neighborhood over another because of factors such as income, ethnicity or religion. Comparisons of differential effects can also use groups based on individual differences or personality factors. For example, the influence of intentions to engage in healthy behaviors on actual behavior might be strongest for people who score high on personality-level conscientiousness.

The study by Godin et al. (2010) that we considered earlier in this chapter contains one example of such an interactive or moderated effect. Godin et al. showed that, in addition to the mediation of intentions and perceived behavioral control on behavior, education level *moderated* the effect of intentions to engage in physical activity on subsequent physical activity levels: intentions were weaker predictors of physical activity among the less educated participants than among the more educated. This is quite important because it suggests that interventions designed to increase intentions to engage in physical activity in a sample or population (as is common in many health promotion messages) will be less effective for those with less education compared to those with more education. It could be the case that among those with less education an intervention targeting intentions to engage in physical activity needs to also target some of the tangible barriers to physical activity.

Concerning health behaviors generally, a key environmental variable has been **socio-economic status (SES)**. SES refers to the social standing of an individual or group in the social hierarchy, and is measured by factors such as relative material deprivation, income, education and occupational classification. Low SES is consistently associated with both increased morbidity and mortality rates (Adler et al., 1994; Centers for Disease Control and Prevention, 2011). In addition, research has demonstrated parallel differences in engagement with a variety of health behaviors as a function of SES (Blaxter, 1990). For example, health risk behaviors such as smoking and alcohol dependency tend to be higher for low SES groups compared to high SES groups, and health protective behaviors such as physical activity and healthy eating tend to be lower. In fact, research has suggested the link between SES and mortality is attributable to differences in engagement with various health behaviors (Stringhini et al., 2010).

One pertinent question is whether SES also moderates the effects of *cognitions* on health behaviors. Findings from Conner et al. (2013) suggest this to be the case. They found that the relationship between intentions to engage in a specific health behavior and subsequent performance was moderated by participants' level of SES: lower SES weakened the intention-behavior relationship across three studies, examining smoking, breastfeeding and physical activity. Schüz et al. (2021) found a similar pattern for COVID-19 related behavioral intentions and reported protection behaviors. Specifically, although the relationship between intentions to perform COVID-19 protective behaviors was significant for all participants, it was significantly stronger for higher SES participants than for lower SES participants.

Other types of moderation effects have been detected. For example, O'Brien (2012), using a longitudinal design of US adults over 10 years, found that SES (operationalized as the number of years of education) was (as expected) a strong predictor of changes in chronic illness (including diabetes, lupus, cancer, etc.) over time, such that less educated respondents reported significantly greater increases in chronic illnesses. However, control beliefs (including both personal mastery and personal constraints/obstacles) interacted with SES in predicting changes in reported chronic illness. When control beliefs were weak, there was a significant difference between low SES and high SES respondents. However, when control beliefs were strong, no differences were found between low and high SES groups. Another way to look at their findings is to consider that the greatest increases in chronic illness were reported among respondents with both low SES and weak control beliefs.

POLICY-BASED APPROACHES TO BEHAVIOR CHANGE

In relation to policy-based approaches to behavior change we will now examine how work on making behaviors illegal (e.g., not wearing seatbelts), changing pricing (e.g., for alcohol and tobacco) and requiring health warnings (e.g., texting and driving, smoking) have been shown to be effective means of changing health behaviors. In this section we will examine the direct behavioral outcomes of public policies, and we also a subset or corollary of the policy-based approach, which is typically referred to as the *Social Marketing* approach to behavior change.

The approaches that fall under the category of policy-based interventions are generally of two types. They will either be based on an informational strategy, or based on changing the market environment itself. Informational approaches are focused on getting people to think more about their choices, or to be aware of the benefits of certain choices or the dangers of other choices (see also the "empowerment" approach; Feufel et al., 2011).

One drawback to these approaches is that they may not reliably result in behavior change even though people may become more knowledgeable, aware or persuaded about the consequences of certain behaviors. The other type of strategy involves changing the market environment directly. These may be seen as more difficult, expensive and intrusive (see Brambila-Macias et al., 2011), but tend to be quite effective in producing changes to behavior and other desired psychological outcomes. In this section, we will review some important areas of health behavior where changes to policies have had measurable impacts.

SEAT BELTS

Over the past few decades the mandatory use of seat belts in motor vehicles has increased to the point where most developed countries now have compulsory seat belt laws. There are variations to these laws, both across countries as well as within them. In the US, for example, each state has its own seat belt laws. Currently, the only US state without compulsory seat belts for adults is New Hampshire, whose state motto is, appropriately, "Live Free or Die!"

The introduction of seat belt laws has reduced fatalities and related outcomes in the UK (Rutherford, 1985) and the US (Cohen & Einav, 2003). It is unclear, however, what psychological mechanisms might be at work generally in producing greater compliance with seat belt laws. It could be the case that seat belt laws have a direct effect on behavior. Alternatively, such laws may change cognitive processes, which in turn affect behavior. For example, Stasson and Fishbein (1990) reported that perceived risk (of injury/death) does not have a direct effect on seatbelt usage. Instead, that behavior is predicted proximally by intentions to use a seatbelt. In their study, intentions were best predicted by perceived risk and social norms. Sutton and Eiser (1990) also showed that fear arousal and perceived risk predicted seatbelt use intentions, but that over time intentions became less important and past behavior (i.e., automatic tendencies or habits) emerged as the main predictor of seatbelt use. Regardless of the exact mechanisms, policies and laws requiring the use of seat belts increase seat belt usage and ultimately prevent injuries and save lives.

TEXTING AND DRIVING

In the UK, using a handheld device has been illegal since 2003, but of the UK vehicle fatalities caused by distractions in 2012, nearly 20% of those were due to mobile phone usage. Although there are not (yet) many long-term studies examining the effectiveness of mobile phone restrictions, there are some studies that shed some light on the issue. One such study (Ehsani et al., 2014; see also Highway Loss Data Institute, 2010) reported an

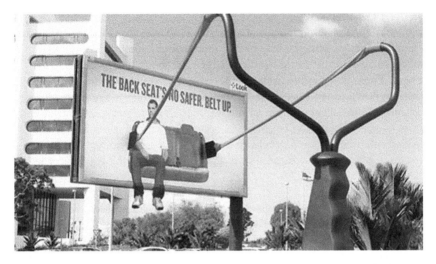

FIGURE 8.3 A whimsical but jarring advertisement for wearing a seat belt.
Credit: Carscoops.

increase in crashes following the introduction of a 2010 texting restriction law put into place in the US state of Michigan. Ehsani et al. speculate that this result may be due to an unintended consequence of the law, which is that people will likely deliberately conceal their mobile phone use behavior while driving so as to avoid being seen by others, especially by police officers/law enforcement. Thus, by keeping their mobile phones out of sight, their driving vision impairments and distractions are exacerbated.

However, larger-scale studies tell a different story. For example, Ferdinand et al. (2014) used a specialized vehicle fatality reporting system to examine the rate of fatal vehicle accidents across 10 years in the US, comparing states with and without texting restrictions or bans. They found a difference overall in fatalities between states with primary bans on texting (drivers can be stopped and fined because they are using their mobile phones), compared to states with secondary bans (drivers must be stopped for some other infraction first, then may be issued a fine for mobile phone usage). Specifically, secondary bans on texting had no effect on traffic fatalities, whereas primary bans did have an effect on reducing fatalities. In fact, the primary bans were found to have the strongest life-saving impact on the sector of the population most at-risk for texting-related accidents and deaths: young people.

Thus, generally-speaking, although mobile phone use bans may produce a shift in behavior from overt to covert in some cases, such laws do have a positive effect on reducing accidents and on saving lives. However, researchers should examine the social and cognitive mechanisms by which better, less distracted driving behavior can be encouraged.

DRUNK DRIVING

There are various policies, laws and blood alcohol content (BAC) limits in countries around the world, some of which are much more stringent than others. These limits range from an upper limit of around 0.08% (e.g., US, Canada) down to 0% (e.g., Brazil, United Arab Emirates). There are also variations in these laws within countries, such as more stringent restrictions on younger drivers or on commercial operators. The penalties for drunk driving offenses also vary widely. In some US states, for example, all first-time offenders are required to install an ignition-lock breathalyzer in their vehicle.

Because drunk driving has been a serious public health problem for a long time, a variety of policy- and law-based solutions have been tested and implemented over the years. For example, Fell and Voas (2006) examined the outcomes of 14 different studies on the effectiveness of BAC-limit laws, around the US and in Europe and Australia, and concluded that having lower BAC limits (e.g., from 0.08 to 0.05 or lower) does serve to reduce the number of vehicle accidents, injuries and deaths. Some of the more effective laws, apart from BAC laws described above, include license bans/suspension, publicized sobriety checkpoints, alcohol ignition locks, minimum drinking age laws and zero tolerance laws (see Goodwin et al., 2015).

PRICE HIKES, WARNING LABELS AND HEALTH LABELS

Tobacco

Over the years, there have been many tests of whether price or tax increases on certain products have their desired effects. Much of this research focuses on the price of tobacco and its effects on smoking behavior. Bader et al. (2011) reviewed many such studies in relation to smoking and found that the majority of studies reviewed indicated that increasing the price of tobacco products reduced both the prevalence of youth smoking behavior as well as the amount of tobacco that they consumed. The evidence is more mixed concerning the initiation or uptake of smoking behavior; however, some studies found some impact on preventing smoking, whereas others found no effect at all. One concern with raising prices or taxes on certain products is that such a policy risks being socially regressive, or more punishing to the finances of poorer people. That is, they must spend a greater proportion of their total income on raised prices, compared to wealthier people. Thus, Bader et al. examined whether price increases on tobacco products had differential effects on low SES versus higher SES groups of consumers. In fact, the majority of studies reviewed showed an equal or better impact of price increases on low SES groups compared to the general population. However, one of the unintended consequences of price increases is that lower SES groups tend to show more demand for smuggled cigarettes when prices go up (e.g., Wiltshire et al., 2001).

In another review of the effects of excise taxes/duties on cigarette smoking, Sharbaugh et al. (2018) examined data from 2001–2015 across all 50 US states and territories, comprising responses from about 5.5 million people during that time. Across all respondents, tax increases were significantly associated with reductions in smoking prevalence. In contrast with the Bader et al. (2011) results, however, the effects were actually weakest for the very lowest SES respondent group (< $25,000 per year income).

Food and drink

With taxes and price-hikes on sugared products being implemented in both the UK and in the US, the key question of course is whether and how they work in favor of public health. Researchers in both countries (e.g., Brownell & Frieden, 2009; Michie, 2016) argue for a tax on sugar-sweetened beverages because such a policy would almost certainly improve health and reduce obesity. Such beverages are seen as a leading cause of obesity, and reductions in sugar beverage intake are clearly associated with improved health over time (see Vartanian et al., 2007). One point of uncertainty in this research so far concerns which alternative foods people would buy instead of sugary drinks. Cartwright (2014) argues that warning label policies are good for academics and people who think rationally about the relationships among consumption of calories, weight gain and associated diseases. However, warning labels are perhaps unlikely to have much of an impact on people who struggle with weight gain for a variety of reasons. One of the ethical considerations for warning labels about obesity is that such labels may lead to further stigmatization and moral judgment of people who choose to consume such products.

Concerning the issue of the effectiveness of warning labels on behavioral choice, van Epps and Roberto (2016) conducted a representative online study to test whether warning labels for sugar-sweetened beverages can influence beverage choices. They gathered responses from over 2,200 adolescents aged 12–18 years. They key independent variable was the type of label accompanying different drinks. They compared a condition with no warning label to a condition with just a calorie indicator label, and to four different types of health warnings telling the prospective consumer that sugary drinks were linked to weight gain, obesity, diabetes and tooth decay. The main outcome in this study was a hypothetical choice of beverage from a vending machine. Warning labels, compared to control and calorie-only labels, generally and significantly reduced the percentage of participants choosing sugar-sweetened beverages.

Using an experimental methodology but in a real-world retail setting with actual purchase behavior, Hall et al. (2022a) had parents of children between 2 and 12 come to the study appointment at the University of North Carolina (UNC), where they were accompanied to a local UNC Mini Mart (convenience store). Their job was to select a drink and a snack for their child, as well as one household item. They would be paid $40 for their participation, and the cost of one of the three items (unobtrusively always the drink) would be subtracted from their $40. Participants were randomly assigned to the warning label condition or the control condition. In the warning label condition, the sugary drinks were all prepared ahead of time with either a type-2 diabetes warning label along with a photo of a necrotizing foot or a heart disease warning along with a photo of a realistic human heart. In the control condition, prominent bar codes were placed instead of warning labels. In the pictorial warning labels condition, only 28% bought a sugary drink for their child. By contrast, in the control/bar code condition, 45% bought a sugary drink.

Because increasing taxes on sugary drinks is a recent phenomenon, there is relatively little data concerning the actual behavioral purchasing habits of consumers, not to mention the longer-term health effects of such policies. Some early findings are encouraging, however. In California, voters in two neighboring cities (San Francisco and Berkeley) voted in 2014 on proposals to add a sugar tax to beverages sold in those cities (see Charles, 2016). Voters in Berkeley approved the tax, whereas voters in San Francisco rejected the proposal. This "natural experiment" yielded some important, if preliminary data. Compared to baseline data, in which residents in both cities reported drinking about 1.5 sugary, fizzy drinks per day, the sugar tax

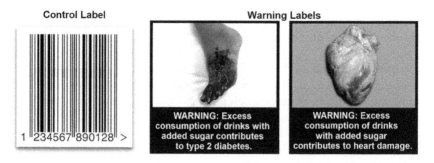

FIGURE 8.4 The warning labels and control images used in Hall et al.'s (2022a) field experiment assessing purchase behavior.

Hall, M.G., Grummon, A.H., Higgins, I.C.A., Lazard, A.J., Prestemon, C.E., Avendaño-Galdamez, M.I. et al. (2022). The impact of pictorial health warnings on purchases of sugary drinks for children: A randomized controlled trial. *PLoS Med, 19*(2): e1003885. https://doi.org/10.1371/journal.pmed.1003885

seems to have had its intended effects. Residents in Berkeley reported about 20% lower consumption of sugary drinks (and an increase in reported water consumption) following the introduction of the tax, whereas reported consumption of sugary drinks in San Francisco did not change over time. Three years after the "experiment" began, Lee et al. (2019) reported that significant reductions in sugary drinks were maintained over time. Of course, it remains to be seen whether such taxes in the UK and the US will have their desired effects on behavior and health over the longer term, and not just on raising money for government programs. Promisingly, Cabrera Escobar et al.'s (2013) review of the effects of price hikes or taxes on sugar-sweetened beverages across the world found that such policies tend to reduce obesity and BMI, and that they may be effective policies generally, despite their "regressive" nature. There is no doubt that many researchers will continue to collect data on this issue to understand not just what the patterns of behavior are, but why and under what conditions they occur.

In contrast to warning labels, there is an emerging research program focusing on the effects of health labels that may be misleading or irrelevant to the actual nutrition of the food itself. This idea is illustrated in a scene in the 1997 comedy film *Romy and Michele's High School Reunion*, in which Romy claims to have invented a new fat-free diet and that for six days she had only eaten gummy bears, jelly beans and candy corns. Hall et al. (2022b) examined the effects of labels of "fruit drinks" that contain nutrition-related claims ("fruit drinks" defined as fruit-flavored drinks that contain additional sugar) on purchase choices when compared to 100% juice drinks or to water. The nutrition-related claims were "No artificial sweeteners," "100% All Natural" and "100% Vitamin C." A control beverage had no label apart from "fruit drink." Participants were parents of young children (ages 1–5) who reported that their child had consumed a "fruit drink" in the previous week. They were asked to make two drinks selections in a virtual grocery store. In the first selection task, they selected between a grape-flavored drink with one of the three labels or control (randomly assigned) and a 100% grape juice drink, and in the second task they selected between an apple-flavored drink with one of the three labels or control (randomly assigned) and pure water. When participants selected between a grape-flavored fruit drink and 100% grape juice (task 1), those who saw any of the three nutrition-related claims on the beverage were significantly more likely to select the fruit drink compared to those in the no-claim control condition. In the second task, those who saw the labels "No artificial sweeteners" and "100% All Natural" (but not "100% Vitamin C") were significantly more likely than those in the no-claim control condition to select the apple-flavored drink. These findings show that such nutrition-related claims on product labels can lead to a misunderstanding about the healthiness of beverages.

In the same broad category of health-related labels, as of the spring of 2022 cafés, restaurants and takeaways (with more than 250 employees) in the UK must provide calorie labels on their menus (Churchill, 2021). Is there sufficient evidence in the research literature to suggest that such labels work, warranting a nationwide implementation of such an intervention? Using an experimental method, Hammond et al. (2013) randomly assigned participants (who would receive a free meal) to get a Subway sandwich under four menu conditions: no nutritional information; calorie amounts only; calorie amounts presented in "traffic lights" (see earlier in the chapter); or calorie, fat, sodium and sugar amounts presented in "traffic lights." They found no difference in the calorie content of meals ordered across conditions, but they did find that participants in the calories-only condition actually consumed (assessed by weighing the meal before and after consumption) significantly fewer calories than did those in the no-information control condition. This might seem like good, albeit somewhat weak, evidence in favor of using calorie labels on menus. However, there have been some reviews of the literature concerning the effects of calorie labeling. Kiszko et al. (2014) reviewed all such studies and found that although there are some weak effects, the studies with the best research designs (i.e., they have comparison groups, they use real-world purchasing behavior, etc.) showed no effects on reducing the number of calories ordered at purchase. Bleich et al. (2017) also reviewed the literature and noted that the positive effects of calorie labels seems to be weak and few in number. They also pointed out the dearth of good RCT designs in field settings, suggesting the need for more systematic and rigorous intervention research.

As an alternative to calorie-only labels, another class of health-related labels are called Physical Activity Calorie Equivalent (PACE) labels, which indicate to consumers how much energy would need to be exerted in order to expend the energy consumed in the product. In a review of the literature examining the effects of PACE labels, Daley et al. (2020) found that across the 15 studies included, PACE labels resulted in fewer calories selected, compared to control labels. However, as Reynolds et al. (2022) note, most of the studies included in that review were potentially at risk for bias, and only one of the studies (Bleich et al., 2012) was conducted in a naturalistic field setting. Following this, Reynolds et al. conducted a large study in a naturalistic study, using 10 worksite cafeterias (with almost 20,000 total employees included) across England for several weeks. Compared to baseline purchases, the introduction of the PACE labels only reduced calorie purchases by about 5kcal per transaction, which was not significant. However, they found quite a bit of variation between the different cafeteria sites. Four cafeterias decreased their calorie purchases significantly compared to baseline, whereas one cafeteria increased their calorie purchases significantly. Five were unchanged. This variability indicates that there are possible untested moderating factors that may be operating to produce positive effects in some sites.

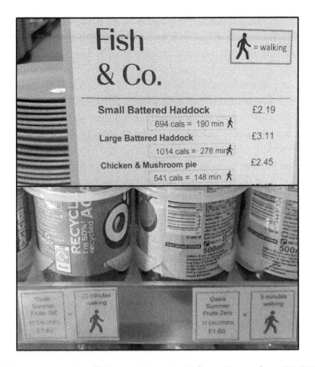

FIGURE 8.5 An example of Physical Activity Calorie Equivalent (PACE) labels.

Reynolds, .JP., Ventsel, M., Hobson, A., Pilling, M.A., Pechey, R., Jebb, S.A., et al. (2022). Evaluation of physical activity calorie equivalent (PACE) labels' impact on energy purchased in cafeterias: A stepped-wedge randomized controlled trial. *PLoS Med, 19*(11): e1004116. https://doi.org/10.1371/journal.pmed.1004116

SOCIAL MARKETING APPROACH TO BEHAVIOR CHANGE

As an increasingly popular method of health promotion, social marketing tries to influence behavior by offering people tangible and social benefits, by reducing barriers and constraints that may block them physically or emotionally, and by using persuasion in targeted or personalized ways to create behavior change. It is a model that differs from traditional health promotion programs, which tend to simply instruct people on how to behave. Instead, social marketing is about getting people to "buy" the better behavior because it is desirable and worth their time, energy or resources (Grier & Bryant, 2005).

The core of the social marketing approach is applying known and proven techniques of influence in consumer behavior to encourage or promote change in health behaviors (see Andreasen, 2002). The ideal outcome is that individuals make more healthy choices for their own benefit as well for the benefit of society as a whole. According to this approach, researchers and practitioners should examine and understand the values and beliefs that motivate and underlie a variety of health behaviors, so that those values and beliefs can be targeted in creating messages or interventions that have the greatest likelihood of effecting change. Although you will undoubtedly recognize this as similar to other models and theories discussed in this book so far, proponents of the social marketing approach argue that it is distinct in some key ways.

According to Andreasen (2002), there are six criteria that should be met for an intervention to qualify as social marketing. First, the intervention must focus on behavior change (rather than intentions or attitudes) in its design and evaluation. Second, social marketing should focus on the motives and needs of the target audience, including both pretesting ideas and monitoring them as they are implemented. Third, interventions should be tailored to specific segments of the population (e.g., based on ethnicity, sex, language, etc.), without assuming that a general intervention can be implemented for all members of a population. Fourth, the intervention should be based on exchange theory, emphasizing the rewards of behavior change and lowering the costs of compliance. Fifth, the intervention should utilize the four Ps of traditional marketing: *Product* (rewards, benefits), *Price* (cost, effort), *Place* (ease of access) and *Promotion* (relevance to the target audience). Finally, the intervention should be designed around an understanding of the competition for an individual's behavior change choices. That is, the behavior change strategy should focus on minimizing the likelihood of other possible behaviors, including current behaviors.

Social marketing strategies and interventions have been developed and used in a variety of countries and cultures, and for an array of health behaviors. One innovative program utilizing this approach was designed to increase of the use of insecticide-treated mosquito nets in Tanzania (Kikumbih et al., 2005) through social promotion of this behavior using stickers, flags, shirts and billboards. The campaign increased the usage of mosquito nets in the intervention area, compared to a control area of the country.

In a social marketing campaign involving nearly 3,000 Canadian university students, Scarapicchia et al. (2015) aimed to increase self-efficacy, outcome expectancies, behavioral intentions to exercise and ultimately changes in moderate to vigorous physical activity. You probably recognize these constructs from the theories discussed in earlier chapters. Their campaign contained social marketing elements emphasizing the benefits of exercise, including stress reduction, enjoyment and academic achievement. These messages were disseminated in postcards, posters, online social media, in classrooms and via face-to-face interactions with peer "ambassadors" from the campaign. Overall, their findings supported the model that they proposed based on the social marketing principles as well as the theoretical framework guiding the choice of measured variables. Specifically, awareness of the campaign predicted greater outcome expectancies (e.g., "Regular physical activity helps me manage stress"), which were associated with greater perceived self-efficacy (e.g., "I am confident that I can regularly do 30 minutes or more of moderate physical activity per day most days of the week."). In turn self-efficacy predicted both stronger intentions to be physically active as well as higher self-reported participation in moderate and vigorous physical activity.

In addition to a focus on increasing healthy behaviors, several studies aim to reduce or prevent harmful behaviors. Glider et al. (2001), using a social marketing intervention that included school newspaper advertisements, awareness activities and interviews in the local radio and television media, reduced alcohol-related behaviors in random samples of the university population at two different time points, before and after the deployment of the intervention. They also saw changes in perceived campus norms, including a significant decrease in the percentage of students who believe that most students have five or more drinks at parties, and that drinking alcohol makes sexual opportunities more likely. However, the study was limited as it did not employ a control group.

Rather than the mediated-type effect demonstrated by Glider et al., a similar intervention conducted in Australia found a moderated effect. In this study, Dietrich et al. (2015) randomly assigned 20 high schools to an alcohol social marketing intervention and another 20 schools to serve as no-exposure controls and found differential effects of social marketing across different segments of the population studied: abstainers, bingers and moderate drinkers. For example, participation in the intervention resulted in a significant reduction in intentions to binge drink, but only among the bingers. For them, their changed knowledge about and attitudes toward drinking impacted their subsequent intentions to binge drink. The same pattern was not observed for the abstainers and moderate drinkers, but their baseline intentions to binge drink were already quite low to begin with.

In an early review of social marketing interventions, Gordon et al. (2006) found the approach to be effective in increasing fruit and vegetable consumption, reducing fat intake and improving people's attitudes toward healthy eating; the findings were more heterogeneous for physical activity, with several studies showing a positive effect on exercise and several showing no effects (but was seemingly effective for changing people's awareness, knowledge or attitudes about exercise); and reasonably successful for substance misuse such as smoking and illicit drug use (although social marketing was less effective in smoking cessation than in preventing or reducing smoking behavior). Gordon et al. also reported that social marketing interventions can be effective across a range of different target groups and in different settings, such as in schools, churches, workplaces and even in supermarkets.

LIMITATIONS TO THE SOCIAL MARKETING APPROACH

There are a number of limitations to this approach. First, Kubacki et al. (2015) noted that, despite a focus in the literature on six key benchmark criteria (discussed earlier in this chapter; see Andreasen, 2002), few studies employ all six criteria.

Second, some critics (e.g., Langford & Panter-Brick, 2013) argue that social marketing focuses too much on individual agency and individual behavior, without taking into account the very real structural constraints of many populations, especially disadvantaged populations that are often the most in need of health interventions. For example, when individuals in disadvantaged populations or areas become motivated to change via social marketing campaigns, they often cannot because of resource constraints. In the end, they may have even worse outcomes because they can feel powerless to act, and ashamed or stigmatized for not changing their behavior.

Third, and as a related point, because many of the principal factors influencing health behavior are social and political, public health campaigns (including those using social marketing), should include attempts to change public policy so that the barriers and constraints on opportunities can be reduced or removed for everyone. Such a sentiment is not inconsistent with the major theorist, integrated model of behavior change (Fishbein et al., 2001, see Chapter 2), in which constraints are a major factor in determining behavior change.

Fourth, although the studies testing social marketing can possess good external validity, they tend to suffer from a lack of internal validity. Such studies employ their methods in the real world, outside of the laboratory, so they cannot typically randomly assign participants to conditions or get representative, random samples of their populations. Caution is warranted because these approaches tend to combine several variables or interventions together, and they lack strong theoretical frameworks. This makes it difficult for scientists and consumers to have a clear sense of which factors are responsible for any observed effects, or of why they occurred in the first place. On the other hand, applying techniques in a problem-focused way is often done with the goal of solving some social problem – in this case improving individual and public health. Thus, we may see a sacrificing of strict internal validity to research when lives are at stake.

Finally, if these strategies are seen to be effective, then they will likely require long-term investments by communities and their respective governments. This is because such interventions must compete against a constant array of countervailing forces encouraging us to engage in unhealthy behaviors.

SCIENCE OF HEALTH BEHAVIOR CHANGE: IN ACTION

In Action Box Action 8.1 considers a pair of observational studies by Collins et al. (2019). In these studies, the authors examined the impact of social norms versus health messages on vegetable purchases. Two different university canteen locations had either a social norms message or the health message displayed on posters. Vegetable purchases were observed at a baseline phase, during the intervention phase (when the posters were displayed) and then post-intervention. The theory suggests that social norms will act as direct modelling influences on eating behavior, so the authors expected that participants would purchase more vegetables with their meals when presented with information suggesting that other students regularly do so.

SCIENCE OF HEALTH BEHAVIOR CHANGE: IN ACTION 8.1

Study: Collins et al., 2019. Two observational studies examining the effect of a social norm and a health message on the purchase of vegetables in student canteen settings
Aim: To examine the effects of social norms versus health messages on vegetable purchases. Method: Two university canteen locations were chosen and displayed prominent posters with either a health message relating to vegetable consumption (i.e., vegetables lower the risk of heart disease) or a social norm about vegetable consumption (i.e., most students choose to eat vegetables with their meal). Researchers observed which meals were purchased and assessed whether the meal contained a portion of vegetables.

Observations were made at three time points: pre-intervention, during the intervention period and post-intervention. A similar design was used in both studies.

Results: In study 1, the purchase of meals with vegetables increased significantly from baseline to both intervention and post-intervention stages in the social norms condition, but did not increase in the health message condition. However, the baseline rate of vegetable consumption was already higher in the health messages condition. In study 2, significant increases from baseline to intervention phase were observed in both conditions. Unlike study 1, purchases of vegetables dropped back to baseline levels at post-intervention in the social norms condition, but remained elevated at post-intervention in the health message condition.

Authors' conclusion: Social norms can have an effect on vegetable consumption, although the effects on longer-term eating behavior are somewhat ambiguous given the inconsistency across studies. Health messages can also have an impact.

THEORY & TECHNIQUES OF HEALTH BEHAVIOR CHANGE		
BCTs	INTERVENTION: Based on Michie et al.'s (2013) taxonomy: Health message: 5.1 Health consequences; 7.1: Prompts/cues;Social norms message: 6.2 Social comparison; 7.1: Prompts/cues	
	CONTROL: None	
Critical Skills Toolkit		
3.1	Does the design enable the identification of which BCTs are effective?	Yes to some degree. Any differences between the intervention and control groups would be attributable to either the prompt and/or the normative message (and social comparison that it could lead to) for the social norms condition. The effects of the health message would be attributable to the information on health consequences and/or prompt.

4.1	Is the intervention based on one theory or a combination of theories (if any at all)?	The social norms intervention targeted social norms on the basis that previous research has indicated the importance of this for behavior. In this sense, it is based on the concept of what Michie and Prestwich (2010) term predictors rather than a formal theory. There was no clear theory upon which the health message intervention was based.
	Are all constructs specified within a theory targeted by the intervention?	N/A
	Are all behavior change techniques explicitly targeting at least one theory-relevant construct?	For the social norms condition, to some degree, yes. This intervention is a face valid manipulation of social norms. It is not clear what constructs are targeted by the health-based message.
	Do the authors test why the intervention was effective or ineffective (consistent with the underlying theory)?	No. Mediation analyses were not conducted. Exit surveys were collected from a relatively small sub-sample of observed participants, but these were primarily for obtaining demographic information and whether the posters were correctly recalled.
4.1	Does the study tailor the intervention based on the underlying theory?	No. The intervention is the same for everybody within a particular condition (it did not differ based on varying scores on measures of theory-relevant constructs at baseline).
2.1, 2.2	What are the strengths/limitations of the underlying theory?	No formal theory is specified as the basis of the intervention. There is some evidence-base to support this type of norms-based approach to health behavior change, however.

THE METHODOLOGY OF HEALTH BEHAVIOR CHANGE		
5.3	Methodological approach	The study adopted an observational design (see Critical Skills Toolkit 5.3).
5.2, 5.5	Are the measures reliable and valid?	The main outcome variable, purchase of meals with vegetables (study 1) or vegetable sides (study 2), was measured by observation from two independent researchers. The intra-class correlation (reliability between judges) was high in both studies.
5.5	May other variables have been manipulated other than the independent variable?	Some risk of bias. Participants were not randomly assigned to canteen locations. The differences observed between locations may have been due to some self-selection bias.
	Non-random allocation of participants to condition	Some risk. Participants were not randomized to locations/conditions, and some baseline differences in vegetable purchases were observed between locations.
	Blinding & Allocation Concealment	Unclear risk. There was no evidence of blinding or allocation concealment in the procedure. There was also some risk of demand effects given the presentation of previous participants' eating behavior. The information could have suggested the appropriate or sanctioned amount of vegetables to be eaten. However, such information is by definition what social norms convey.
ANALYZING HEALTH BEHAVIOR CHANGE DATA		
6.2	Was the sample size calculated a-priori?	The sample size was calculated a-priori and these were calculated based on anticipated small effects. However, many more observations were collated than the number of observations planned a-priori.

Fig. 6.1	Was the hypothesis tested with an appropriate statistical test?	Yes.
5.5, 6.4	Incomplete outcome data	The authors did not report the removal of any data.
5.5	Selective outcome reporting	Unclear given the protocol was not pre-published, however, all of the measures reported in the Method section were analyzed and reported in the Results section.
4.2	Lack of variability (non-sig. effects only)	Not applicable. Significant differences across groups emerged.
6.3	Non-linear relationship (non-sig. effects only)	Not applicable. Significant differences across groups emerged.
REPLICABILITY: Are the effects likely replicable?		
BIB 5.4	The case for	Some consistency in findings across two studies indicating that some of the findings might be more replicable than others.
BIB 5.4	The case against	Differences across conditions at baseline meant differences across groups were not compared; self-selection into condition; no preregistration or data availability/sharing statement; while there was an a-priori sample size calculation, the actual number of observations exceeded the planned number and effects were small; risk of selective outcome reporting, blinding and allocation concealment were unclear. Some of the findings varied across the two studies (e.g., the effectiveness of the health message).

SUMMARY

In the first part of this chapter, we examined some direct environmental factors that influence behavior, including positive reinforcements, nudging and choice architecture interventions. We then explored some indirect or mediated effects of the environment on health behavior, such as when environmental factors lead to changes in cognition, which in turn affect behavior. Interactive or moderated effects were then examined, including when the effects of environmental factors are different depending on the type or group of persons in question. In the second part of the chapter, we explored a series of policy-based approaches to changing behavior, followed by a consideration of the social marketing approach to behavior change.

FURTHER READING

French, J., & Gordon, R. (2015). *Strategic Social Marketing*. Sage. This popular book introduces and critically evaluates the value of the social marketing approach to changing behaviour and solving social problems.

Hardin, G. (1968). The tragedy of the commons. *Science*, *162*, 1243–1248. This philosophical paper is an early introduction to the social dilemma of freedom of choice when resources are limited.

Kahneman, D. (2011). *Thinking, Fast and Slow*. New York: Farrar, Straus, and Giroux. Nobel Prize winner Daniel Kahneman uses his decades of experience in the psychology of decision-making to explore the various influences on our choices. Includes a discussion of System 1 and System 2 thinking.

Thaler, R., & Sunstein, C. (2021). *Nudge: The Final Edition*. London: Penguin. *Nudge* is easy and amusing to read, but deals with the serious topic of decision-making and its consequences in the real world, including areas such as health, finance, COVID-19 and climate change.

GLOSSARY

Choice architecture: Part of Nudge Theory, suggesting that we can alter the environment in which decisions are made to make certain choices more or less likely.

Direct effect: Simple case where changes in behavior are explained by changes in the environment.

Indirect/mediated effect: Where changes in behavior are explained

by changes in the ways that individuals view the behavior which in turn are caused by changes in the environment.

Moderated effect: Where the relationship between cognitions and behavior is explained by changes in the environment (e.g., living in a deprived area reducing the impact of your intentions to not smoke on your subsequent smoking behavior).

Norm Activation Model: Emphasizes the idea that behavior can be adopted not because of the expected outcomes of performance, but for more internalized, moral reasons.

Psychological reactance: Proposed by Brehm (1966), reactance is an unpleasant motivational state that arises when we feel that our freedom is being constrained or threatened. The typical response is to push back, resist the perceived control or otherwise behave to restore our sense of freedom.

Socio-economic status (SES): Refers to the social standing of an individual or group in a social hierarchy and is measured by factors such as relative material deprivation, income, education and occupational classification.

System 1 thinking: Refers to non-reflective, automatic or impulsive influences on behavior.

System 2 thinking: Refers to more effortful, conscious, deliberative and reflective thought processes impacting behavior.

REFERENCES

Adler, N.E., Boyce, T., Chesney, M.A. et al. (1994). Socioeconomic status and health. The challenge of the gradient. *American Psychologist, 49*, 15–24.

Andreasen, A.R. (2002). Marketing social marketing in the social change marketplace. *Journal of Public Policy & Marketing, 21*, 3–13.

Bader, P., Boisclair, D., & Ferrence, R. (2011). Effects of tobacco taxation and pricing on smoking behavior in high-risk populations: a knowledge synthesis. *International Journal of Environmental Research and Public Health, 8*, 4118–4139.

Blaxter, M. (1990). *Health and lifestyles.* London: Tavistock.

Bleich, S.N., Economos, C.D., Spiker, M.L. et al. (2017). A systematic review of calorie labeling and modified calorie labeling interventions: impact on consumer and restaurant behaviour. *Obesity, 25*, 2018–2044.

Bleich, S.N., Herring, B.J., Flagg, D.D., & Gary-Webb, T.L. (2012). Reduction in purchases of sugar-sweetened beverages among low-income black adolescents after exposure to caloric information. *American Journal of Public Health, 102*, 329–335.

Bosveld, W., Koomen, W., & Pligt, J. (1994). Selective exposure and the false consensus effect: The availability of similar and dissimilar others. *British Journal of Social Psychology, 33*, 457–466.

Brambila-Macias, J., Shankar, B., Capacci, S. et al. (2011). Policy interventions to promote healthy eating: a review of what works, what does not, and what is promising. *Food and Nutrition Bulletin, 32*, 365–375.

Brehm, J.W. (1966). *A theory of psychological reactance.* New York, NY: Academic Press.

Brownell, K.D., & Frieden, T.R. (2009). Ounces of prevention—the public policy case for taxes on sugared beverages. *New England Journal of Medicine, 360*, 1805–1808.

Burger, J.M., Bell, H., Harvey, K. et al. (2010). Nutritious or delicious? The effect of descriptive norm information on food choice. *Journal of Social and Clinical Psychology, 29*, 228–242.

Burger, J.M., & Shelton, M. (2011). Changing everyday health behaviours through descriptive norm manipulations. *Social Influence, 6,* 69–77.

Cabinet Office (2012). Applying behavioural insights to reduce fraud, error and debt. HMSO: London.

Cabrera Escobar, M.A., Veerman, J.L., Tollman, S.M., et al. (2013). Evidence that a tax on sugar sweetened beverages reduces the obesity rate: a meta-analysis. *BMC Public Health, 13,* 1072.

Cartwright, M.M. (2014, June 15). Soda Warning Labels: Rated "F" for Futility: Why warning labels on sugary beverages will not impact obesity. https://www.psychologytoday.com/blog/food-thought/201406/soda-warning-labels-rated-f-futility-0

Centers for Diseases Control and Prevention. (2011). CDC health disparities and inequalities report – United States, 2011. *Morbidity and Mortality Weekly Reports, 60,* 1–113.

Centers for Diseases Control and Prevention. (2016). *Measles Cases and Outbreaks.* http://www.cdc.gov/measles/cases-outbreaks.html

Charles, D. (2016). Berkeley's Soda Tax Appears to Cut Consumption of Sugary Drinks. http://www.npr.org/sections/thesalt/2016/08/23/491104093/berkeleys-soda-tax-appears-to-cut-consumption-of-sugary-drinks

Christakis, N. A., & Fowler, J.H. (2008). The collective dynamics of smoking in a large social network. *New England Journal of Medicine. 358,* 2249–2258.

Chung, D., Christopoulos, G.I., King-Casas, B. et al. (2015). Social signals of safety and risk confer utility and have asymmetric effects on observers' choices. *Nature Neuroscience, 18,* 912–916.

Churchill, J. (2021). Calorie labelling on menus to be introduced in cafes, restaurants and takeaways. https://www.gov.uk/government/news/calorie-labelling-on-menus-to-be-introduced-in-cafes-restaurants-and-takeaways

Cialdini, R.B., Reno, R.R., & Kallgren, C.A. (1990). A focus theory of normative conduct: Recycling the concept of norms to reduce littering in public places. *Journal of Personality and Social Psychology, 58,* 1015–1026.

Codling, S., Mantzari, E., Sexton, O., et al. (2020). Impact of bottle size on in-home consumption of wine: a randomized controlled cross-over trial. *Addiction, 115,* 2280.

Cohen, A., & Einav, L. (2003). The effects of mandatory seat belt laws on driving behavior and traffic fatalities. *Review of Economics and Statistics, 85,* 828–843.

Collins, E.I., Thomas, J.M., Robinson, E. et al. (2019). Two observational studies examining the effect of a social norm and a health message on the purchase of vegetables in student canteen settings. *Appetite, 132,* 122–130.

Conner, M., McEachan, R., Jackson, C. et al. (2013). Moderating effect of socioeconomic status on the relationship between health cognitions and behaviors. *Annals of Behavioral Medicine, 46,* 19–30.

Cruwys, T., Platow, M.J., Angullia, S.A., et al. (2012). Modeling of food intake is moderated by salient psychological group membership. *Appetite, 58,* 754–757.

Cubbin, C., Sundquist, K., Ahlen, H. et al. (2006). Neighborhood deprivation and cardiovascular disease risk factors: protective and harmful effects. *Scandinavian Journal of Public Health, 34,* 228–237.

Daley, A.J., McGee, E., Bayliss, S. et al. (2020). Effects of physical activity calorie equivalent food labelling to reduce food selection and consumption: systematic review and meta-analysis of randomised controlled studies. *Journal of Epidemiology & Community Health, 74,* 269–275.

Dietrich, T., Rundle-Thiele, S., Schuster, L. et al. (2015). Differential segmentation responses to an alcohol social marketing program. *Addictive Behaviors, 49,* 68–77.

Ehsani, J.P., Bingham, C.R., Ionides, E., & Childers, D. (2014). The impact of Michigan's text messaging restriction on motor vehicle crashes. *Journal of Adolescent Health, 54,* S68–S74.

Faith, M.S., Rose, E., Matz, P.E. et al. (2006). Co-twin control designs for testing behavioral economic theories of child nutrition: methodological note. *International Journal of Obesity, 30,* 1501–1505.

Fell, J.C., & Voas, R.B. (2006). The effectiveness of reducing illegal blood alcohol concentration (BAC) limits for driving: evidence for lowering the limit to. 05 BAC. *Journal of Safety Research, 37,* 233–243.

Ferdinand, A. O., Menachemi, N., Sen, B. et al. (2014). Impact of texting laws on motor vehicular fatalities in the United States. *American Journal of Public Health, 104,* 1370–1377.

Feufel, M.A., Antes, G., Nelson, D. et al. (2011). How to achieve better health care: Better systems, better patients, or both? In G. Gigerenzer, & J.A.M. Gray (Eds.), *Better doctors, better patients, better decisions: Envisioning healthcare 2020* (pp. 117–134). Cambridge: MIT Press.

Fischer, M., & Lotz, S. (2014). Is soft paternalism ethically legitimate? The relevance of psychological processes for the assessment of nudge-based policies. *Cologne Graduate School Working Paper Series (05-02).*

Fishbein, M., Triandis, H.C., Kanfer, F.H. et al. (2001). Factors influencing behaviour and behaviour change. In A. Baum, T.A. Revenson, & J.E. Singer (Eds.), *Handbook of Health Psychology* (pp. 3–17). Mahwah, NJ: Lawrence Erlbaum Associates.

Fu, F., Rosenbloom, D.I., Wang, L., & Nowak, M.A. (2011). Imitation dynamics of vaccination behaviour on social networks. *Proceedings of the Royal Society of London B: Biological Sciences, 278,* 42–49.

Glider, P., Midyett, S.J., Mills-Novoa, B. et al. (2001). Challenging the collegiate rite of passage: A campus–wide social marketing media campaign to reduce binge drinking. *Journal of Drug Education, 31,* 207–220.

Godin, G., Conner, M., & Sheeran, P. (2005). Bridging the intention-behavior "gap": The role of moral norm. *British Journal of Social Psychology, 44,* 497–512.

Godin, G., Conner, M., Sheeran, P. et al. (2010). Social structure, social cognition, and physical activity: A test of four models. *British Journal of Health Psychology, 15,* 79–95.

Goodwin, A., Thomas, L., Kirley, B. et al. (2015). *Countermeasures that work: A highway safety countermeasure guide for State highway safety offices, Eighth edition.* (Report No. DOT HS 812 202). Washington, DC: National Highway Traffic Safety Administration.

Gordon, R., McDermott, L., Stead, M., & Angus, K. (2006). The effectiveness of social marketing interventions for health improvement: what's the evidence? *Public Health, 120,* 1133–1139.

Grant, A.M., & Hofmann, D.A. (2011). It's not all about me: Motivating hand hygiene among health care professionals by focusing on patients. *Psychological Science, 22,* 1494–1499.

Grier, S., & Bryant, C. (2005). Social marketing in public health. *Annual Review of Public Health, 26*, 319e339.

Haines, M.P., Barker, G., & Rice, R. (2003). Using social norms to reduce alcohol and tobacco use in two midwestern high schools. In H.W. Perkins (Ed.) *The social norms approach to preventing school and college age substance abuse: A handbook for educators, counselors, and clinicians* (pp. 235–244). San Francisco: Jossey-Bass, 2003.

Hall, M.G., Grummon, A.H., Higgins, I.C. et al. (2022a). The impact of pictorial health warnings on purchases of sugary drinks for children: A randomized controlled trial. *PLoS Medicine, 19*, e1003885.

Hall, M.G., Lazard, A. J., Higgins, I.C. et al. (2022b). Nutrition-related claims lead parents to choose less healthy drinks for young children: a randomized trial in a virtual convenience store. *American Journal of Clinical Nutrition, 115*, 1144–1154.

Hammond, D., Goodman, S., Hanning, R., & Daniel, S. (2013). A randomized trial of calorie labeling on menus. *Preventive Medicine, 57*, 860–866.

Hanks, A.S., Just, D. R., Smith, L.E., & Wansink, B. (2012). Healthy convenience: nudging students toward healthier choices in the lunchroom. *Journal of Public Health*, fds003.

Hardin, G. (1968). The tragedy of the commons. *Science, 162*, 1243–1248.

Highway Loss Data Institute (2010). Texting laws and collision claim frequencies. *Highway Loss Data Institute Bulletin, 27*(11).

Hill, D.J., White, V.M., & Scollo, M.M. (1998). Smoking behaviours of Australian adults in 1995: trends and concerns. *Medical Journal of Australia, 168*, 209–213.

Hollands, G.J., Bignardi, G., Johnston, M. et al. (2017). The TIPPME intervention typology for changing environments to change behaviour. *Nature Human Behaviour, 1*, 0140.

Johnson, E.J., & Goldstein, D. (2003). Do defaults save lives? *Science, 302*(5649), 1338–1339.

Jung, J.Y., & Mellers, B.A. (2016). American attitudes toward nudges. *Judgment And Decision Making, 11*, 62–74.

Kahneman, D. (2011). *Thinking, Fast and Slow*. New York: Farrar, Straus, and Giroux.

Kenworthy, J.B., & Miller, N. (2001). Perceptual asymmetry in consensus estimates of majority and minority members. *Journal of Personality and Social Psychology, 80*, 597–612.

Kikumbih, N., Hanson, K., Mills, A. et al. (2005). The economics of social marketing: the case of mosquito nets in Tanzania. *Social Science & Medicine, 60*, 369–381.

Kiszko, K.M., Martinez, O.D., Abrams, C., & Elbel, B. (2014). The influence of calorie labeling on food orders and consumption: a review of the literature. *Journal of Community Health, 39*, 1248–1269.

Krueger, J., & Clement, R. W. (1994). The truly false consensus effect: an ineradicable and egocentric bias in social perception. *Journal of Personality and Social Psychology, 67*, 596–610.

Kubacki, K., Rundle-Thiele, S., Pang, B., & Buyucek, N. (2015). Minimizing alcohol harm: A systematic social marketing review (2000–2014). *Journal of Business Research, 68*, 2214–2222.

Langford, R., & Panter-Brick, C. (2013). A health equity critique of social marketing: where interventions have impact but insufficient reach. *Social Science & Medicine, 83*, 133–141.

Lee, I., Blackwell, A.K., Hobson, A. et al. (2023). Cigarette pack size and consumption: a randomized cross-over trial. *Addiction*, 118, 489–499.

Lee, M.M., Falbe, J., Schillinger, D. et al. (2019). Sugar-sweetened beverage consumption 3 years after the Berkeley, California, sugar-sweetened beverage tax. *American Journal of Public Health*, *109*, 637–639.

Mantzari, E., & Marteau, T.M. (2022). Impact of sizes of servings, glasses and bottles on alcohol consumption: a narrative review. *Nutrients*, *14*(20), 4244.

Metcalfe, J.J., Ellison, B., Hamdi, N. et al. (2020). A systematic review of school meal nudge interventions to improve youth food behaviors. *International Journal of Behavioral Nutrition and Physical Activity*, *17*, 1–19.

Michie, C. (2016). Childhood obesity: enough discussion, time for action. *British Journal of Diabetes*, *16*, 4–5.

Miller, G.F., Gupta, S., Kropp, J.D. et al. (2016). The effects of pre-ordering and behavioral nudges on national school lunch program participants' food item selection. *Journal of Economic Psychology*, *55*, 4–16.

O'Brien, K.M. (2012). Healthy, wealthy, wise? Psychosocial factors influencing the socioeconomic status–health gradient. *Journal of Health Psychology*, *17*, 1142–1151.

Pechey, R., Bateman, P., Cook, B., & Jebb, S. A. (2022). Impact of increasing the relative availability of meat-free options on food selection: two natural field experiments and an online randomised trial. *International Journal of Behavioral Nutrition and Physical Activity*, *19*, 1–11.

Petrescu, D.C., Hollands, G.J., Couturier, D.L. et al. (2016). Public acceptability in the UK and USA of nudging to reduce obesity: the example of reducing sugar-sweetened beverages consumption. *PLoS One*, *11*(6), e0155995.

Piernas, C., Harmer, G., & Jebb, S.A. (2022). Removing seasonal confectionery from prominent store locations and purchasing behaviour within a major UK supermarket: Evaluation of a nonrandomised controlled intervention study. *PLoS Medicine*, *19*, e1003951.

Pilling, M., Clarke, N., Pechey, R. et al. (2020). The effect of wine glass size on volume of wine sold: a mega-analysis of studies in bars and restaurants. *Addiction*, *115*, 1660–1667.

Potter, C., Pechey, R., Clark, M. et al. (2022). Effects of environmental impact labels on the sustainability of food purchases: Two randomised controlled trials in an experimental online supermarket. *PLoS One*, *17*, e0272800.

Potter, C., Pechey, R., Cook, B. et al. (2023). Effects of environmental impact and nutrition labelling on food purchasing: An experimental online supermarket study. *Appetite*, *180*, 106312.

Prestwich, A., Kellar, I., Conner, M. et al. (2016). Does changing social influence engender changes in alcohol intake? A meta-analysis. *Journal of Consulting and Clinical Psychology*, *84*, 845–860.

Rachlin, H. (2015). Choice architecture: A review of why nudge: The politics of libertarian paternalism. *Journal of the Experimental Analysis of Behavior*, *104*, 198–203.

Reynolds, J.P., Ventsel, M., Hobson, A. et al. (2022). Evaluation of physical activity calorie equivalent (PACE) labels' impact on energy purchased in cafeterias: A stepped-wedge randomised controlled trial. *PLoS Medicine*, *19*, e1004116.

Riskos, K., Dekoulou, P., Mylonas, N., & Tsourvakas, G. (2021). Ecolabels and the attitude–behavior relationship towards green product purchase: a multiple mediation model. *Sustainability*, *13*, 6867.

Robinson, E., Thomas, J., Aveyard, P., & Higgs, S. (2014). What everyone else is eating. A systematic review and meta-analysis of the effect of informational eating norms on eating behavior. *Journal of the Academy of Nutrition and Dietetics*, *114*, 414–429.

Rutherford, W.H. (1985). The medical effects of seat-belt legislation in the United Kingdom: a critical review of the findings. *Archives of Emergency Medicine*, *2*, 221.

Scarapicchia, T.M., Sabiston, C.M., Brownrigg, M. et al. (2015). MoveU? Assessing a social marketing campaign to promote physical activity. *Journal of American College Health*, *63*, 299–306.

Schüz, B., Conner, M., Wilding, S. et al. (2021). Do socio-structural factors moderate the effects of health cognitions on COVID-19 protection behaviours? *Social Science and Medicine*, *285*, 114261.

Schwartz, S.H. (1977). Normative influence on altruism. In L. Berkowitz (Ed.), *Advances in Experimental Social Psychology*, *10* (pp. 221–279). New York: Academic Press.

Schwartz, S.H., & Howard, J.A. (1984). Internalized values as moderators of altruism. In E. Staub, D. Bar-Tal, J. Karylowski, & Reykowski (Eds.), *Development and maintenance of prosocial behavior* (pp. 229–255), New York, NY: Plenum.

Sharbaugh, M.S., Althouse, A.D., Thoma, F.W. et al. (2018). Impact of cigarette taxes on smoking prevalence from 2001–2015: A report using the Behavioral and Risk Factor Surveillance Survey (BRFSS). *PLoS One*, *13*, e0204416.

Silvia, P.J. (2006). Reactance and the dynamics of disagreement: Multiple paths from threatened freedom to resistance to persuasion. *European Journal of Social Psychology*, *36*, 673–685.

Smith, D.V., & Delgado, M.R. (2015). Social nudges: Utility conferred from others. *Nature Neuroscience*, *18*, 791–792.

Stasson, M., & Fishbein, M. (1990). The relation between perceived risk and preventive action: A within-subject analysis of perceived driving risk and intentions to wear seatbelts. *Journal of Applied Social Psychology*, *20*(19), 1541–1557.

Stok, F.M., De Ridder, D.T., De Vet, E., & De Wit, J.B. (2014). Don't tell me what I should do, but what others do: The influence of descriptive and injunctive peer norms on fruit consumption in adolescents. *British Journal of Health Psychology*, *19*, 52–64.

Strack, F., & Deutsch, R. (2004). Reflective and impulsive determinants of social behavior. *Personality and Social Psychology Review*, *8*(3), 220–247.

Stringhini, S., Sabia, S., Shipley, M. et al. (2010). Association of socioeconomic position with health behaviors and mortality. *Journal of the American Medical Association*, *303*, 1159–1166.

Sunstein, C.R. (2015). Nudges, agency, and abstraction: A reply to critics. *Review of Philosophy and Psychology*, *6*(3), 511–529. doi:10.1007/s13164-015-0266-z

Sunstein, C.R. (2017). Nudges that fail. *Behavioural Public Policy*, *1*, 4–25.

Sutton, S.R., & Eiser, J.R. (1990). The decision to wear a seat belt: The role of cognitive factors, fear and prior behaviour. *Psychology & Health*, *4*, 111–123.

Thaler, R., & Sunstein, C. (2008). *Nudge: Improving decisions about health, wealth and happiness*. London: Penguin.

Thaler, R., & Sunstein, C. (2021). *Nudge: The final edition*. New Haven, CT: Yale University Press.

Thorndike, A.N., Riis, J., Sonnenberg, L.M., & Levy, D.E. (2014). Traffic-light labels and choice architecture: Promoting healthy food choices. *American Journal of Preventive Medicine*, *46*(2), 143–149.

Van Epps, E.M., & Roberto, C.A. (2016). The influence of sugar-sweetened beverage warnings: a randomized trial of adolescents' choices and beliefs. *American Journal of Preventive Medicine*, *51*, 664–672.

Vartanian, L.R., Schwartz, M.B., & Brownell, K.D. (2007). Effects of soft drink consumption on nutrition and health: a systematic review and meta-analysis. *American Journal of Public Health*, *97*(4), 667–675.

Wiltshire, S., Bancroft, A., Amos, A., & Parry, O. (2001). "They're doing people a service"—Qualitative study of smoking, smuggling, and social deprivation. *BMJ*, *323*, 203–207.

Wrigley, N. (2002). "Food deserts" in British cities: policy context and research priorities. *Urban Studies*, *39*, 2029–2040.

Yau, A., Berger, N., Law, C. et al. (2022). Changes in household food and drink purchases following restrictions on the advertisement of high fat, salt, and sugar products across the Transport for London network: A controlled interrupted time series analysis. *PLoS Medicine*, *19*, e1003915.

9

CHAPTER 9
TECHNOLOGY-BASED APPROACHES TO HEALTH BEHAVIOR CHANGE

OVERVIEW

In this chapter we will cover a variety of theoretical approaches to the application of technology. We consider an array of technological advances that have been employed to change behavior. Technological advances, including the development of smartphones, provide a platform through which to change the health behaviors of individuals and groups at any point on any given day. We examine the use of computers, the internet, smartphone applications (or *apps*), wearable devices and other modern technologies in the context of health behavior change.

USING CLASSIC AND SOCIAL/HEALTH COGNITION MODELS

In their review of internet-based interventions for health behavior change, Webb et al. (2010) concluded that interventions that made greater use of theory were more likely to be effective. The trouble is that many of these types of interventions do not employ theory (e.g., Azar et al., 2013) and those that do, typically do not target all constructs within the chosen theory (e.g., Hale et al., 2015). However, there is vast potential for theory to contribute to informing what should be incorporated within these types of interventions (e.g., which behavior change techniques to use) and many technology-based interventions are or could be at least theory-inspired.

In a review of how theory has been applied to digital health interventions, Morrison (2015) highlights the role of many theories covered elsewhere in this book. For instance, the Elaboration Likelihood Model (see Chapter 7) proposes that more personally-relevant messages are more likely to be centrally processed by recipients. Thus, message tailoring is a potentially useful element of technology-driven health behavior change. Similarly,

DOI: 10.4324/9781003302414-10

stage-type models such as the Transtheoretical Model (see Chapter 2) lend themselves nicely to tailoring within information technology-based, electronic health (**eHealth**) and mobile health (**mHealth**) interventions. Indeed, this theory has been applied widely to inform technology-based interventions for behaviors such as physical activity (see LaPlante & Peng, 2011).

Self-Determination Theory (SDT; Ryan & Deci, 2000; see also Chapter 2) posits that increasing autonomous motivation, for example by providing choice rather than external pressure, maximizes the likelihood that behavior change is initiated and maintained in the future. Thus, employing strategies to promote a sense of choice within the architecture of technology-based interventions should maximize effectiveness. Choi et al. (2014) conducted a content analysis of smartphone smoking apps, in which they searched for elements that were conceptually related to SDT. The important concepts from this theory are autonomy, competence and relatedness to others. Of the more than 300 apps identified as being designed for smoking cessation, only about 10% of randomly selected apps had all three theoretical components.

Gamification, which involves the application of game-like features such as incentives, prizes, points, rewards and competitions to non-game contexts, has been increasingly utilized within web-based platforms (see Chapter 3). For example, mobile apps like Fitbit provide badges for physical activity achievements, while apps such as MySugr provide progress tracking and rewards for successfully managing diabetes. The many aspects of gamification employed to make the behavior targeted in the intervention more fun is also consistent with SDT given its tenet that intrinsically rewarding behaviors are more likely to be maintained in the long term. And, of course, the use of incentives and rewards is very much in keeping with classic behaviorist models/operant conditioning (see Chapter 2) – rewarding behavior contingent on its performance should help to promote future, regular performance of the target behavior.

A BRIEF HISTORY OF TECHNOLOGICAL AIDS TO HEALTH BEHAVIOR

In the early days of health and lifestyle apps (beginning around 2009), the majority of interventions and studies were concerned primarily with using the new technology to track and monitor behaviors, which as you know by now is an important part of self-regulation and behavior change (see for example, Chapter 3). Even in those early days, researchers (e.g., Cummiskey, 2011) noted that the Apple App store already had many thousands of apps designed for health and fitness. It took a few more years before interventions were designed to help people make changes, such as eating healthier, quitting smoking or reducing alcohol intake. Many of these interventions were not grounded in any behavioral change theory, but some were. For example, some attempted to leverage the power of social norms, or other forms of social influence (e.g., Gasser et al., 2006). Others focused on making health information and encouragement more available or cognitively accessible to users (e.g., Consolvo et al., 2008).

One early review of smartphone apps designed for behavioral health (see Luxton et al., 2011) overviewed the different kinds of targeted behaviors, which ranged from developmental, cognitive and mood disorders to substance use, eating and sleep disorders. Luxton et al. concluded that although such technology has emerged as an important component of behavioral health care, much work is still needed to ensure that healthcare policies and evidence-based practices keep up with the rapid acceleration of the technology. In their review of experimental studies testing internet-based interventions to improve health by promoting physical activity, healthy eating or reductions in smoking or drinking, Webb et al., (2010) reported that the benefits of internet-based interventions, on average, were small. However, studies that also incorporated text messages within their internet-based interventions yielded larger effects, highlighting the utility of this approach. In any case, one of the advantages of internet and mobile health apps is that they fit nicely within person-centered models of health-care. These models emphasize individual involvement, autonomy and self-management in the direction and practice of health behaviors (see Handel, 2011). For example, mobile apps are especially useful for making users aware of their physical activity levels (Winter et al., 2012), and for giving support and encouragement in engaging in specific behavioral changes.

In the medical field, smartphone apps are typically found within three categories: clinical decision-making tools, enabling peripheral devices and patient education (Mertz, 2012). Clinical decision-making tools provide information and in doing so act, essentially, as a modern-day library. The supercomputer named "Watson," developed and built by IBM, made headlines when it won the $1 million first prize on the television show *Jeopardy!* in 2011. IBM has indicated that one of the primary future applications of the Watson project is to facilitate medical decision-making. One can imagine a future smartphone app that is connected, via the internet, to the vast databases that are becoming available to medical practitioners.

The second category involves using smartphones as a hub for peripheral devices that include heart rate monitors, blood glucose monitors and even

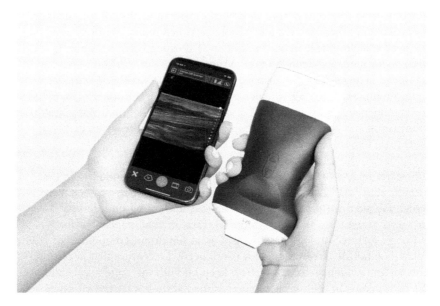

FIGURE 9.1 Portable handheld ultrasound devices now work with modern smartphones.

blood alcohol concentration calculators. There is even an app and connecting device for using a smartphone as a personal, low-cost ultrasonic monitoring device. This can accompany some of the rising number of pregnancy and maternity-relevant apps (see Tripp et al., 2014).

The final category of apps focuses on educating, encouraging and helping people to change their behaviors to become healthier. For example, Ahlers–Schmidt et al. (2010) noted that the majority of parents would like to receive text message reminders about immunizations for their children, and are likely to have mobile phones (see also Peck et al., 2014). We will discuss several of these interventions throughout this chapter.

As the technology for mHealth has accelerated in the past few years, a recent phenomenon has emerged, called just-in-time-adaptive-interventions (JITAI; see Nahum-Shani et al., 2018). JITAIs are a type of intervention that adapts support to users over time and as a function of their changing status and ideally delivers support or information at the time when it is most needed or most useful. Examples of JITAIs include Apple watch wearers getting a reminder to stand and move, or getting a notification if an irregular heart rhythm is detected. Hardeman et al. (2019) reviewed 19 papers studying JITAIs (primarily targeting sedentary behavior and physical activity), and noted that while such research is fairly new, several of the studies are theory-based and utilize specific, effective BCTs, including getting feedback, action planning and goal setting. Unfortunately, as an emerging field, more evidence is needed to support the effectiveness of JITAIs in promoting healthy behaviors.

APPLICATIONS

Marcolino et al. (2018) reviewed the field of mHealth intervention research and found mHealth apps to be effective across a range of health conditions (e.g., asthma, pulmonary conditions, heart failure, glycemic control, weight loss, tobacco use, etc.) and for the delivery of health care services. For example, they highlight the positive impact of text message reminders for improving clinic attendance, similar to phone call reminders but for less cost. In this section, we consider various technology-based solutions and interventions for behaviors important for physical health: alcohol consumption, smoking, physical activity and diet.

ALCOHOL CONSUMPTION

There are many new (and not so new) internet and smartphone tools for helping people who want to cut back on alcohol. Websites can be used to help curb drinking by providing feedback to users about how their drinking compares to their peers (to promote awareness of potentially high levels of drinking), whether their drinking is likely to be causing them harm (to motivate people to reduce their drinking to reduce their risk of alcohol-related harm) and how much their drinking is costing them (to promote awareness of the tangible costs of drinking). Smartphone apps have many of the same functions. DrinkControl is one such app that tracks how much a user drinks, how many calories those drinks represent and how much money has been spent on drinks.

There is some scientific evidence to support the use of websites and smartphone apps to change this behavior. For example, the Check Your Drinking (CYD) screener has been tested in a handful of experiments. Cunningham et al. (2009) conducted a randomized controlled trial comparing the use of CYD to a no-intervention control group. Those in the CYD condition reduced their problem drinking by around six drinks per week at six-months follow-up, compared to approximately a one drink per week reduction in the control group. Cunningham (2012) randomly assigned problem drinkers to the CYD website or to an extensive online help website that applied cognitive behavioral therapy and relapse prevention for drinking. Those in the CYD group reduced their problem drinking over time, but the effects were even stronger for those in the extended internet-based intervention condition.

With the advent of smartphone apps to help control alcohol and drinking behavior, research has now focused on comparing the effectiveness of web vs. app-based tools. In one such investigation, Gonzalez and Dulin (2015) compared a smartphone app monitoring intervention to an internet-based motivational intervention. Although their study was limited in sample size, they found that those in the self-administered smartphone app conditions had significantly more days abstinent from alcohol over six weeks compared to those receiving the internet-based intervention.

Garnett et al. (2015) noted that there is great potential for smartphone apps to engage users with evidence-based techniques, but that there is little research examining which behavior change techniques can be effective in such a medium. They argue that the behavior change techniques with the greatest likelihood of helping smartphone users reduce their alcohol intake are goal-setting, self-monitoring, planning deliberate action and giving goal-relevant feedback. Dulin et al. (2014) found that when drinkers used apps with a variety of theory-based features, they reported that the most useful features were those that helped them to monitor consumption, manage their cravings and identify the cues or triggers that made them most likely to drink. Participants in their study also showed a significant decrease in dangerous alcohol consumption during the study period.

In Crane et al. (2018), participants were not recruited for the study and then given an app, but were drinkers seeking an app for help with their drinking and were only recruited when they sought help. Their app, called *Drink Less*, was designed around several theories and behavior change techniques (BCTs) discussed earlier in this book. Participants were randomly assigned to one of five modules: normative feedback, cognitive bias re-training, identity change, action planning or self-monitoring/feedback. The greatest reductions in alcohol consumption were found in the normative feedback, cognitive bias re-training and self-monitoring/feedback conditions. These three interventions should sound familiar to you by now. The normative feedback intervention focused on providing "participants with personalized information about how their drinking compared with other people of their age group and gender in the UK" (p. 7), which is a kind of descriptive norm that we discussed in Chapter 8. The cognitive bias re-training intervention focused on changing automatic attitudes toward alcohol via an approach-avoid game, which is targeting system 1 thinking that was also discussed in Chapter 8. Self-monitoring and feedback should also be quite familiar to you by now as well, as these are reasonably effective BCTs discussed in Chapter 3.

Despite the benefits of such alcohol-related smartphone apps, caution is warranted with their use. For example, as Weaver et al. (2013) noted, apps that track consumption and BAC levels are not very accurate for a variety of reasons, and many apps that can be found in the app stores actually encourage drinking behavior. There is a good chance that if you were to open your smartphone's app store right now and search for alcohol, you would find that a majority of them will facilitate drinking behavior (e.g., get wine delivery, how to mix any drink, learn drinking games, etc.) rather than help to discourage or control it. On the other hand, there is evidence to support the idea that people who are committed to monitoring and controlling their drinking behavior can be helped in some ways by smartphone apps. Monk et al. (2015) showed that alcohol consumption recorded into a smartphone app by users during their drinking sessions was quite different from their retrospective reports of drinking, such as during the day after. Such apps could be useful for more accurate self-monitoring of alcohol consumption.

BURNING ISSUE BOX 9.1

HOW GOOD ARE INTERNET-BASED INTERVENTIONS FOR PROBLEM DRINKING? (CUNNINGHAM & VAN MIERLO, 2009)

1. *Is it fair to assume that they are effective?* Many alternative approaches to problem drinking are based on brief face-to-face interventions. How well internet-based interventions work compared to face-to-face interventions needs to be tested; one cannot assume that the internet-based intervention will work as well. Using face-to-face delivery, the healthcare professional can pick up on body language, tone of voice and hesitation in speech that can help inform delivery of the intervention. Such verbal or non-verbal cues can be difficult to integrate within online systems and this may reduce how effective they are.
2. *Temptation.* When you're receiving an intervention face-to-face, it's hard to get away! When using an online intervention, escape is possible with just one click. As a result, people may not complete all of the elements of the intervention and this may make the online intervention less effective (especially when used in the real world, outside the lab).
3. *Where should the intervention be tested?* The researcher could get people into the lab to test out the online intervention. The advantage of this approach is that participants are more likely to do what they're supposed to do (e.g., less likely to click away from the online intervention to check the latest football scores) and any

technical issues can be resolved face-to-face, but this is problematic as testing the online intervention in the lab is moving away from the beauty of it being used outside of the lab. If you evaluate the intervention outside of the lab then you run the risk of temptation, technical issues putting the user off visiting the site, and people generally not using the online intervention as intended. Delivering the intervention in the lab increases internal validity (the strength of control and being used as intended) but reduces external validity (how the results can be generalized to users in real-world settings outside of the lab).

4. *How should the participants be recruited?* Trials that recruit people online, while more closely mirroring the real world, typically use pre-post designs without control groups. As a consequence, the people entering the trial and using the online intervention may be people who would have reduced their drinking anyway. This is particularly true given the high motivation required to complete the online intervention and avoid the other temptations on offer through the internet. Recruiting people online to complete measures twice (before and after the intervention) can be extremely difficult leading to high risk of participants dropping out of the study and thus not returning to complete the follow-up measures to see how their drinking behavior (or other behaviors) have changed.

5. *More evidence is needed to support online interventions.* This is particularly true of studies conducted outside the lab, which mirror more closely how the intervention might be delivered outside the context of an experiment.

6. *Do online interventions work for everybody?* They may work for everybody but they may not. For example, they may work only for people experienced in using computers and the internet; they may work only for volunteers than for problem drinkers directly requested to use the site.

7. *Which parts of the online intervention work?* Online interventions are often complex and involve many different types of behavior change techniques. Without fully-crossed factorial designs the effectiveness of each specific behavior change technique cannot be determined.

8. *How does the intervention work?* By identifying the psychological determinants of drinking (such as motivation and self-efficacy, one's confidence in being able to reduce drinking) and testing whether these determinants change or not can help to inform how the online intervention can be modified to make it more effective. For example, if the intervention only changes motivation and not

> self-efficacy then the addition of behavior change techniques most likely to boost self-efficacy (such as modeling; Bandura, 1998) could make the intervention more effective in reducing problem drinking. There is a need for studies to evaluate whether the intervention changes psychological determinants of behavior. This can help explain why an intervention was effective or ineffective and suggest ways in which the intervention can be improved.

TOBACCO USE

Sometimes the development of technology can outpace evidence-based practice and awareness. For example, in Van Agteren et al.'s (2016) focus groups of Australian smokers and health professionals, both groups of participants showed enthusiasm for technology-based apps to quit smoking because they emphasize personal agency in quitting over pharmacology and counselling-based approaches. However, both groups also showed low experience and awareness of such interventions. Recent app-based interventions share a common theme in focusing on individual agency and self-determining their own choices and behavior. For those who want to cut back on or give up cigarettes, there are also several websites (e.g., smokefree.gov), which provide both expert advice on quitting as well as social support networks. There are also dozens of smartphone apps to help users stop smoking.

As well as issues around general lack of awareness, a recent review of the evidence for smartphone quit apps (Cobos-Campos et al., 2020) notes that while there are not that many RCT studies assessing the effectiveness of quit apps, the data so far do not suggest that they are effective compared to other methods. Relatedly, Staiger et al. (2020) reviewed the effectiveness of apps for reducing the consumption of alcohol, tobacco and drugs. Their conclusions were similar to those of Cobos-Campos et al., that the effectiveness of such apps is not very compelling at this time. In Staiger et al.'s review, only about one-third of the included studies showed a significant reduction in substance use either during or after the intervention period.

As an example of this type of intervention, Ubhi et al. (2015) evaluated abstinence rates in over 1,100 quitting smokers who used a smartphone app to quit, compared to a comparable national British sample of those who attempted to quit unaided. The app-based intervention employed gamification-type features such as rewarding users with "stars" and "hearts" on their phone for abstinent days, as well as information about how much money had been saved thus far during the period of abstinence. They found a small but significant effect, such that users of the app reported better abstinence rates

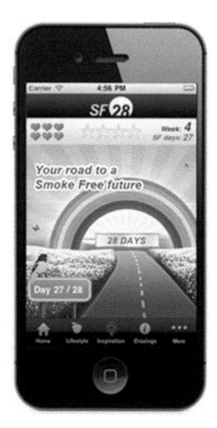

FIGURE 9.2 This is an example of the smartphone app used in Ubhi et al.'s (2015) smoking cessation study.

© Ubhi, Harveen Kaur, Michie, S., Kotz, D., Wong, W-Ch, & West, R. (2015). *Journal of Medical Internet Research*, 16.01.2015. (http://www.jmir.org)

than unaided controls. This research design was not experimental, however, so there is a need for randomized controlled trials (RCT, see Chapter 5).

In contrast with quitting smartphone apps, other quit interventions are delivered only via SMS. This kind of intervention is easy, less-expensive and requires low-bandwidth, and so may be deployed for a greater range of populations. As an example of such an intervention, Free et al. (2011) randomly assigned nearly 6,000 British smokers to either an intervention or a control condition. In the intervention condition (called the text2stop intervention), they received five texts per day for the first five weeks, then three texts per week for another 26 weeks. These texts were personalized and emphasized the damages of smoking and the benefits of quitting. For example, on "quit day" they received a text saying, "This is it! – QUIT DAY, throw away all your fags. TODAY is the start of being QUIT forever, you can do it!" If participants ever felt a craving, they could send a "crave" text and receive a text saying, "Cravings last less than five minutes on average. To help distract yourself, try sipping a drink slowly until the craving is over." In the control condition, participants received one text every two weeks with a simple thanks for their participation in the study. Those in the text2stop condition had a significantly higher rate of abstinence from smoking at six months, compared to the control condition.

Whittaker et al. (2016) conducted a review and meta-analysis of research examining mobile phone-based interventions for smoking cessation, most of which used text messaging as the medium. Although there was a fair amount of heterogeneity in the outcomes, the pooled results showed a significant positive effect, meaning that compared to controls, those in the text messaging intervention conditions were more successful at quitting. More recently, Palmer et al. (2018) conducted a similar review, and found effectiveness versus controls (e.g., getting the same information in a brochure) for quitting smoking and abstinence. The results of these two reviews are noteworthy because the outcomes in these studies are not self-reports – they are biochemically verified in participants by testing their carbon monoxide levels in laboratory or clinical settings.

As with apps for reducing alcohol intake, in more recent years the research designs for testing the effectiveness of quit-smoking apps sometimes directly compare text messaging or internet-based interventions to those employing smartphone app usage. Buller et al. (2014) randomly assigned their smokers to a smartphone app condition or to a text messaging service condition to aid them in quitting tobacco. They found no strong differences between the conditions; using either service increased abstinence at 12 weeks, as long as participants actually used the service. Those who used the mobile services had a 47% rate of abstinence, compared to 20% for those who didn't follow through on their use. Buller et al. noted that the smartphone app, while theoretically-grounded, was more complicated and difficult to use. By contrast, the text messages came to their normal text messaging inbox, requiring less effort or complication. Although these authors did not report differential rates of abstinence for those who fully complied with the smartphone app versus the text messaging service, there are theoretical reasons to suspect that the greater level of effort required by the smartphone app might yield better outcomes. Cognitive dissonance theory (Festinger, 1957; Kenworthy et al., 2011) proposes that when greater effort is required to achieve something, we cognitively justify that time and effort spent, resulting in a greater commitment to the decision. For example, Axsom and Cooper (1985) randomly assigned women at a weight loss clinic to a high effort or a low effort condition while undertaking weight loss counselling. Those in the high effort condition were asked to complete a series of cognitively demanding tasks whenever they came to the clinic. In the low effort condition, they completed much easier versions of the same tasks during their clinic visits. Those in the high effort condition lost significantly more weight, which was apparent at three months, six months and one year following initial treatment. The argument for why such findings were obtained is that the participants became more committed to the decision to lose weight after exerting greater amounts of effort to obtain the goal, compared to those who exerted less effort. Perhaps this principle of **effort justification** could be incorporated into smoking cessation programs as well.

Mindfulness and technology-aided smoking cessation

You have no doubt encountered the concept of mindfulness emerging as part of modern applied philosophy and meditation practices. There are several forms of cognitive behavior therapy (CBT) for behavior change that involve the notion of mindfulness. Some of these CBT techniques are now being incorporated into technology-based solutions for behavior change. With respect to smoking cessation, the general formula for an intervention is to get mobile-based mindfulness training. In this context, mindfulness means developing a non-judgmental awareness of one's discomfort and cravings for tobacco, accepting those affective states and drives. One is also taught to practice creating psychological distance between oneself and one's cravings. Then, the focus is on behaving according to one's values and specific plans. Thus, for research purposes abstinence is the primary outcome, but reductions in cravings and other negative emotions are of secondary importance to the mindfulness training.

In an early examination of these ideas, Jonathan Bricker et al. (2014) tested a smartphone app for smoking cessation using techniques from their model, called ACT (Acceptance and Commitment Therapy). This work was important because it used a double-blind, randomized controlled trial design. The techniques from ACT involve training users to be willing to accept smoking cravings, and to be aware of and accept negative feelings and thoughts, while at the same time committing to values-based behavior change. The app based on ACT was compared to a comparison app using an existing technique used by the US National Cancer Institute. The app employing ACT techniques had better quit rates than the comparison group. Because this was a small-sample pilot test, there was not enough power for firm conclusions. However, there have been other tests of these ideas.

Heffner et al. (2015), for instance, tested an ACT-based app called SmartQuit. In their study, they found that the features that best predicted smoking cessation were (a) practicing the skill of letting urges and cravings pass, and (b) concretely planning to deal constructively with having urges or experiencing lapses. In this sense, the approach overlaps in many ways with the Relapse Prevention Model (see Chapter 2). In a similar exploration of these techniques, Zeng et al. (2016) tested a smartphone app-based intervention that is similar to mindfulness in that it also encourages awareness and acceptance of aversive internal states (craving) without using smoking to reduce those feelings. In their study, those who fully adhered to the app training components on a regular basis were four times more likely to quit smoking than those who did not adhere fully. The training components were having a quit plan, completing eight daily training modules, practicing the skill of letting 10 smoking urges pass, and visiting the online coach (which provided social support and other practical exercises). Drawing firm conclusions on the basis of such analyses is problematic: those who engage more with the intervention might well be those who are most motivated to change. As a consequence, differences between the conditions might reflect a useful intervention, a more motivated/likely to change sample or a combination of the two.

PHYSICAL ACTIVITY, DIET AND WEIGHT LOSS

Most developed or developing countries in the modern era are experiencing an epidemic of obesity. Obesity can generally be traced to the disruption of a simple formula of behavioral energy balance, or behaving in such a way as to disrupt the equilibrium between the energy taken in from food and the energy expended on daily activities. Although there are some other contributing factors (genetics, environmental conditions, etc.), poor diet and inactivity – things that are largely within our personal control – are the primary causes of people becoming overweight or obese (see Popkin et al., 2012).

In addition to traditional means of self-regulation in diet and exercise, smartphone apps can also be useful for creating and maintaining exercise regimens and for monitoring the intake of calories. Fitness or activity apps take advantage of the built-in GPS capabilities and accelerometers of smartphones and allow users to track the number of steps taken, their speed, distance and progress toward other goals. Apps like Runkeeper or Nike Run Club also interface with social media websites, so you can share your workouts with friends and get feedback and encouragement from them as well. Apps are now capable of communicating with each other to integrate data about a person's physical activity, sleep patterns and diet. For example, the app Myfitnesspal can be used to track calories consumed, and it can also accept exercise data from the Runkeeper app, weight data from a Bluetooth-enabled scale, and steps taken from a Fitbit device. Jared, one of the authors of this book, has been using Myfitnesspal in conjunction with Runkeeper for several years now. The calories that he burns by cycling and jogging are synced up automatically from his Runkeeper app to his Myfitnesspal app, increasing his daily number of allowable food calories consumed. By staying at or below the daily limit of calories consumed (referred to as energy balance), he was able to lose more than 20 pounds in

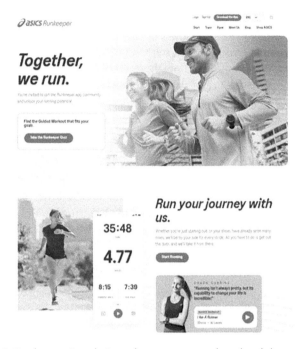

FIGURE 9.3 Runkeeper's website, where users can download the app, register for training and find other functions.

about 100 days and maintain it ever since by regular monitoring and balancing of calories consumed and calories burned!

Is it just Jared who benefits from this type of intervention? Given the relatively recent development of smartphone apps for tracking food intake, it is a reasonable question to ask how well they do in helping people to monitor and control their calorie consumption. Semper et al. (2016) reviewed some studies that had examined this question, with a focus on studies with good research designs. For the majority of the studies that they reviewed, the apps were shown to be effective in their intended purpose, which was to facilitate efforts to lose weight. However, it is important to note here that although the apps were shown to be effective tools, they often did not produce a significant difference in weight loss from their respective control groups, which were either websites or traditional paper diaries of food intake. But the apps did tend to result in greater adherence to a self-monitoring program, compared to other methods, signaling their convenience. So, since participants using the smartphone apps dropped out of their regimens at a lower rate compared to other methods, this is encouraging for the future of apps in personal healthcare, especially given the growing ubiquity of smartphones.

In a more recent review and meta-analysis of research examining the effects of mobile phone apps for weight loss, Islam et al. (2020) found and examined 12 eligible studies. Across those studies, there was a significant difference between the app intervention groups and control conditions on both weight loss and well as reductions in BMI. Similarly, in a review and meta-analysis of eHealth interventions for children and adolescents who are overweight or obese, Azevedo et al. (2022) found a small but significant effect favoring the outcomes in the eHealth intervention groups; their BMI reduction was greater than for those in the control conditions.

More broadly, Milne-Ives et al. (2020) reviewed the research examining mobile app interventions with RCT methodologies. The outcomes of interest were a range of behaviors, including physical activity, diet, drug and alcohol use, and mental health. Regarding physical activity, of the 25 RCT studies that were included, only eight reported significant positive findings favoring the mobile app interventions. The authors suggest more closely examining which BCTs can and should be included in apps to make them more effective.

Concerning the prevalence and use of physical activity apps, Bort-Roig et al. (2014) reviewed the evidence for the effectiveness of mobile devices to track and change behavior and noted few employed RCT designs and large samples. They also found that the strategies employed generally tended not to be theory-based. However, there were some elements identified that were deemed to be useful in encouraging more physical activity. These elements included user-created physical activity profiles, the setting of concrete goals, getting social support and building social networks, receiving feedback in real time about one's activities, and having online consultation with experts. However, many of these techniques are typically delivered in combination with other techniques and thus it is not always easy to identify effective behavior change techniques.

In a recent study, through a carefully crafted design, we managed to isolate the effect of manipulating competition on physical activity within a web-based intervention (Prestwich et al., 2017). In this study, physically inactive adults were randomized to one of three web-based conditions: a group encouraged to self-monitor their steps and who received basic feedback (self-monitoring group); a second, identical group who were additionally exposed to additional feedback to instigate competition (competition group), or a control group. Participants in the competition group increased their step counts over the 4-week intervention period significantly more than those in the control group and those in the self-monitoring group. Making people feel like they were in a competition, by showing participants a continually updated "leaderboard" with those achieving the most daily steps appearing near the top and those with the least appearing towards the bottom, boosted steps via improvements in various types of motivation.

Wearable devices for fitness tracking are not new. In the 1960s a Japanese researcher named Yoshiro Hatano invented a device called *manpo-kei*, which translates as "10,000 steps." Hatano and his research team were concerned about the rise of obesity in Japan, and determined that the average Japanese person walked only about 4,000 steps per day. They advocated increasing that number to 10,000 and the *manpo-kei* was to help in that endeavor. The first FitBit came out in 2009. Today, almost all of us carry a device with an accelerometer and a GPS tracker, whether that device is a smartphone, a smartwatch or both. In a meta-analysis of the effects of wearable devices on weight loss, BMI and waist circumference, Yen and Chiu (2019) showed that overall interventions with wearable devices produced more beneficial outcomes – moderate to large effect sizes – for all three dependent variables, compared to controls. The effect for weight loss was especially significant for those with chronic diseases (e.g., diabetes, breast cancer), and the effect for BMI was stronger for obese individuals compared to healthy weight individuals. In a similar review of wearable devices and their effects on weight loss and other variables, Wang et al. (2022) examined only those studies that focused on children and adolescents. As in Yen and Chiu's review, Wang et al. found that wearable device interventions had significant effects (versus controls) on body weight, BMI and body fat. They did not find an overall effect for waist circumference, however. The effect for BMI was also stronger in overweight and obese children and adolescents, compared to those of healthy weight.

BURNING ISSUE BOX 9.2

ADVANTAGES AND DISADVANTAGES OF INTERNET AND APP-BASED APPROACHES TO HEALTH BEHAVIOR CHANGE

Advantages

1. Reach. (a) They can change health behaviors in a wide range of people given many people have access to internet; (b) they can be used by people who are reluctant to access local services involving face-to-face contact; (c) based on these points, they could be used as a means of potentially reducing health inequalities (but see related disadvantage on smartphones).
2. Can be used to change health behaviors at any time.
3. They are a useful means of encouraging people to actively engage with their behavior change.

4. Generally low cost (e.g., compared to interventions delivered face-to-face).
5. Internet and mobile app approaches are potentially effective, at least in the short term (Afshin et al., 2016).
6. Potentially cost-effective given relatively low cost and potential to effectively change behavior.
7. Behavior change techniques and other features can be tailored to the needs of the individual.
8. Well positioned to provide ongoing support over the longer term, especially if the content is engaging and easy-to-use.
9. It can be a more convenient and easy means to screen people for different illnesses (including those related to mental health). Linked to this, it can also reduce human data entry errors.
10. People tend to be more honest, especially about issues of a personal or sensitive nature, when disclosing online compared to face-to-face settings.
11. Reliability and validity of measures comparable to non-online methods (e.g., Donker et al., 2010).
12. With the growing ubiquity of smartphone-based health app usage, there is a corresponding potential for data aggregation, meaning that companies and governments can look for broader population patterns (for things like foods consumed, calories burned, physical activity levels, BMI, etc.) as a function of different demographic categories and locations. This could make it easier and more efficient to create targeted interventions for certain groups (but see related disadvantage regarding ethics and privacy).

Disadvantages

1. Many (if not most) health apps have not yet been peer reviewed by health professionals, so the theoretical and practical value of such apps can be questionable.
2. Most apps are not developed based on evidence-based models or on tested and validated theories of behavior change.
3. There are few tests of internet, and mobile app-based interventions over the longer-term (e.g. past one year; e.g., Afshin et al., 2016) although this is a broader problem applicable to non-technology focused health behavior change research.
4. The majority of these studies are done in high-income countries (Afshin et al., 2016), sometimes referred to as WEIRD countries (Henrich et al., 2010), an abbreviation for Western, Educated, Industrialized, Rich, and Democratic. It remains to be seen how

well Internet and smartphone tools can generalize to non-WEIRD countries and cultures.

5. Higgins (2016) notes that individuals must own a smartphone and have reliable and adequate cellular or Wi-Fi data plans, limiting access to those who can afford it.

6. Needs to be well-designed and user-friendly.

7. Certain populations are still largely left out of the targeted client base, including the elderly who may not use a smartphone, and people with certain physical or intellectual disabilities that prevent them from engaging with standard smartphone apps.

8. There are complex ethical issues linked to issues such as maintaining privacy (see Clarke & Steele, 2015). In addition, some individuals may become upset after completing an online behavior change intervention or screening questionnaire (e.g., upon realizing that they may have symptoms) and their subsequent behaviors are out of researchers' control.

9. Relatedly, there is a risk that app developers, most of which are unregulated, may misuse personal data without users' knowledge or consent, such as selling it to third parties (see Jiya, 2015). Users also risk identity theft when collected data are not safeguarded properly.

10. Risk of **false positives/false negatives**. Deciding whether the cut-off scores for app-based screenings are the same as for traditional measures is not straightforward (Houston et al., 2001). Taking action on a screening score that is too low indicates a false positive and potentially wasted resources. Setting the cut-off scores too high, by contrast, can result in false negatives, or not acting on patients who may be in life-threatening situations.

11. Inaccurate app information may be relatively harmless in some cases (e.g., when a step counter slightly overestimates the number of steps a user takes) but could be dangerous (e.g., a food nutrient estimation tool underestimates the sugar, sodium or cholesterol content of foods, leading users to consume potentially harmful levels).

12. Encouraging even greater use of technological solutions, especially increased use of the internet, does little to curb the risk of internet addiction.

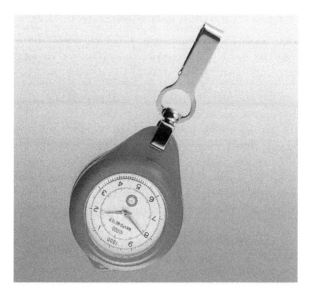

FIGURE 9.4 This is an early pedometer called *manpo-kei*, developed in Japan in the 1960s.

SCIENCE OF HEALTH BEHAVIOR CHANGE: IN ACTION

In Action Box 9.1 considers a randomized clinical trial by Gustafson et al. (2014) in which patients being treated for alcohol use disorders were randomly assigned to a treatment-as-usual condition or to treatment-as-usual supplemented by a smartphone app focusing on constructs from Self-Determination Theory (SDT; see Deci & Ryan, 2002). Their aim was to reduce the number of risky drinking days in their participants, who were patients leaving a treatment facility for alcohol use disorder. In the intervention condition, the smartphone app that participants used was designed to encourage the SDT constructs of autonomy, competence and relatedness to others. This was done via a variety of smartphone features. Proponents of the theory suggest that if individuals can gain competence, leverage intrinsic and autonomous motivation for behavior change, and foster social support and encouragement from others, their behavior should change and be more long-lasting.

SCIENCE OF HEALTH BEHAVIOR CHANGE: IN ACTION BOX 9.1

Study: Gustafson et al. 2014. A Smartphone Application to Support Recovery From Alcoholism: A Randomized Clinical Trial	

Aim: To reduce the number of risky drinking days in patients leaving a residential alcohol use disorder treatment facility.
Method: Participants were randomly assigned to treatment as usual, or treatment as usual with a smartphone app focusing on Self-Determination Theory (SDT) constructs.
Results: At 4- and 12-months following discharge from the facility, participants in the smartphone-aided condition reported significantly fewer average risky drinking days than did those in the treatment as usual condition.
Authors' conclusion: Usual treatment for alcohol use disorders can be supplemented with SDT-based smartphone features.

THEORY & TECHNIQUES OF HEALTH BEHAVIOR CHANGE

BCTs	INTERVENTION: Treatment as usual, plus a smartphone app with features based on SDT.Based on Michie et al.'s (2013) taxonomy: 2.2 Feedback about sobriety behavior; 3.1 General social support; 3.2 Practical social support; 3.3 Emotional social support; 6.1 Modeling of behavior; 6.2 Social comparison; 6.3 Information about others' approval; 8.2 Behavior substitution; 11.2 Regulation of negative emotions; 12.3 Avoidance of the behavior	
	CONTROL: Treatment as usual	
Critical Skills Toolkit		
3.1	Does the design enable the identification of which BCTs are effective?	*No. The smartphone app condition contained several BCTs and a full-factorial design was not used to identify the active components.*
4.1	Is the intervention based on one theory or a combination of theories (if any at all)?	*Notwithstanding the overlaps with the Relapse Prevention Model noted in an accompanying paper to the main trial paper, the authors report that the intervention is based on SDT.*

	Are all constructs specified within a theory targeted by the intervention?	*To some degree: SDT's focus on autonomy does not seem to be explicit in any of the smartphone app features apart from measuring autonomous motivation in questionnaires, although autonomy using the smartphone app is generally implied in the intervention condition. Competence and relatedness to others seem to be specifically targeted.*
	Are all behavior change techniques explicitly targeting at least one theory-relevant construct?	*No. Some of the BCTs are not linked to a theory-relevant construct.*
	Do the authors test why the intervention was effective or ineffective (consistent with the underlying theory)?	*Yes. The authors tested mediation and showed that perceived competence at four months mediated the relationship between the intervention and risky drinking days at 8 months. Other theory-relevant constructs did not show evidence of mediating the outcomes.*
4.2	Does the study tailor the intervention based on the underlying theory?	*No. Irrespective of their scores on SDT-related constructs, intervention participants could access the same BCTs within the intervention.*
TC 2.12	What are the strengths/limitations of the underlying theory?	*See Theory Critique 2.12.*
THE METHODOLOGY OF HEALTH BEHAVIOR CHANGE		
5.1, 5.4, 5.5, 5.6	Methodological approach	*Randomized controlled trial with self-report measures (see Critical Skills Toolkits 5.1 and 5.4–5.6).*
6.1	For experimental designs: Is the study between-subjects, within-subjects or mixed?	*Mixed design because participants were allocated to one of two conditions (between-subjects) and then completed measures at multiple time-points (within-subjects). For advantages & disadvantages of this design, see Critical Skills Toolkit 6.1.*

5.2, 5.5	Are the measures reliable & valid?	*The main outcome variables were not previously validated.*
5.5	May other variables have been manipulated other than the independent variable?	*The authors note that the treatment group completed regular measures that the comparison group did not and this could cause a question-behavior type effect (see Chapter 7).*
	Non-random allocation of participants to condition	*Low risk. Participants were randomized to conditions on a 1:1 ratio using a computer program, in blocks of 8.*
	Blinding & Allocation Concealment	*High risk. Both participants and physicians were aware of allocation to conditions.*
ANALYZING HEALTH BEHAVIOR CHANGE DATA		
6.2	Was the sample size calculated a-priori?	*Yes, the sample size calculated a-priori, based on an estimated effect size.*
Fig. 6.1	Was the hypothesis tested with an appropriate statistical test?	*Yes*
5.5, 6.4	Incomplete outcome data	*Study completion was not different between the conditions. The data were analyzed on an intention-to-treat basis.*
5.5	Selective outcome reporting	*The study's design and measures were registered at clinicaltrials.gov. However, the preregistration referred to some measures not reported in this article (e.g., cravings, days of abstinence) and some measures (e.g., competence) were not preregistered.*
4.2	Lack of variability (non-sig. effects only)	*Not applicable. The participants in the intervention condition reported fewer risky drinking days compared to the control condition.*
6.3	Non-linear relationship (non-sig. effects only)	*Not applicable, effects significant.*

REPLICABILITY: Are the effects likely replicable?		
Burning Issue Box 5.4	The case for	*The sample size was planned a-priori; the study was pre-registered (but there are some deviations from the pre-registration as noted elsewhere in this Action Box); intention-to-treat analyses used.*
Burning Issue Box 5.4	The case against	*The comparison group, "usual care," will likely vary across settings making direct replication attempts more difficult; has a between-subjects design element; there were method-ological limitations (such as lack of blinding) that may have worked in favor of the intervention; many effects were just below the p < .05 threshold.*

SUMMARY

This chapter examined emerging technological aids in the service of health behavior change, with a focus on the internet, smartphones and other modern technologies. We reviewed how a range of theories of behavior change can and should be incorporated into technological advances in health interventions. We covered the technological tools that have been developed for helping people to curb alcohol consumption, quit smoking and change their diets and physical activity levels. At the same time, we examined some relevant research evaluating the effectiveness of those approaches. We noted that many internet and smartphone apps lack a strong theoretical basis, and that in the future program developers and behavior change professionals should spend more time and energy collaborating for the benefit of users.

FURTHER READING

Bort-Roig, J., Gilson, N. D., Puig-Ribera, A. et al. (2014). Measuring and influencing physical activity with smartphone technology: a systematic review. *Sports Medicine*, 44(5), 671–686. This paper reviews several studies examining the effectiveness of smartphone interventions to promote physical activity. Discusses the limitations and potential of such applications.

Hekler, E. B., Michie, S., Pavel, M. et al. (2016). Advancing Models and Theories for Digital Behavior Change Interventions. *American Journal of Preventive Medicine*, *51*(5), 825–832. Attempts to guide the use of theory in building digital interventions for health behaviour. Focuses on variations between individuals and on changes to behaviour over time.

Higgins, J. P. (2016). Smartphone applications for patients' health and fitness. *The American Journal of Medicine*, *129*(1), 11–19. Written from a physician's perspective, this paper gives an overview of smartphone apps that can be useful in helping patients to reach their goals, including those for diet, exercise and stress management.

Staiger, P. K., O'Donnell, R., Liknaitzky, P. et al. (2020). Mobile apps to reduce tobacco, alcohol, and illicit drug use: systematic review of the first decade. *Journal of Medical Internet Research*, *22*(11), e17156. Reviews recent research concerning the effectiveness of mobile apps in reducing a variety of unhealthy behaviors.

GLOSSARY

Effort justification: A concept from Cognitive Dissonance theory describing a change in attitudes, commitment or loyalty toward something, which comes about due to increased time, energy and effort spent toward it.

eHealth: Refers to using information technology (e.g., internet, gaming, robotics, virtual reality, etc.) to promote health behaviors.

False negative: When a test result indicates that some conditions has not been met or fulfilled, when in actuality it has. This is also referred to as a *Type II error*.

False positive: When a test result indicates that some condition has been met or fulfilled, when in actuality it has not. This is also referred to as a *Type I error*.

Gamification: Refers to the use of game-like features such as incentives, prizes, points, rewards, status, connectedness and competitions to promote non-game behaviors, such as health behaviors.

mHealth: Refers to wireless or mobile apps and devices, including the use of social media, to promote and deliver health-related information and services.

Self-Determination Theory: This theory concerns the degree to which our actions are intrinsically- or self-motivated. Proponents argue that there are three general, intrinsic, psychological motivations, namely autonomy, competence and relatedness to others.

REFERENCES

Afshin, A., Babalola, D., McLean, M. et al. (2016). Information technology and lifestyle: a systematic evaluation of internet and mobile interventions for improving diet, physical activity, obesity, tobacco, and alcohol use. *Journal of the American Heart Association*, 5(9), e003058.

Ahlers-Schmidt, C.R., Chesser, A., Hart, T. et al. (2010). Text messaging immunization reminders: feasibility of implementation with low-income parents. *Preventive Medicine*, 50(5), 306–307.

Axsom, D., & Cooper, J. (1985). Cognitive dissonance and psychotherapy: The role of effort justification in inducing weight loss. *Journal of Experimental Social Psychology*, 21, 149–160.

Azar, K.M., Lesser, L.I., Laing, B.Y. et al. (2013). Mobile applications for weight management: Theory-based content analysis. *American Journal of Preventive Medicine*, 45, 583–589.

Azevedo, L.B., Stephenson, J., Ells, L. et al. (2022). The effectiveness of e-health interventions for the treatment of overweight or obesity in children and adolescents: A systematic review and meta-analysis. *Obesity Reviews*, 23(2), e13373.

Bandura, A. (1998). Health promotion from the perspective of social cognitive theory. *Psychology & Health*, 13, 623–649.

Birkhoff, S., & Moriarty, H. (2016). Smartphone mobile health apps interventions across various populations: an integrative review of the literature. *Nursing Research*, 65, e26–e27.

Bort-Roig, J., Gilson, N.D., Puig-Ribera, A. et al. (2014). Measuring and influencing physical activity with smartphone technology: a systematic review. *Sports Medicine*, 44, 671–686.

Bricker, J.B., Mull, K.E., Kientz, J.A. et al. (2014). Randomized, controlled pilot trial of a smartphone app for smoking cessation using acceptance and commitment therapy. *Drug and Alcohol Dependence*, 143, 87–94.

Buller, D.B., Borland, R., Bettinghaus, E.P. et al. (2014). Randomized trial of a smartphone mobile application compared to text messaging to support smoking cessation. *Telemedicine and e-Health*, 20, 206–214.

Choi, J., Noh, G.Y., & Park, D.J. (2014). Smoking cessation apps for smartphones: content analysis with the self-determination theory. *Journal of Medical Internet Research*, 16, e44.

Clarke, A., & Steele, R. (2015). Smartphone-based public health information systems: Anonymity, privacy and intervention. *Journal of the Association for Information Science and Technology*, 66, 2596–2608.

Cobos-Campos, R., Sáez de Lafuente, A., Apiñaniz, A. et al. (2020). Effectiveness of mobile applications to quit smoking: Systematic review and meta-analysis. *Tobacco Prevention & Cessation*, 6, 62.

Consolvo, S., McDonald, D.W., Toscos, T. et al. (2008, April). Activity sensing in the wild: a field trial of UbiFit garden. In *Proceedings of the SIGCHI Conference on Human Factors in Computing Systems* (pp. 1797–1806). ACM.

Crane, D., Garnett, C., Michie, S. et al. (2018). A smartphone app to reduce excessive alcohol consumption: Identifying the effectiveness of intervention components in a factorial randomised control trial. *Scientific Reports*, 8, 1–11.

Cummiskey, M. (2011). There's an app for that smartphone use in health and physical education. *Journal of Physical Education, Recreation & Dance, 82,* 24–30.

Cunningham, J.A. (2012). Comparison of two internet-based interventions for problem drinkers: randomized controlled trial. *Journal of Medical Internet Research, 14,* e107.

Cunningham, J.A. & van Mierlo, T. (2009). Methodological issues in the evaluation of Internet-based interventions for problem drinking. *Drug and Alcohol Review, 28,* 12–17.

Cunningham, J.A., Wild, T.C., Cordingley, J. et al. (2009). A randomized controlled trial of an internet-based intervention for alcohol abusers. *Addiction, 104,* 2023–2032.

Dulin, P.L., Gonzalez, V.M., & Campbell, K. (2014). Results of a pilot test of a self-administered smartphone-based treatment system for alcohol use disorders: usability and early outcomes. *Substance Abuse, 35,* 168–175.

Festinger, L. (1957). *A theory of cognitive dissonance.* Evanston, IL: Row, Peterson.

Free, C., Knight, R., Robertson, S. et al. (2011). Smoking cessation support delivered via mobile phone text messaging (txt2stop): A single-blind, randomised trial. *The Lancet, 378*(9785), 49–55.

Garnett, C., Crane, D., West, R. et al. (2015). Identification of behavior change techniques and engagement strategies to design a smartphone app to reduce alcohol consumption using a formal consensus method. *JMIR mHealth and uHealth, 3*(2), e73.

Gasser, R., Brodbeck, D., Degen, M. et al. (2006, May). Persuasiveness of a mobile lifestyle coaching application using social facilitation. In *International Conference on Persuasive Technology* (pp. 27–38). Springer Berlin Heidelberg.

Gonzalez, V.M., & Dulin, P.L. (2015). Comparison of a smartphone app for alcohol use disorders with an Internet-based intervention plus bibliotherapy: A pilot study. *Journal of Consulting and Clinical Psychology, 83,* 335–345.

Gustafson, D.H., McTavish, F.M., Chih, M.Y. et al. (2014). A smartphone application to support recovery from alcoholism: a randomized clinical trial. *JAMA Psychiatry, 71,* 566–572.

Hale, K., Capra, S., & Bauer, J. (2015). A framework to assist health professionals in recommending high-quality apps for supporting chronic disease self-management: Illustrative assessment of type 2 diabetes apps. *JMIR mHealth and uHealth, 3,* e87.

Handel, M. J. (2011). mHealth (mobile health)—Using apps for health and wellness. *EXPLORE: The Journal of Science and Healing, 7,* 256–261.

Hardeman, W., Houghton, J., Lane, K., et al. (2019). A systematic review of just-in-time adaptive interventions (JITAIs) to promote physical activity. *International Journal of Behavioral Nutrition and Physical Activity, 16,* 1–21.

Heffner, J.L., Vilardaga, R., Mercer, L.D. et al. (2015). Feature-level analysis of a novel smartphone application for smoking cessation. *The American Journal of Drug and Alcohol Abuse, 41,* 68–73.

Henrich, J., Heine, S.J., & Norenzayan, A. (2010). The weirdest people in the world? *Behavioral and Brain Sciences, 33,* 61–83.

Higgins, J.P. (2016). Smartphone applications for patients' health and fitness. *The American Journal of Medicine, 129,* 11–19.

Islam, M. M., Poly, T. N., Walther, B. A., & Li, Y. C. J. (2020). Use of mobile phone app interventions to promote weight loss: meta-analysis. *JMIR mHealth and uHealth, 8*(7), e17039.

Jiya, T. (2015). A realisation of ethical concerns with smartphone personal health monitoring apps. *ACM SIGCAS Computers and Society, 45*, 313–317.

Kenworthy, J.B., Miller, N., Collins, B.E. et al. (2011). A trans-paradigm theoretical synthesis of cognitive dissonance theory: Illuminating the nature of discomfort. *European Review of Social Psychology, 22*, 36–113.

LaPlante, C., & Peng, W. (2011). A systematic review of e-Health interventions for physical activity: An analysis of study design, intervention characteristics, and outcomes. *Telemedicine and e-Health, 17*, 1–15.

Luxton, D.D., McCann, R.A., Bush, N.E. et al. (2011). mHealth for mental health: Integrating smartphone technology in behavioral healthcare. *Professional Psychology: Research and Practice, 42*, 505–512.

Marcolino, M.S., Oliveira, J.A.Q., D'Agostino, M. et al. (2018). The impact of mHealth interventions: systematic review of systematic reviews. *JMIR mHealth and uHealth, 6*, e23.

Mertz, L. (2012). Ultrasound? Fetal monitoring? Spectrometer? There's an app for that! *IEEE Pulse, 3*, 16–21.

Milne-Ives, M., Lam, C., De Cock, C. et al. (2020). Mobile apps for health behavior change in physical activity, diet, drug and alcohol use, and mental health: systematic review. *JMIR mHealth and uHealth, 8*, e17046.

Monk, R.L., Heim, D., Qureshi, A., & Price, A. (2015). "I have no clue what I drunk last night." Using smartphone technology to compare in-vivo and retrospective self-reports of alcohol consumption. *PLoS One, 10*, e0126209.

Morrison, L.G. (2015). Theory-based strategies for enhancing the impact and usage of digital health behaviour change interventions: A review. *Digital Health, 1*, 2055207615595335.

Nahum-Shani, I., Smith, S.N., Spring, B.J. et al. (2018). Just-in-time adaptive interventions (JITAIs) in mobile health: key components and design principles for ongoing health behavior support. *Annals of Behavioral Medicine, 52*, 446–462.

Palmer, M., Sutherland, J., Barnard, S. et al. (2018). The effectiveness of smoking cessation, physical activity/diet and alcohol reduction interventions delivered by mobile phones for the prevention of non-communicable diseases: a systematic review of randomizedsed controlled trials. *PLoS One, 13*, e0189801.

Peck, J.L., Stanton, M., & Reynolds, G.E. (2014). Smartphone preventive health care: Parental use of an immunization reminder system. *Journal of Pediatric Health Care, 28*, 35–42.

Popkin, B.M., Adair, L.S., & Ng, S.W. (2012). Global nutrition transition and the pandemic of obesity in developing countries. *Nutrition Reviews, 70*, 3–21.

Prestwich, A., Conner, M., Morris, B. et al. (2017). Do web-based competitions promote physical activity? Randomized controlled trial. *Psychology of Sport & Exercise, 29*, 1–9.

Ryan, R. M., & Deci, E. L. (2000). Self-determination theory and the facilitation of intrinsic motivation, social development, and well-being. *American Psychologist, 55*, 68–78.

Semper, H.M., Povey, R., & Clark-Carter, D. (2016). A systematic review of the effectiveness of smartphone applications that encourage dietary self-regulatory strategies for weight loss in overweight and obese adults. *Obesity Reviews, 17*, 895–906.

Staiger, P.K., O'Donnell, R., Liknaitzky, P. et al. (2020). Mobile apps to reduce tobacco, alcohol, and illicit drug use: systematic review of the first decade. *Journal of Medical Internet Research, 22*, e17156.

Tripp, N., Hainey, K., Liu, A. et al. (2014). An emerging model of maternity care: smartphone, midwife, doctor? *Women and Birth*, *27*, 64–67.

Ubhi, H.K., Michie, S., Kotz, D. et al. (2015). A mobile app to aid smoking cessation: preliminary evaluation of SmokeFree28. *Journal of Medical Internet Research*, *17*, e17.

Van Agteren, J., Carson, K., Jayasinghe, H., & Smith, B. (2016). The barriers and facilitators to effective use of a smartphone application for smoking cessation by health professionals and smokers. *Respirology*, *21*, 42.

Wang, W., Cheng, J., Song, W., & Shen, Y. (2022). The effectiveness of wearable devices as physical activity interventions for preventing and treating obesity in children and adolescents: systematic review and meta-analysis. *JMIR mHealth and uHealth*, *10*(4), e32435.

Weaver, E.R., Horyniak, D.R., Jenkinson, R., Dietze, P., & Lim, M.S. (2013). "Let's get wasted!" and other apps: characteristics, acceptability, and use of alcohol-related smartphone applications. *JMIR mHealth and uHealth*, *1*(1), e9.

Webb, T.L., Joseph, J., Yardley, L., & Michie, S. (2010). Using the internet to promote health behavior change: A meta-analysis of the impact of theoretical basis, use of behavior change techniques, and mode of delivery on efficacy. *Journal of Medical Internet Research*, *12(1)*, e4.

Whittaker, R., McRobbie, H., Bullen, C., Rodgers, A., & Gu, Y. (2016). Mobile phone-based interventions for smoking cessation. *Cochrane Database of Systematic Reviews*, (4), CD006611

Winter, S.J., Hekler, E.B., Grieco, L. A., Chen, F., Pollitt, S., Youngman, K., & King, A.C. (2012). Teaching Old Dogs New Tricks: Perceptions of SmartPhone-naïve midlife and older adults about using SmartPhones and SmartPhone applications to improve health behaviors. *Annals of Behavioral Medicine*, *43*(1), s41.

Yen, H.Y., & Chiu, H.L. (2019). The effectiveness of wearable technologies as physical activity interventions in weight control: A systematic review and meta-analysis of randomized controlled trials. *Obesity Reviews*, *20*(10), 1485–1493.

Zeng, E.Y., Heffner, J. L., Copeland, W.K., Mull, K.E., & Bricker, J.B. (2016). Get with the program: Adherence to a smartphone app for smoking cessation. *Addictive Behaviors*, *63*, 120–124.

10

CHAPTER 10
FUTURE DIRECTIONS

OVERVIEW

The science underpinning health behavior change is clearly at a relatively early stage of development. Much more remains to be learned. Highlighting all possible future directions in the area of health behavior change, therefore, is a challenging task. So, in this chapter, we focus our attention on three broad themes: 1) What factors influence intervention success and how should these be characterized? 2) How can health behavior change be achieved on a widespread, global stage to tackle current and emergent health issues? 3) Given the need to address critical questions well enough and quickly enough, how can the science of behavior change develop more quickly?

IDENTIFYING AND CHARACTERIZING FACTORS THAT INFLUENCE INTERVENTION SUCCESS

In this book, we have covered various factors that can influence how successful an intervention is for health behavior change. An obvious component of this is the content of the intervention (see, for example, Chapter 3) and possibly the underlying theory (see, in particular, Chapters 2 and 4), how the intervention is tailored to individuals or groups (see Chapters 3 and 4) and the characteristics of individuals receiving the intervention such as their socio-economic status (see Burning Issue Box 7.9). In addition, intervention effectiveness could be improved by delivering it with greater intensity or for more time, or via interventionists with specific characteristics such as high credibility or expertise (see, for example, the Elaboration Likelihood Model covered in Chapter 7).

There are other factors that are likely to be important in achieving health behavior change but have been covered comparatively less within the

DOI: 10.4324/9781003302414-11

existing literature. For instance, Prestwich et al. (2017) demonstrated that interventions to reduce smoking in patients awaiting elective surgery were more effective when delivered by nurses suggesting that who, and possibly how, an intervention is delivered can influence how effective it is. The mode of delivery, setting and characteristics of the target behavior itself are other examples of factors that could modify the success of a behavioral intervention and represent important areas for future research (see Burning Issue Box 10.1 and also Dombrowski, O'Carroll & Williams, 2016). Certain ways of delivering interventions might influence not only the effectiveness of the intervention but also their cost effectiveness. For example, Beard et al. (2022), based on a review of interventions covering a range of behaviors including smoking, diet and sexual health, reported that high intensity interventions were *less* cost-effective than low intensity interventions, while interventions targeting groups or groups and individuals were more cost-effective than interventions targeting individuals.

Taxonomies, like the ones used for behavior change techniques, are now starting to emerge for other aspects of an intervention and will continue to evolve. For example, Marques et al. (2021) have developed a classification system of the ways in which a behavior change intervention is delivered (i.e., its mode of delivery). This can be used in conjunction with behavior change technique taxonomies to identify which is the most effective way of delivering specific behavior change techniques. These different types of taxonomies are being brought together within a broader Behavior Change Intervention Ontology (BCIO; Michie et al., 2020) to ultimately try to identify what behavior change techniques work best for which people, in which contexts and through what means/modes.

BURNING ISSUE BOX 10.1

WHICH FACTORS INFLUENCE THE SUCCESS OF A BEHAVIORAL INTERVENTION?

Factor	Examples
Content	Behavior change techniques.
Theory	Whether the behavior change techniques are consistent with the underlying theory; are all appropriate theoretical constructs targeted? Which theory was applied?
Mode of delivery	Is the intervention delivered directly to participants face-to-face or through a mediated form (e.g., computer; post)? Delivered *by* a group vs. an individual; delivered *to* a group vs. to an individual.

Factor	Examples
Intensity/duration	How many sessions were delivered over what time frame? How long was each session? What was the total amount of contact? Over what period of time did participants have access to intervention content? Did the intervention intensity increase, decrease or remain stable over time?
Interventionist	Age; years of experience; level of training; profession; whether they are part of the research team or whether they have been trained by the research team; credibility.
Participants	Behavior levels before intervention; their underlying cognitions and feelings; their level of support (from other people and/or aspects of the environment); demographics such as socio-economic status, age, sex.
Tailoring	What features of the intervention (e.g., content, mode of delivery, intensity/duration) were tailored, and on what basis (e.g., characteristics of the participants, setting etc.)? How was the underlying theory used to tailor the intervention?
Setting	Is the setting familiar vs. unfamiliar to the participants and/or interventionist? Medical vs. non-medical? Educational vs. non-educational? Home based or not?
Cost	Financial cost; time cost; do the benefits outweigh the costs?
Acceptability	Is the intervention acceptable to those delivering it (interventionists), those receiving it (target population) and those endorsing it (e.g., policymakers)? Are there ethical issues and can these be adequately resolved?
Scalability	Are the resources (e.g., financial, people) required to deliver the intervention on a larger scale available and sufficient? To how many people, groups, countries, conditions, etc. can the intervention be applied and at what cost?
Sustainability	How will the target population continue to receive intervention content over the long-term? Is this achievable? Are there any barriers (e.g., cost, materials, other resources, desire to sustain the intervention)?

Factor	Examples
Behavior	One-off behavior (e.g., immunization) vs. repeated behavior (e.g., exercise; diet); health promoting vs. health risk vs. detection; level of ease/difficulty; habitual vs. non-habitual; whether the behavior generates short-term vs. long-term costs/benefits.
Fidelity	Were the other important characteristics (e.g., content, theory, mode of delivery, intensity/duration) utilized as intended? If not, how did they differ? What proportion of participants was affected?
Measurement	Is the behavior assessed while the intervention is still being delivered or after the intervention has stopped? Does the measure capture behavior throughout the assessment period or just at specific stages? Is the measure reliable? Is the measure valid?
Comparison group	On which features (e.g., content, mode, intensity/duration) does the comparison group differ from the intervention and how do they differ? Over what period of time did the intervention and comparison groups differ?
Risk of bias	Can specific risks of bias (e.g., lack of randomization; lack of blinding) account for the intervention effects? Is the intervention effective when risk of bias is low?

Characterizing different elements of health behavior interventions in ways that have been achieved for behavior change techniques is likely to be challenging. For example, an issue faced by users of the most comprehensive taxonomy of behavior change techniques produced to date (by Michie et al., 2013) is that they can struggle to use it reliably. Rather disappointingly, results from Wood et al. (2015) suggests this taxonomy is generally not used reliably before, or even after, training. Moreover, in these evaluations, only some of the BCTs were used rather than all 93 BCTs. If the studies were repeated using the full 93-item taxonomy, it seems likely that the reliability may drop further. For taxonomies that comprise fewer techniques, reliability may be better. However, direct comparisons of these different taxonomies are needed to establish the most reliable option. Given the least reliable option could be the taxonomy with the most techniques, there may need to be some trade-off between reliability and comprehensiveness (number of behavior change techniques) in identifying the most appropriate taxonomy. The most appropriate taxonomy may also differ for different behaviors with taxonomies designed for smoking (Michie, Hyder, Walia & West, 2011), for instance, more likely to be suitable for smoking research than more general taxonomies that were designed for use across different behaviors (e.g., Michie et al., 2013). Taxonomies for mode of delivery, setting, types of behavior or other factors outlined in Burning Issue Box 10.1 would face similar challenges in ensuring they can be used reliably. Furthermore, it is likely that these classification systems will be used in conjunction with one another, and it is unknown at this stage what the impact on coding reliability might be when these are used in conjunction especially given more coder demands may lead to a higher rate of coding errors.

Part of the reason for the difficulty in reliably coding behavior change techniques and other intervention elements using relevant taxonomies is that they are contingent on clear reporting of the intervention in publications (including protocols) and/or the reviewers accessing the actual intervention materials. Unfortunately, this reporting can often be substandard, and intervention materials are often not easily available, if at all. It is hoped that, over time, the use of taxonomies will actually improve reporting of intervention content to minimize the impact of these issues in the future. Furthermore, ensuring they are machine readable means that, in principle, computers may be able to code information about intervention content at a rapid rate (Ganguly et al., 2019).

Characterizing specific features of interventions can be useful when attempting to synthesize the available evidence through systematic review and/or meta-analysis (see Chapters 5 and 6) as it can be used to identify features in which certain studies are sufficiently similar and other studies that differ. These studies can then be grouped and compared to identify whether the presence or absence of a particular feature influences the success of an intervention.

However, Ogden (2016) has argued that taking this approach is overly simplistic as well as problematic if the evidence that is being synthesized is weak, reported badly and/or based on what was intended to be done within the intervention rather than what was actually done (i.e., the fidelity of the intervention). Thus, Ogden (2016) argues that the time to use approaches such as behavior change techniques may be in the future rather than now. General issues with taxonomies are highlighted in Burning Issue Box 10.2.

A further complication is that interventions tend to comprise multiple behavior change techniques and are compared against control groups that differ by more than just one behavior change technique. As such, within

BURNING ISSUE BOX 10.2

ISSUES WITH BEHAVIOR CHANGE TECHNIQUE TAXONOMIES

1. A taxonomy provides lists and definitions of various behavior change techniques, aiming to provide a shared language to be used by all. As there are a growing number of taxonomies, however, there is potential for "different languages." This can be in at least two forms: i) different taxonomies comprise different definitions of the same technique; ii) different taxonomies partly overlap with one another, sharing some techniques but not others. In short, attempts to systematize and to improve consistency has led to other issues relating to systematization and consistency.
2. Their use is contingent on high quality reporting/accessibility of actual intervention materials. However, applying taxonomies should improve reporting quality over time to partly address this issue.
3. Although taxonomies usually intend to capture techniques that cannot be reduced into other techniques, this is not always the case (see the main text for an illustrative example).
4. Evidence suggests that some taxonomies may be difficult to use even after training (Wood et al., 2015). Over time, training computers to code techniques reliably could address this issue to some extent.
5. To maximize their use, other aspects of interventions such as mode of delivery, dose (i.e., how often participants were exposed to interventions) and setting should be taken into account simultaneously with the behavior change techniques delivered.
6. Taxonomies such as the BCTTv1 focus on techniques that target individuals rather than those that can be delivered at other levels of a socio-ecological framework such as families, organizations and communities (Tate et al., 2016).
7. Taxonomies have often been used to code behavior change techniques in different studies before applying a technique called meta-regression to identify which techniques are associated with higher levels of behavior change. However, because the studies included in these reviews can vary in several ways (e.g., different measures, doses, durations) and they typically test complex interventions comprising of multiple behavior change techniques, the evidence generated from these reviews may provide only weak signals regarding what may work and what might not.

Moreover, if certain behavior change techniques only ever occur alongside other techniques, it can be impossible to know if the technique only works because of the co-occurring technique. Thus, the results from such reviews can be misleading.

8. More complex statistical approaches based on individuals are needed to better account for tailoring of behavior change techniques to specific individuals and/or actual delivery of behavior change techniques to different individuals (given interventions are not always delivered as consistently as planned).

9. Related to a number of the points raised above, Ogden (2016) criticizes the use of taxonomies (and the approach of systematization more broadly) by arguing that they aim to code what is intended to be delivered as depicted in protocols. According to Ogden (2016) this is problematic because it is several steps away from what individual patients actually do (e.g., what is in the protocol might not be delivered by all interventionists, it might not be done consistently, those who receive it may not pay attention to it, etc.).

10. Ogden (2016) also criticizes the use of taxonomies for potentially painting a picture of what should be used, possibly stifling creativity in the form of discouraging use of techniques not included in taxonomies and/or discouraging use of different techniques for different people in different situations.

11. While a behavior change technique taxonomy focuses on *what* was delivered and thus, by extension, recommendations regarding what to deliver, they are not capable (by themselves) to enable consideration of/recommendations for *how* to deliver the interventions or how to train others to deliver these techniques (Hilton & Johnston, 2017).

standard randomized trials, one cannot identify whether differences between an intervention and control group are partly due to the presence or absence of a particular behavior change technique. Moreover, when synthesizing evidence using taxonomies such as BCTTv1, there are risks that certain BCTs will be confounded with other BCTs (i.e., a specific BCT may *appear* to be effective, but not actually be, simply because it is typically delivered alongside a different BCT that is effective) and other intervention features. There is no doubt that interventions are very complex and that intervention content is only one component that can influence the success of an intervention (see Burning Issue Box 10.1). Reviews that synthesize studies that vary in lots of ways including the presence or absence of different behavior change techniques, delivered through different modes, intensities, settings and to different populations, are therefore "statistically noisy" and difficult to use to identify a clear signal regarding whether a specific behavior change technique works or not.

Taking partial account of the potential risk of confounds is possible, for example through relatively advanced statistical techniques such as multivariate meta-regressions (see for example, Prestwich et al., 2014a, and Prestwich et al., 2016). We agree with Ogden (2016); however, that the task of synthesizing evidence through taxonomies will be easier and more fruitful in the future when there are more studies conducted that are well reported and of higher quality. An alternative solution has also been offered more recently.

This alternative approach to reviewing studies that comprise multiple behavior change techniques is to conduct primary studies testing single behavior change techniques and then systematically review and, where possible, meta-analyze such studies. Armitage et al. (2021) propose this approach in the form of Centres for Understanding Behavior Change (CUBiC), a worldwide, collaborative venture to consider a whole host of behavior change techniques for how effective they are, for which behaviors and people, in what contexts, which mechanisms of action (determinants) that they change and how their effects can be improved (combined with which behavior change techniques, delivered in which form, etc.). Hopefully, the scientific evidence will continue to grow at a rapid rate in the future to help identify what works and under what circumstances.

ACHIEVING HEALTH BEHAVIOR CHANGE ON A GLOBAL STAGE

Scalability (how well an intervention can be delivered on a larger, mass scale), acceptability (the extent to which people are willing to try the intervention, use the intervention, endorse or tolerate it), sustainability (how well an intervention can achieve success in the longer term) and equity (how equal the effects of an intervention will be across groups) represent vital factors (in addition to intervention effectiveness) that influence the potential wider impact that an intervention can achieve at the level of the wider population. Such factors are crucial the world over but are particularly important in lower-income countries which face issues such as environmental hazards (e.g., droughts, land degradation) and increases in chronic, non-communicable disease such as cardiovascular disease and cancer with relatively few resources. Achieving widespread behavior change to facilitate better health across large populations is a global, grand challenge for now and in the future. Regarding equity, issues around culture and socioeconomic differences are important.

CULTURE

To achieve health behavior change on a global stage, interventionists need to consider culture, the customs, ideas, values and behaviors of a group of people, and how interventions can be delivered in culturally relevant and valued ways. At the heart of health behavior change is the need to identify and subsequently change factors (or determinants) that influence health behavior. As such, it is important to first consider the role of culture and behavior change theory. Are the determinants of health behavior, and the theories that encompass them, the same or work similarly, across cultures?

Theories and models that have been used to understand, predict and change health behaviors tend to be (implicitly) universal assuming that they work in equivalent ways across cultures. Maybe they do. Belief-based models, such as the Theory of Planned Behavior, in principle, account for (at least some) cultural influence by seeing the role of culture as being something more distal (further away) from behavior than the determinants specified in the model such as attitudes and intentions. For instance, a person's culture could influence their beliefs about a behavior that influences factors like their attitudes and subjective norms. However, while many models have studies providing at least some support in different areas across the world, the bulk of the evidence is based on samples drawn from Western societies. As such, we can be more confident about how such theories work in Western societies and less confident about how they work elsewhere.

Although at least part of the influence of culture is likely to be mediated by more proximal determinants (e.g., norms) specified in particular models, its influence on behavior may not be fully mediated by the constructs within a model. Moreover, culture may prevent changes in determinants translating to changes in behavior. For instance, a sexual health program, *MEMA kwa Vijana* ("Good things for young people"), was evaluated in nearly 10,000 adolescents in Tanzania. Although the intervention improved knowledge and attitudes, it only positively impacted one of five behavioral measures and tended not to positively influence health outcomes (e.g., HIV incidence) with weaker effects in women than men. Ross et al. (2007) argue these findings could be due to cultural norms implying men have greater power than women in the context of sex which may make it particularly difficult for women to change their sexual behaviors.

There is additional evidence that culture can moderate the influence of particular determinants on behavior. For instance, subjective norms to donate bone marrow may more strongly relate with intentions in some cultures (e.g., Chinese) than others (e.g., American) possibly because of the relative importance of social influences on decisions to donate in line with cultural norms (Bagozzi & Van Loo, 2001).

One additional factor to consider is that determinants may not be understood or "exist" in different cultures. Recently, Andrew was supervising three Chinese students on a project related to identifying different subtypes of motivation. As the project required recruiting participants from China, the materials developed and previously tested in UK samples needed to be translated from English into Chinese. Within the project, Andrew ran a task where he said words related to motivation (e.g., desire to do, intend to do, committed to doing, long to do) and the students each had to say the equivalent word in Mandarin at the same time. This sometimes led to different words and in the case of "long to do it" an equivalent word could not be found.

Socio-ecological models have also been developed that take into account the interrelationships between an individual, groups, social, cultural, physical and political environment-level factors that can all influence health and related behaviors. In this way, cultural differences are acknowledged along with the argument that targeting people at the level of the individual is insufficient; instead, consideration of the wider influences on behaviors, including culture, needs to be considered in health behavior change efforts. Explicitly, what might work for one set of individuals may not work elsewhere given differences in cultures and other broader influences on behavior.

As you will have learned throughout this book, behavior change techniques represents a critical element of interventions to help change behavior and thus considering how to change health behaviors on a global stage warrants examination of the question of whether behavior change techniques work similarly across cultures.

However, there's a further aspect to help move from the theoretical (what should we target and how?) to the applied (what should the intervention be like *in practice*?). The intervention mapping approach describes this aspect as developing a practical application that maintains effectiveness and fits the relevant population, context *and culture*. On this basis, an important consideration is to ensure that the (collection of) behavior change techniques are designed and produced in a way that is relevant to and consistent (and not inconsistent) with cultural values and norms. A good way to achieve this is through co-creation in which the various stakeholders work together to design and produce an intervention (see Chapter 5). Other approaches to developing and evaluating behavior change interventions, covered in Chapter 4, could be considered too. For example, the Theory Coding Scheme highlights the issue of tailoring and the need to refine theory based on evidence (so to the four-step approach) while the experimental medicine/operating conditions framework highlights moderators (culture could moderate the influence of interventions on determinants and behavior, as well as the relationship between determinants and behavior).

SOCIOECONOMIC DIFFERENCES

Just as the role of culture could be mediated by determinants of health behaviors (with differences in determinants across cultures) and/or moderating (influencing whether changes in determinants can be translated to changes in behavior), socioeconomic differences could have the same role. For instance, individuals from lower socioeconomic groups could have lower levels on key determinants of behavior (e.g., motivation, self-efficacy) or that high levels of these key determinants are less likely to be translated into action due to various barriers linked to socioeconomic status (e.g., financial). These factors could explain socioeconomic differences in behaviors such as healthy eating or attendance at health screenings (see also Burning Issue Box 7.9).

It also important to highlight that health behavior interventions can cause inequity if availability, uptake, engagement or fidelity differs across socio-economic groups. For instance, green space (that could prompt more physical activity) tends to be more available in less deprived areas. Moreover, non-targeted interventions risk having greater uptake, engagement and fidelity in higher rather than lower socio-economic groups. Price-based interventions (such as increasing taxation on cigarettes or unhealthy foods) could help reduce health inequalities across the highest to lowest income groups, as such interventions have been shown to lead to greater reductions in low- rather than high-income groups. Marteau et al. (2021) highlights the impact of these types of approaches on health inequalities and the need to fundamentally alleviate poverty.

LONG-TERM CHANGE AND MULTIPLE BEHAVIOR CHANGE

An important area of focus is the most effective means to change health behaviors and maintain any change. Maintenance of change is important because for many health promotion behaviors such as physical activity or healthy eating the health benefits only accrue after long-term performance of these behaviors. Increasingly studies focus on impacts on behavior change over longer time intervals with 6- and 12-month follow-up periods now quite common. Further research might usefully look at the ways in which current interventions might be supplemented to promote long-term change. Strategies that are likely to be low-cost, scalable, acceptable and sustainable, like implementation intentions and other strategies to prompt habit formation (e.g., see Chapter 3) may be particularly helpful. There are many issues to be addressed in relation to these techniques. For instance, the long term effects of implementation intentions may be enhanced if they are repeated at regular intervals (e.g., Conner & Higgins, 2010). However, one factor that is likely to be key is maintaining the motivation to engage in the behavior because we know that implementation intentions are more effective for those with strong motivation to perform the behavior.

Another efficient way to achieve greater changes in health behaviors is to consider how change on one health promotion behavior (e.g., exercise) is independent or related to changes in other health behaviors (e.g., drinking alcohol). If change in one health promoting behavior diffuses to other related behaviors this may allow synergy among interventions. However, if individuals compensate for improvements in one health promoting health behavior by doing less of another or more of the health risking behaviors (e.g., rewarding yourself for going running by having a few more alcoholic drinks) then we may need to think more carefully about the impact on overall health of specific health behavior interventions. Evidence suggests that while attempting to change a small number of behaviors together may be beneficial, trying to tackle many health behaviors simultaneously can lead less change overall (Wilson et al., 2015). Nevertheless, some interventions have been shown to lead to changes in multiple health behaviors even through minimal approaches such as completion of certain measures (Wilding et al., 2019) and encouraging goal prioritization (Conner et al., 2021).

So, impact on a global stage could be achieved by delivering interventions with the right qualities linked to characteristics such as scalability and acceptability and ensuring that interventions target constructs relevant to behaviors of specific groups of people in culturally appropriate ways, remaining mindful of the risk of widening health inequalities. We also highlight that tackling multiple health behaviors simultaneously may be an efficient approach, albeit complex. Critically, however, in the face of a number of known and current unknown health challenges across low- and middle-income countries, in particular, but also in high-income countries, there is a need for the science of health behavior change to continue its momentum and preferably to speed-up its development. We turn to this issue next.

———————————

ACCELERATING THE RATE OF SCIENTIFIC PROGRESS

WITH BETTER THEORIES AND TECHNIQUES

Evidence regarding the effect of using theory on intervention success is rather mixed (Prestwich et al., 2015). While some reviews suggest that using theory increases intervention success (e.g., Webb et al., 2010) other reviews suggest little or no benefit in terms of intervention success (e.g., Prestwich et al., 2014b). Part of the reason for this may be the quality of theories upon which the interventions are based. Many theories are built on correlational data. This approach has a number of inherent weaknesses (e.g., see Chapter 5) and hinder attempts to establish which theories are useful. In addition, theories are not often directly compared to help determine which theories work best in different situations. In the future, there will need to be more experimental tests of theories to provide a stronger basis for establishing which theories work best, for whom and in which situations. For some theories there are few, if any, experimental tests. For example, tests of integrated theories such as Fishbein et al. (2001) are needed (see Chapter 2), to identify whether these combined theories are superior to (and as usable as) individual theories. In relation to dual process models (e.g., Strack & Deutsch, 2004, see Chapter 2), more studies are needed that attempt to manipulate both reflective and impulsive systems to create more sustained change than merely targeting either reflective or impulsive systems.

In addition, Sheeran et al. (2017) highlight the issue that few studies attempt to identify the situations under which aspects of theories *fail*. For example, highlighting situations when self-efficacy does not influence behavior could be a means to improve the precision and specificity of models/theories that highlight the role of self-efficacy in influencing behavior. This type of mindset may represent an important approach for future research.

WITH BETTER REPORTING, MEASURES AND METHODS

In the future, methodological statements such as the **CONSORT** (for randomized controlled trials) and **PRISMA** (for systematic reviews) guidelines, as well as the consistent use of preregistration (see Chapter 5), will be adopted more widely across the field of health behavior change, encouraging the standard reporting of key methodological and statistical information for randomized controlled trials and systematic reviews, respectively. Similarly, use of BCT taxonomies, as well as similar approaches to help ensure use of theory is clearly reported (Prestwich et al., 2015), will also improve the reporting of techniques and theories. Clear reporting makes it easier to identify what has and what has not been tested and thus gaps in knowledge can be more easily detected. An online paper authoring tool has been developed by West (2020) to aid the reporting of randomized controlled trials ensuring that all relevant information is clearly and consistently presented. This tool produces a record that is machine readable in the hope that this will facilitate the rapid synthesis of evidence across studies. Over time, tools such as this could be more widely adopted.

Furthermore, as Sheeran et al. (2017) note, there are several issues with measurement of constructs within theories. These include: relying on self-reports which are subject to a range of bias; measuring constructs at a single moment in time when the construct is more dynamic and variable over time (i.e., an individual may strongly intend to exercise at one point in the day but if assessed at a different time in the day, may not intend to exercise at all); lack of standardization such that different researchers use different measures to assess the same construct (see also Spruijt-Metz et al., 2015).

There have been calls for core outcome sets (COS) in which a minimum set of measures are always applied and reported in studies related to a particular domain/health condition (e.g., rheumatology). These core outcome sets need input from a range of stakeholders, including patients/participants and healthcare professionals using consensus methods (see Chapter 5), to ensure that the measures taken are important and meaningful to them. Once a decision has been made regarding what to assess, the next part is to decide how to assess the outcome. Just as there have been attempts to standardize the use of BCTs, there have been steps taken to encourage researchers to use standard, reliable measures of constructs. Approaches such as the Patient-Reported Outcomes Measurement Information System (PROMIS; Carle et al., 2015), COnsensus-based Standards for the selection of health Measurement INstruments (COSMIN) and the Grid-Enabled Measures (GEM) (Moser et al., 2011) initiatives are useful resources to help identify high quality measures. These approaches, as well as in assisting in reliability, validity and relevance of the measures to users, would help in comparing the effectiveness of different interventions across studies in the future as well as in the synthesis of results in systematic reviews. COS also help reduce the risk of reporting bias because the particular set of outcomes should always be reported for studies in a particular domain. The Core Outcome Measures in Effectiveness Trials (COMET) is an initiative that encourages and supports the development of COS and provides a database of various COS across different domains.

There have also been recent advances in measures that do not rely on self-report such as the neurological measures that we highlight in the next section of this chapter plus mobile technology that permit continuous

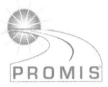

FIGURE 10.1 Researchers are encouraged to use standard, reliable measures of constructs from health behaviour models such as the *Patient-Reported Outcomes Measurement Information System* (PROMIS).

assessment of constructs in real time. These constructs are not just limited to behavior (e.g., physical activity assessed through accelerometers, diet choices through purchase transactions) but also individual's thoughts and feelings (via social media, self-reports via apps, physiological measures, etc.) and their environment (e.g., via **mobile sensing**).

Methodologically, adopting better practices such as preregistration, a priori sample sizes and embracing open science will help speed up progress in the field. Issues around replicability and how these can be addressed have been overviewed elsewhere in this text (e.g., Burning Issue Box 5.4) and represent important ways to move the science of health behavior change forward.

WITH CONSIDERATION OF BIOLOGICAL AND NEUROLOGICAL INFLUENCES

There are many kinds of interaction effects that researchers should explore, and undoubtedly will in the years to come. For example, some researchers have examined how environmental influences interact with genetic influences to predict a variety of behaviors. Griffin et al. (2015) studied the moderating effect of one such genetic factor: the dopamine receptor D4 gene (DRD4). This gene is a good candidate gene because it is assumed to influence individuals' (especially adolescents) vulnerability to social influence because of the role that dopamine plays in reward sensation. Griffin and colleagues found that although peer pressure for antisocial behaviors (such as cheating or petty theft) had a significant influence on alcohol use, this effect was even stronger in those participants who had the DRD4 genotype, compared to those who did not (for a similar discussion concerning sexual behavior, see Kogan et al., 2014).

BURNING ISSUE BOX 10.3

WHAT DOES SOCIAL NEUROSCIENCE BRING TO HEALTH BEHAVIOR CHANGE?

1. *Social neuroscience helps assess processes that are difficult to assess otherwise.*
    At its core, social neuroscience attempts to identify individual differences in social behaviors (including those related to health) by identifying biological differences (typically brain activity or genetic) across individuals. Moreover, the tools of social neuroscience that provides metabolic and electrophysiological images of activity in the brain can provide detailed information, as it emerges, regarding when and where social cognition is occurring.
2. *It can provide unique answers to behavioral problems.*
    For example, people who have difficulty in self-regulating their behavior, including levels of physical activity, have a different neurobiology than those that are more successful (Hall et al., 2008).
3. *It helps develop more comprehensive theories of social and health behavior and this helps behavioral scientists better predict behavior.*
    By identifying that activity in specific brain regions correlate with behavior, over-and-above self-report measures (e.g., Falk et al., 2011; Reuter et al., 2011), social neuroscience can help develop more comprehensive models and theories of behavior. These models would incorporate constructs reflecting neural activity alongside constructs available to introspection such as one's intentions to perform a particular behavior. As measures of neural activity in specific regions of the brain can explain unique variance in behavior, theories that incorporate neural activity should lead to better, more reliable predictions of how individuals or groups are likely to behave.
4. *It helps develop effective behavior change interventions.*
    By identifying that activity in specific regions of the brain are linked to changes in health behavior work by researchers such as Falk (Falk et al., 2010; Falk et al., 2011) and others (e.g., Imhof et al., 2020) could help lead to the development of more effective behavior change interventions. Specifically, by identifying health-based messages, or other types of interventions, that are more likely to increase activity in regions of the brain linked to positive changes in health behavior (regions of the medial prefrontal cortex) one could be more confident that these interventions are likely to lead to actual health behavior change.

WITH COMPUTER SCIENCE

With the ability to assess so many important influences on behaviors, as well as behavior itself, researchers have access to a vast amount of data that can be used to understand the dynamic processes underlying an individual's behavior. This data can then be used to develop new forms of personalized interventions. Moreover, by aggregating data across individuals, computational models of human behavior can be developed and later tested across large samples of individuals and across many complex environments (Spruijt-Metz et al., 2015). Such models require significant volumes of data that are difficult to accumulate across studies given issues with reporting and measures (see the previous section). However, with enhanced data sharing and development of common languages via, for example, taxonomies of BCTs, data across hundreds of studies, at the level of the individual, could be shared and combined to overcome issues regarding limited data.

Systematic reviews (see Chapter 5) represent a useful way of combining data at the study level but as the number of publications escalates rapidly, conducting systematic reviews is becoming more burdensome. Fortunately, **text mining** is a technique in which computers can be used to identify automatically the studies most likely to be eligible for a particular review. Different text mining techniques are emerging but current estimates are that using text mining as opposed to humans can lead to a time-saving of up to 70% (O'Mara-Eves et al., 2015).

The Human Behaviour Change Project, led by Susan Michie at UCL, has also made use of computer science by building an artificial intelligence system that will continually scan the behavior change literature and extract relevant information. The aim of this work is to identify which behavior change interventions work and relevant modifying factors such as how personal characteristics, settings and behavior type influence this success. By making use of computer science, the project has the ability to synthesize and analyze volumes of data that are beyond the capabilities and time resources of even the most efficient and best systematic review teams (see also Larsen et al., 2017). Moreover, the system could be used to potentially make sufficiently accurate predictions regarding how effective certain combinations of intervention elements (e.g., behavior change techniques, settings, modes of delivery) will be in terms of behavior change for specific populations (Ganguly et al., 2021). Such approaches can be useful when there is a limited evidence base where few, if any equivalent, studies have been conducted. In addition, it could help inform policy decisions regarding what can be done to improve population behavior and health.

While artificial intelligence (AI) can play in a role in utilizing big data to identify evidence and make predictions, it can also be used as a means to

Building the science of behaviour
change through machine learning

FIGURE 10.2 The *Human Behaviour Change Project* (HBCP) will make use of an artificial intelligence system to scan the behavior change literature for relevant information.

support behavior change interventions. For instance, chatbots powered by AI can be used to engage and build relationships with users using natural language that, in turn, can be used to change health behaviors (see Zhang et al., 2020, for a review of such approaches to change diet and physical activity).

WITH ADAPTIVE DESIGNS

Adaptive designs make use of data collated during the study to inform what pre-specified changes (e.g., to sample size; to study conditions such as to switch conditions and to drop conditions); to end the trial early; recruiting participants most likely to respond) can be made based on analyses conducted mid-study. Pre-specified here means changes to the course of the study that are planned *before* the study starts rather than being made up on the spot *during* the study. There are various benefits in terms of efficiency, ensuring a study is powered, increasing the proportion of participants exposed to the most effective treatments and reducing the proportion allocated to ineffective treatments.

An example of an adaptive design is the Sequential Multiple Assignment Randomized Trial (SMART; Lei et al., 2012) which offers a flexible and efficient way to test the individual and combined effects of specific techniques relative to using full-factorial designs (see Critical Skills Toolkit 3.1). In a SMART design, participants are randomized to different interventions at multiple stages. In the first stage, participants are typically randomized to one of two conditions. At the next stage (e.g., a week later), participants are classified as responders (e.g., their behavior changes) and non-responders (e.g., their behavior does not change and/or they have missed intervention sessions). The responders and non-responders are then separated and randomized again to different interventions or the same intervention. This process is repeated at multiple stages. Consequently, the approach maximizes the likelihood of behavior change (i.e., it should be a more efficacious approach) and it permits the examination of different combinations of techniques. Such adaptive designs offer interesting insights into which intervention techniques should be most effective for whom and in what doses. These insights however should be further tested in standard RCTs.

With the rise in digital interventions and their ability to deliver intervention components using "push" (when an individual receives an intervention component automatically, just at the right time when the individual most needs it, based on certain criteria such as their location or time of day) and "pull" (when a user actively accesses the component anytime, as they wish) elements, micro-randomized trials (MRT) have emerged as a design to help inform which elements are useful and when as well as identifying when it is best to not intervene (Klasnja et al., 2015). In an MRT, participants can be randomized at hundreds of decision points in the study to try to identify the causal effect of specific components in specific contexts on particular outcomes (e.g., motivation, behavior). These decision points can be chosen by the experimenters or by the individual participants themselves.

To avoid overly burdening participants with too many elements, particularly when these are intensive, in an MRT, the probability of being assigned to a particular group does not need to be equal and can be set-up such that participants are more likely to be assigned to the less burdensome options (Qian et al., 2022). For ethical and safety reasons, options to "do nothing" and not deliver intervention components at certain times (e.g., sending notifications through when an individual is driving) is a neat feature of such designs. Likewise, if an individual is already doing the behavior at a specific time (e.g., doing physical activity), not delivering intervention components (e.g., prompts to walk more) at this time, can also be incorporated in the study design.

Moreover, MRTs can incorporate exploratory moderator tests by collating data on things such as location, day of the week and weather to help determine when best to deliver intervention components in the final product/intervention. A challenge with MRTs, however, is determining how long after each randomization point the outcome (e.g., behavior) will be assessed such that the participant has a chance to act on the intervention component but not too late such that detecting the effect of the manipulation has decayed or becomes too noisy or interferes with tests of later components. A further challenge is determining how many components an individual should be exposed to over a specific period of time (e.g., day) to optimize the trade-off between effectiveness and overly burdening the participants.

WITH MORE SOPHISTICATED USE OF STATISTICS

Newer statistical approaches are being developed and used by behavioral scientists to address important questions. For example, rather than simply look at pools of studies collated through systematic review and then via meta-analysis or meta-regression techniques (see Chapters 5 and 6) infer which individual, specific BCTs are effective, Dusseldorp et al. (2014) used an approach called "meta-CART (classification and regression trees)" to identify which combinations of BCTs are effective. On the basis of their review, Dusseldorp et al. concluded that combining providing information about the health-behavior link and prompt intention formation was the most effective approach while combining feedback on performance without providing instructions was the least effective. Other statistical developments within meta-analyses, include the use of meta-analytic path analyses to test specific paths stipulated by theories of health and social behavior using data across multiple studies. This approach has been applied, for example, to validate aspects of the Theory of Planned Behavior (Hagger et al., 2016). Outside of meta-analysis, other statistical approaches will continue to evolve too, especially in the area of multilevel modeling. Recent developments include structural equation methods to assess moderation in multilevel models (Preacher et al., 2016).

Sequential analysis can consider events within sessions to see how one person's behavior can impact another person. For example, Jacques-Tiura et al. (2017) looked at how counsellor's language impacted whether caregivers of overweight/obese adolescents used motivational statements to change. They found, for instance, that caregiver change talk (e.g., "I would like to plan our meals better") was more likely when preceded by counsellors' reflections of change talk (e.g., "What's slipped that you want to get back to?"). Such approaches can be used more widely in the future to consider how healthcare providers and digital systems can prompt statements from patients reflecting motivation to change. Moreover, computer science and natural language processing techniques can speed up coding which, otherwise, can be fairly laborious.

As individuals do not operate in isolation, they interact with others within groups and within organizations, communities and environments, alternative analytical approaches can be used to account for these different interactions. Systems science approaches such as agent-based modelling can enable this and allows researchers to simulate the effect of manipulating one or more elements or variables (such as banning junk food advertising or smoking in different public places) on the entire system. As these approaches become better understood, they could be utilized more often, particularly in the earlier phases of research prior to actual testing of such manipulations in more definitive trials.

On a broader level, researchers will be more likely to be required to publish their planned statistical methods within a study protocol in advance of actually conducting the study and to publish datasets alongside their scientific publication. Given that datasets can be analyzed using various statistical methods (e.g., ANOVA, ANCOVA, regression), publishing the protocol in advance minimizes the likelihood of selecting the statistical test that is most likely to produce a significant effect while publishing the dataset allows for the possibility of re-analysis by other research groups. On a related matter, there is a need to standardize approaches to identifying and removing statistical **outliers**, as well as how information relating to these are reported within health behavior change articles.

The trend of behavioral scientists working more and more within multidisciplinary teams will continue. A consequence of this will be that behavioral scientists will become acquainted with and use more sophisticated (and complex!) statistical procedures. Calls for behavioral scientists to work with information and computer scientists have been made (e.g., Larsen et al., 2020) and the Human Behaviour Change Project, noted earlier in this chapter, has brought such groups of researchers together. As such, it provides a good illustration of multidisciplinary working relevant to behavior change that makes use of emerging technology and complex data systems. More collaboration is needed in the future.

SUMMARY

In this chapter we highlighted some key issues for further research to tackle. We are at a stage at which health behavior change research is rapidly accelerating in an attempt to catch up with more traditional sciences, as well as to address important health-related challenges. However, getting the discipline "in-shape" through better reporting, methods, analyses and ultimately theories and techniques is critical, as is the need to consider broader aspects of the intervention that could influence success such as who delivered it and how. We have noted that by working with computer scientists, as well as those with expertise in relation to methods, statistics, the environment, genetics and neuroscience, behavioral scientists are well positioned to address these issues and to make even more important contributions to health and social-related challenges. Time will tell which directions bear most fruit but undeniably, the future is exciting.

FURTHER READING

Collins, L.M., Baker, T.B., Mermelstein, R.J., Piper, M.E., et al. (2011). The multiphase optimization strategy for engineering effective tobacco use interventions. *Annals of Behavioral Medicine, 41*, 208–226. This paper introduces another adaptive design with some overlap with SMART designs.

Larsen, K., Hekler, E.B., Paul, M., & Gibson, B. (2020). Improving usability of social and behavioral sciences' evidence: A call to action for a national infrastructure project for mining our knowledge. *Communications of the Association for Information Systems, 46*, 1–16. Highlights the issue that there are vast amounts of research related to behavior change but the lack of both a common format to represent this knowledge and automated means to analyze it hinders progress. They highlight the potential benefits of computer and information scientists working with behavioral science researchers to drive change.

Naar, S., Czajkowski, S.M., & Spring, B. (2018). Innovative study designs and methods for optimizing and implementing behavioral interventions to improve health. *Health Psychology*, *37*, 1081–1091. Introduces a range of methods and approaches that are relatively new to the field and/or under-used and highlights their potential role at different phases of research from basic research and early stage intervention development to widespread implementation and policy trials.

Ogden, J. (2016). Theories, timing and choice of audience: some key tensions in health psychology and a response to commentaries on Ogden (2016). *Health Psychology Review*, *10*, 274–276. Offers an interesting counter-position to the movement towards standardized approaches such as behavior change techniques and taxonomies.

Pallmann, P., Bedding, A.W., Choodari-Oskooei, B. et al. (2018). Adaptive designs in clinical trials: why use them, and how to run and report them. *BMC Medicine*, *16*, 29. Overviews different types of adaptive designs and considers methodological, statistical and reporting related issues.

GLOSSARY

CONSORT (Consolidated Standards of Reporting Trials): a set of reporting guidelines for those wishing to transparently report key methodological details from randomized controlled trials. These guidelines have since been extended for other types of studies such as pilot trials.

Mobile sensing: an approach to gathering and presenting data from sensors internal to smartphones such as accelerometers (that could be used to track physical activity) and GPS (to track location).

Outliers: data points that differ substantially from other data-points within the dataset and can unduly influence the results from a study.

PRISMA (Preferred Reporting Items for Systematic Reviews and Meta-Analyses): a set of reporting guidelines for those wishing to transparently report key methodological details from systematic reviews and meta-analyses of randomized controlled trials or other studies testing interventions.

Text mining: a form of computer science used to identify patterns in text, extract key information and support decision making (e.g., whether to include or exclude a particular study for a systematic review).

REFERENCES

Armitage, C.J., Conner, M., Prestwich, A. et al. (2021). Investigating which behaviour change techniques work for whom in which contexts delivered by what means: Proposal for an international collaboratory of Centres for Understanding Behaviour Change (CUBiC). *British Journal of Health Psychology*, *26*, 1–14.

Bagozzi, R.P., Lee, K-H., & Van Loo, M.F. (2001). Decisions to donate bone marrow: The role of attitudes and subjective norms across cultures. *Psychology & Health*, *16*, 29–56.

Carle, A.C., Riley, W., Hays, R.D., & Cella, D. (2015). Confirmatory factor analysis of the Patient Reported Outcomes Measurement Information System (PROMIS) adult domain framework using item response theory scores. *Medical Care*, 53, 894–900.

Conner, M., & Higgins, A.R. (2010). Long-term effects of implementation intentions on prevention of smoking uptake among adolescents: a cluster randomized controlled trial. *Health Psychology*, *29*, 529–538.

Conner, M., Wilding, S., Prestwich, A. et al. (2022). Goal prioritization and behavior change: Evaluation of an intervention for multiple health behaviors. *Health Psychology*, *41*, 356–365.

Dombrowski, S.U., O'Carroll, R.E., & Williams, B. (2016). Form of delivery as a key "active ingredient" in behaviour change interventions. *British Journal of Health Psychology*, *21*, 733–740.

Dusseldorp, E., van Genugten, L., van Buuren, S. et al. (2014). Combinations of techniques that effectively change health behavior: Evidence from Meta-CART analysis. *Health Psychology*, *33*, 1530–1540.

Falk, E.B., Berkman, E. T., Harrison, B. et al. (2010). Predicting persuasion-induced behavior change from the brain. *Journal of Neuroscience*, *30*, 8421–8424.

Falk, E.B., Berkman, E.T., Whalen, D., & Lieberman, M.D. (2011). Neural activity during health messaging predicts reductions in smoking above and beyond self-report. *Health Psychology*, *30*, 177–185.

Fishbein, M., Triandis, H.C., Kanfer, F.H. et al. (2001). Factors influencing behaviour and behaviour change. In A. Baum, T.A. Revenson, & J.E. Singer (Eds.), *Handbook of Health Psychology* (pp. 3–17). Mahwah, NJ: Lawrence Erlbaum Associates.

Ganguly, D., Gleize, M., Hou, Y. et al. (2021). Outcome prediction from behaviour change intervention evaluations using a combination of node and word embedding. *AMIA Annual Symposium Proceedings*, 486–495.

Ganguly, D., Hou, Y., Deleris, L.A., & Bonin, F. (2019). Information extraction of behavior change interventions. *AMIA Joint Summit on Translational Science Proceedings*, 182–191.

Griffin, A.M., Cleveland, H.H., Schlomer, G.L. et al. (2015). Differential susceptibility: the genetic moderation of peer pressure on alcohol use. *Journal of Youth and Adolescence*, *44*(10), 1841–1853.

Hagger, M.S., Chan, D.K.C., Protogerou, C., & Chatzisarantis, N.L.D. (2016). Using meta-analytic path analysis to test theoretical predictions in health behavior: An illustration based on meta-analyses of the theory of planned behavior. *Preventive Medicine*, *89*, 154–161.

Hall, P.A., Elias, L.J., Fong, G.T. et al. (2008). A social neuroscience perspective on physical activity. *Journal of Sport & Exercise Psychology*, *30*, 432–449.

Imhof, M.A., Schmälzle, R., Renner, B., & Schupp, H.T. (2020). Strong health messages increase audience brain coupling. *Neuroimage*, *216*, 116527.

Jacques-Tiura, A.J., Carcone, A.I., Naar, S. et al. (2017). Building motivation in African American caregivers of adolescents with obesity: Application of sequential analysis. *Journal of Pediatric Psychology*, *42*, 131–141.

Klasnja, P., Hekler, E.B., Shiffman, S., et al. (2015). Microrandomized trials: An experimental design for developing just-in-time adaptive interventions. *Health Psychology*, *34*, 1220–1228.

Kogan, S.M., Lei, M.K., Beach, S.R. et al. (2014). Dopamine receptor gene D4 polymorphisms and early sexual onset: Gender and environmental moderation in a sample of African-American youth. *Journal of Adolescent Health*, *55*(2), 235–240.

Larsen, K.R., Michie, S., Hekler, E.B. et al. (2017). Behavior change interventions: the potential of ontologies for advancing science and practice. *Journal of Behavioral Medicine*, *40*, 6–22.

Lei, H., Nahum-Shani, I., Lynch, K. et al. (2012). A "SMART" design for building individualized treatment sequences. *Annual Review of Clinical Psychology*, 8, 21–48.

Marteau, T., Rutter, H., & Marmot, M. (2021). Changing behaviour: an essential component of tackling health inequalities. *BMJ*, *372*, n332.

Michie, S., Hyder, N., Walia, A., & West, R. (2011). Development of a taxonomy of behaviour change techniques used in individual behavioural support for smoking cessation. *Addictive Behaviors*, *36*, 315–319.

Michie, S., Richardson, M., Johnston, M. et al. (2013). The behavior change technique taxonomy (v1) of 93 hierarchically clustered techniques: Building an international consensus for the reporting of behavior change interventions. *Annals of Behavioral Medicine*, *46*, 81–95.

Michie, S., West, R., Finnerty, A.N. et al. (2020). Representation of behaviour change interventions and their evaluation: Development of the Upper Level of the Behaviour Change Intervention Ontology [version 1; peer review: awaiting peer review]. *Wellcome Open Research*, *5*, 123.

Moser, R.P., Hesse, B.W., Shaikh, A.R. et al. (2011). Grid-enabled measures: using Science 2.0 to standardize measures and share data. *American Journal of Preventive Medicine* 40(5):S134–S143.

Naar, S., Czajkowski, S.M., & Spring, B. (2018). Innovative study designs and methods for optimizing and implementing behavioral interventions to improve health. *Health Psychology*, *37*, 1081–1091.

Ogden, J. (2016). Theories, timing and choice of audience: some key tensions in health psychology and a response to commentaries on Ogden (2016). *Health Psychology Review*, *10*, 274–276.

O'Mara-Eves, A., Thomas, J., McNaught, J. et al. (2015). Using text mining for study identification in systematic reviews: a systematic review of current approaches. *Systematic Reviews*, *4*, 5.

Pallmann, P., Bedding, A.W., Choodari-Oskooei, B. et al. (2018). Adaptive designs in clinical trials: why use them, and how to run and report them. *BMC Medicine*, *16*, 29.

Preacher, K.J., Zhang, Z., & Zyphur, M. J. (2016). Multilevel structural equation models for assessing moderation within and across levels of analysis. *Psychological Methods*, *21*, 189–205.

Prestwich, A., Kellar, I., Conner, M. et al. (2016). Does changing social influence engender changes in alcohol intake? A meta-analysis. *Journal of Consulting and Clinical Psychology*, *84*, 845–860.

Prestwich, A., Kellar, I., Parker, R. et al. (2014a). How can self-efficacy be increased? Meta-analysis of dietary interventions. *Health Psychology Review*, *8*, 270–285.

Prestwich, A., Moore, S., Kotze, A. et al. (2017). How can smoking cessation be induced before surgery? A systematic review and meta-analysis of behaviour change techniques and other intervention characteristics. *Frontiers in Psychology*, *8*, 915.

Prestwich, A., Sniehotta, F.F., Whittington, C. et al. (2014b). Does theory influence the effectiveness of health behavior interventions? Meta-analysis. *Health Psychology*, *33*, 465–474.

Prestwich, A., Webb, T.L., & Conner, M. (2015). Using theory to develop and test interventions to promote changes in health behaviour: evidence, issues and recommendations. *Current Opinion in Psychology*, *5*, 1–5.

Qian, T., Walton, A.E., Collins, L.M. et al. (2022). The microrandomized trial for developing digital interventions: Experimental design and data analysis considerations. *Psychological Methods*, *27*, 874–894.

Reuter, M., Frenzel, C., Walter, N.T. et al. (2011). Investigating the genetic basis of altruism: the role of the COMT Val158Met polymorphism. *Social Cognitive and Affective Neuroscience*, *6*, 662–668.

Sheeran, P., Klein, W. M. P., & Rothman, A. J. (2017). Health behavior change: Moving from observation to intervention. *Annual Review of Psychology*, *68*, 573–600.

Spruijt-Metz, D., Hekler, E., Saranummi, N. et al. (2015). Building new computational models to support health behaviour change and maintenance: new opportunities in behavioral research. *Translational Behavioral Medicine*, *5*, 335–46.

Strack, F., & Deutsch, R. (2004). Reflective and impulsive determinants of social behavior. *Personality and Social Psychology Review*, *8*, 220–247.

Webb, T.L., Joseph, J., Yardley, L., & Michie, S. (2010) Using the internet to promote health behavior change: a systematic review and meta-analysis of the impact of theoretical basis, use of behavior change techniques, and mode of delivery on efficacy. *Journal of Medical Internet Research*, *12*, e4.

West, R. (2020). An online paper authoring tool (PAT) to improve reporting of, and synthesis of evidence from, trials in behavioral sciences. *Health Psychology*, *39*, 846–850.

Wilding, S., Conner, M., Prestwich, A. et al. (2019). Using the question-behavior effect to change multiple health behaviors: An exploratory randomized controlled trial. *Journal of Experimental Social Psychology*, *81*, 53–60.

Wilson, K., Senay, I., Durantini, M. et al. (2015). When it comes to lifestyle recommendations, more is sometimes less: A meta-analysis of theoretical assumptions underlying the effectiveness of interventions promoting multiple behavior domain change. *Psychological Bulletin*, *141*, 474–509.

Wood, C.E., Richardson, M., Johnston, M., et al. (2015). Applying the behaviour change technique (BCT) taxonomy v1: a study of coder training. *Translational Behavioral Medicine*, *5*, 134–148.

Zhang, J., Oh, Y.J., Lange, P. et al. (2020). Artificial intelligence chatbots to promote physical activity and a healthy diet: Viewpoint. *Journal of Medical Internet Research*, *22*, e22845.

INDEX

Pages in *italics* refer to figures and pages in **bold** refer to tables.